HEINEMANN
GNVQ

INTERMEDIATE

Health and Social Care

Editor: Neil Moonie

Kip Chan Pensley

Beryl Stretch

Caroline Price

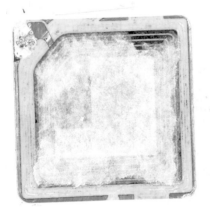

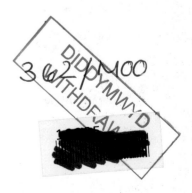

Edexcel
Success through qualifications

COMPULSORY UNITS PLUS OPTIONS

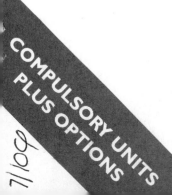

Heinemann Educational Publishers,
Halley Court, Jordan Hill, Oxford OX2 8EJ
A division of Reed Educational & Professional Publishing Ltd

Heinemann is a registered trademark of Reed Educational & Professional Publishing Limited

OXFORD MELBOURNE AUCKLAND JOHANNESBURG BLANTYRE GABORONE
IBADAN PORTSMOUTH NH (USA) CHICAGO

© Neil Moonie, Kip Chan Pensley, Beryl Stretch, Caroline Price 2000

First published 2000
2004 2003 2002 2001
10 9 8 7 6 5 4

A catalogue record for this book is available from the British Library on request.

ISBN 0 435 45600 8

Cover designed by Sarah Garbett

Pages designed by Sarah Garbett

Typeset by TechType, Abingdon, Oxfordshire

Printed and bound in Great Britain by The Bath Press Ltd., Bath

Tel: 01865 888058 www.heinemann.co.uk

Contents

iii

Contents

Introduction

How to use this book

This book has been written as a brand new text for students who are working to the 2000 national standards for Intermediate GNVQ in Health and Social Care. It covers the three compulsory units and six option units for the award.

These units are:

1 Health, social care and early years provision

2 Promoting health and well-being

3 Understanding personal development

4 Introducing human body systems

5 Planning and preparing food for clients

6 Meeting the needs of individuals in care settings

7 Dealing with hazards and emergencies

8 Child development and child care

10 Human behaviour in care settings.

Within each unit, the text is organised under exactly the same headings as the GNVQ units, to make it easy for you to find your way round the unit. By working through the units, you will find all the knowledge and ideas you need to prepare your assessment.

There are also two further options. These are:

9 Using creative activities in care

11 Practical caring skills.

If you decide to choose these options, you will find the full text on the Heinemann GNVQ website www.heinemann.co.uk (user name GNVQ HSC, password Interone for Unit 9 and Intertwo for Unit 11). This website is free.

Assessment

Assessment in the new GNVQ is carried out on the whole unit, rather than by many smaller pieces of work. The methods of assessment are:

- one major assignment, for example, carrying out an investigation into the health and care provision in your local area

- an external test, set and marked by the awarding body, for example, Edexcel.

At the end of each chapter in the book, you will find a **Unit Assessment** section which provides you with practice for both these forms of assessment. The first part is a series of carefully planned tasks or ideas for assignments that can count towards your award. By working through the tasks you will have an opportunity to cover everything you need to obtain a *Pass* grade. Further sections then guide you towards obtaining *Merit* and *Distinction* grades. The second part is a short unit **Test**. This can be used to check your knowledge of the unit and also to prepare for the external test.

Special features of the book

Throughout the text there are a number of features which are designed to encourage discussion and group work, and to help you relate the theory to real work in health and social care. These activities will also help you to build up a portfolio of **key skills** by practising **numeracy**, **communication** and **ICT**. These features are:

Think it over: Thought-provoking questions or dilemmas about people in health and social care. They can be used for individual reflection or group discussion.

Did you know?: Interesting facts and snippets of information about the health and social care sectors.

Try it out: Activities that encourage you to apply the theory in a practical situation.

Try it out

Talk it over: Opportunities for you to discuss your own experience with others.

Talk it over

Case studies: Examples of real (or simulated) clients in health and social care with real needs. Questions on the case studies will enable you to explore the key issues and deepen your understanding of the subject.

Other features, included at the end of the book, are: **Fast facts** – a glossary of key terms; **Suggestions for further reading** – including website addresses; and an **Index**. You can use these reference sections to develop your research skills.

Related titles for Intermediate GNVQ in Health and Social Care:

Student Book without Options (0435 45293 2)

Tutor Resource Pack (0435 45294 0).

Acknowledgements

The author and publisher would like to thank the following individuals and organisations for permission to reproduce tables, photographs and other material:

John Birdsall – page 266
Gareth Boden – pages 29, 253
Bubbles – page 225
ChildLine – pages 17, 166
Corbis – cover
Sally & Richard Greenhill – pages 20, 32
Science Photo Library – page 242

The Stock Market – pages 23 (bottom right), 34 (bottom left), 104
The Stock Market/Zefa – page 26
Stone – pages 23 (top left), 34 (bottom right), 60, 69, 100, 103, 111, 258, 278.

Every effort has been made to contact copyright holders of material published in this book. We would be glad to hear from unacknowledged sources at the first opportunity.

Health, social care and early years provision

This Unit covers the knowledge you will need in order to meet the assessment requirements for Unit 1. It is written in five sections:

Section one explains the organisation of health, social care and early years services. Section two describes the main jobs in health, social care and early years. Section three explores the effective communication skills needed to support others. Section four examines the care value base. Finally section five looks at how codes of practice and charters may influence the delivery of care services.

Advice and ideas for meeting the assessment requirements for the unit and for achieving Merit and Distinction grades are at the end of the unit. Also at the end of the unit is a quick test to check your understanding.

The organisation of health, social care and early years services

This section looks at how health and social care services for adults and children are organised. Care services may be provided in one of three ways (Figure 1.1):

- **Statutory services** have been set up because Parliament has passed a law which requires the services to be provided, for example, accident and emergency departments in hospitals, education services for children or home care services for older people.

- **Private organisations** are run on a profit-making basis and are businesses, for example, private hospitals and residential homes or private children's nurseries.

- **Voluntary organisations** are run on a non-profit making basis, for example, the Woman's Royal Voluntary Services (WRVS), or Barnardo's, an organisation which provides care for children and young people.

However, health and social care is also often provided by people outside these formal agencies and organisations. **Informal care** may be provided by family members, friends and neighbours (see Figure 1.2).

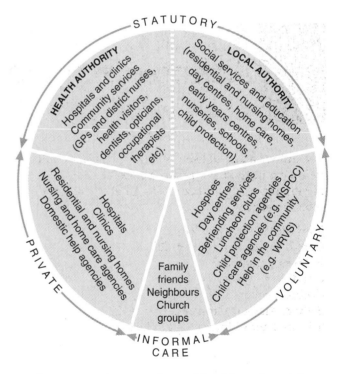

Figure 1.1 An overview of health and social care provision

Statutory sector organisations

The two main providers of statutory services are the National Health Service (**NHS**) and Local Authority services. Statutory services are organised at national, regional and local levels.

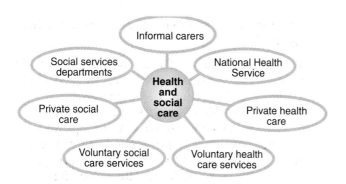

Figure 1.2 The providers of health and social care

National levels of organisation may include key government departments and the Local Government Association. Regional levels include regional services with the NHS, Health and Social Services Boards and special Health Authorities. Local levels include Local Authority social services departments, hospital and community trusts, and GPs (see Figure 1.3).

The government is divided into various departments which have responsibility for specific issues – e.g. the Department of Agriculture, Fisheries and Food; the Department of Foreign and Commonwealth Affairs; and the Department of Defence. The departments concerned with health and social care are the Department of Health, the Department of Social Security (which deals with welfare benefits) and

the Department for Education and Employment. The Home Office has responsibility for overseeing voluntary organisations. There are also specific departments that deal with issues concerning Wales, Scotland and Northern Ireland: the Welsh Office, the Scottish Office and The Northern Ireland Office (see Figure 1.4).

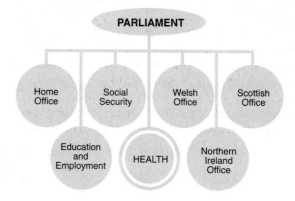

Figure 1.4 Departments of state involved in the provision of health and social care

The Secretary of State for Health in England and the Secretaries of State in Northern Ireland, Scotland and Wales are responsible for all aspects of health and social care provision. The Department of Health (**DOH**) in England has responsibility for:

* making policies in relation to health and social care and issuing guidelines

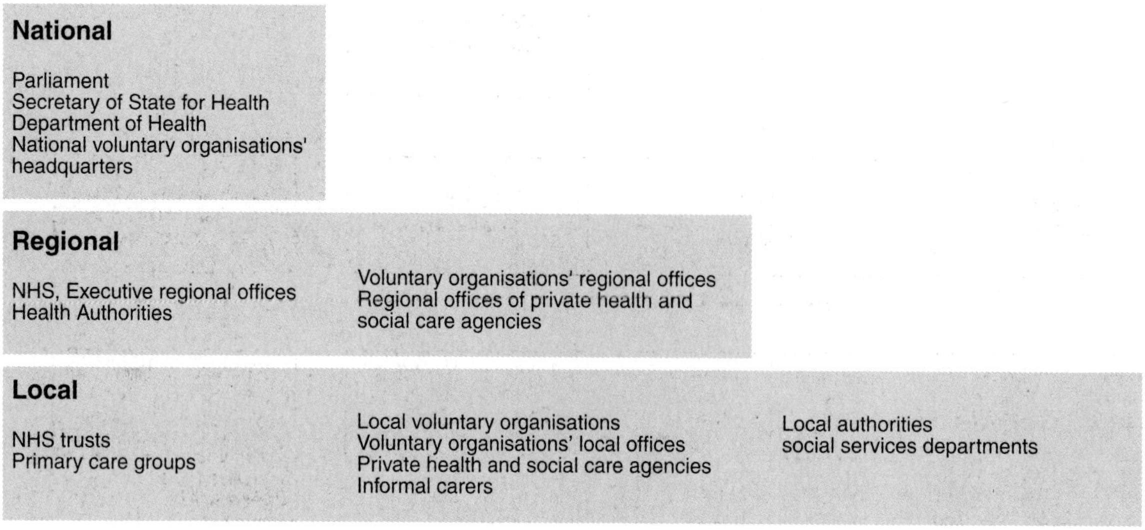

National

Parliament
Secretary of State for Health
Department of Health
National voluntary organisations' headquarters

Regional

NHS, Executive regional offices
Health Authorities

Voluntary organisations' regional offices
Regional offices of private health and social care agencies

Local

NHS trusts
Primary care groups

Local voluntary organisations
Voluntary organisations' local offices
Private health and social care agencies
Informal carers

Local authorities
social services departments

Figure 1.3 National, regional and local levels of health and social care provision

◇ monitoring the performance of Health Authorities and social services departments

◇ allocating resources for the provision of health and social care.

The Scottish Home and Health Department, the Welsh Office and the Department of Health and Social Services in Northern Ireland have similar responsibilities to those of the DOH in England. In Northern Ireland health services and social services are organised as a single agency. This is called a **unified structure** and is outside political control. Four Health Boards provide services at local levels. Although the organisation of health services in Scotland, Wales and Northern Ireland may be different from that in England, the range

and provision of services are much the same (see Figure 1.5).

The Department of Health in England and, within it, the NHS Executive, have the responsibility for deciding what plans need to be made at a national level. There are eight regional offices of the NHS Management Executive in England. These regional offices have a role in monitoring the providers of services in strategic planning. They will be responsible directly to the NHS Chief Executive (see Figure 1.6).

The structure of health services

Before 1948 health services were provided in various ways: some by voluntary organisations,

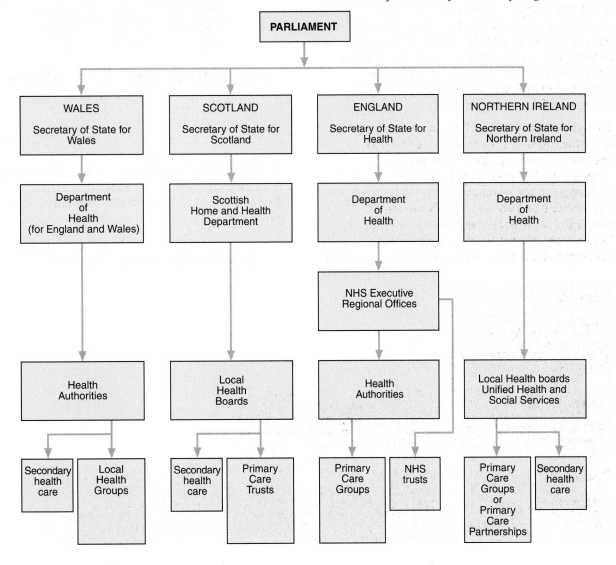

Figure 1.5   The health care structures of England, Wales, Scotland and Northern Ireland

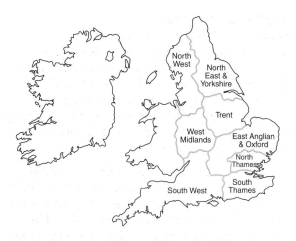

Figure 1.6   The NHS Management Executive: the English regional areas

some by Local Authorities, some by the employers of groups of people, some by private care. There was no co-ordination of services and there were inevitable gaps. Generally people had to pay for their health care. Many poor people were therefore unable to access health care when they needed it. Therefore the NHS came into being in July 1948.

The National Health Service (NHS)

The aim of the National Health Service (NHS) was to provide integrated and co-ordinated health care services to all that were free of charge at the time of use. There were three main parts to the service:

1   **Primary care** services, which include GPs, dentists, opticians and pharmacists.

2   **Secondary and tertiary care** services of the regional and district systems, for example, hospitals and specialist services

3   **Community care** and **public health services**, which had an emphasis on preventative work and health promotion. Early examples of these included vaccination and immunisation programmes against illnesses such as smallpox and whooping cough.

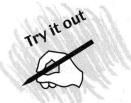

Find out from your local Health Authority about any preventative health care programmes that are being carried out in your area.

Until recently there were only comparatively minor changes in the way the NHS was structured. However the NHS has now undergone major reforms that have been more far-reaching than any other changes undertaken since it was set up in 1948.

These reforms are set out in four government **White Papers**:

1   *Promoting better health* (1987), which concerns primary health care

2   *Working for patients* (1989), which discusses the management and provision of services.

3   *Caring for people* (1989), concerning community care

4   *The New NHS* (1998), which sets out the future of the NHS.

In addition to these White Papers, the **NHS and Community Care Act 1990** had important consequences for the way health and social care agencies are organised. At the centre of the reforms to health and social care was the idea there should be a clear division between purchasing and the provision of services. The idea of **purchasers** and

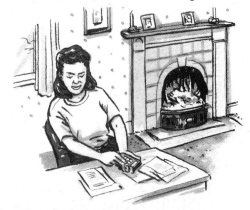

Stella is comparing estimates which she has received from catering firms to do the catering at her sister's 18th birthday party – she is acting as a *purchaser* of a service and the catering firm she chooses will be the *provider* of the service.

providers might best be understood by thinking about obtaining estimates for the catering at a wedding reception or some other large social event. You decide it would be too difficult or expensive to provide the catering yourself, so you contact a number of catering firms to supply you with estimates. Once you have studied the estimates you decide which firm provides the best value for money. You contact this firm again and go ahead to book them to supply the catering. In this situation, you are the **purchaser** of the services. The catering firm you have chosen is the **provider** of the services, and you have chosen your provider by comparing the services offered by others in the same market. NHS and social services departments were therefore split into those departments who have the responsibility for 'buying' services (the purchasers – deciding how the NHS budget should be spent and deciding on the allocation of funds for the provision of different services) and those departments which decide who should provide these services, eg hospitals, dentists and district nurses. In the health service the old District Health Authorities became the purchasers, together with some GP group practices, which became **GP fundholders**. In social services departments, it was the senior managers who became the purchasers. Residential homes, day centres and home care units became the providers.

Health Authorities

Before April 1996 the structure of the administration and provision of health care services within the NHS was quite complicated. This structure included 8 Regional Health Authorities in England (and 3 separate ones in Wales, Scotland and Northern Ireland) 90 Family Health Service Authorities and 186 District Health Authorities (see Figure 1.7).

In April 1996 the Regional Health Authorities were abolished and the District Health Authorities and Family Service Authorities were combined to form 100 new Health Authorities (**HAs**). The Health Authorities are now the main purchasers of care. Each Health Authority has a population of between 125,000 and one million people. The responsibilities of the new Health Authorities reflect on those previously held by the District Health Authorities and Family Health Service Authorities. These include:

- planning services in the Health Authority's area (with national guidelines)
- assessing primary health care needs
- developing services within the area
- **commissioning** (i.e. requesting others to provide, for a fee) primary care

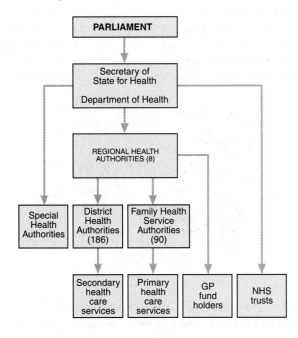

Figure 1.7   The structure of the NHS in England before April 1996

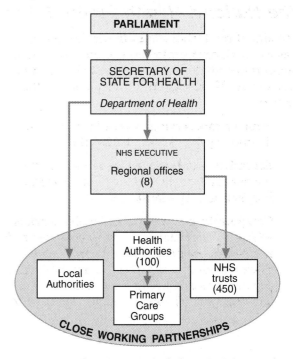

Figure 1.8   The structure of the NHS in England after April 1999

- arranging contracts with acute services, such as hospitals
- managing services provided by GPs, dentists, opticians and pharmacists
- monitoring the quality of services
- providing information to the public about services
- registering and dealing with complaints about the provision of services.

It is expected that, in the future, the Health Authorities will work closely with Primary Care Groups (**PCGs**), **NHS trusts** and Local Authorities (see Figure 1.8).

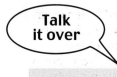

Think it over

Who will the authorities be expected to work closely with in the future?

NHS trusts

National Health trusts are self-governing units within the health service. Trusts are run by a board of directors and are accountable to central government. There are now 450 trusts in England. A trust can either be a hospital, a group of hospitals, community services (such as district nursing) or ambulance services for a particular area.

Talk it over

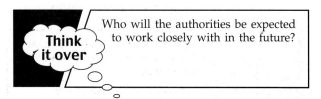

Are there any hospital trusts in your area? What are they called?

A trust is able to:

- decide its own management structure
- employ staff under its own terms and conditions of employment, including salary scales
- buy, own and sell assets, such as land or buildings
- keep surplus money or borrow money
- carry out research
- provide facilities for medical education and other forms of training.

Self-governing trusts receive most of their income from NHS contracts for providing services to Health Authorities and Primary Care Groups. However, they can also treat private patients. All trusts must write annual reports and maintain annual accounts, and they must publish these. This means they are now more accountable to the public in the way they spend their money – and most of their money came from the public in the first place!

Primary care groups

From April 1999 Primary Care Groups (made up of groups of GPs and community nurses) took responsibility for commissioning services within their area. They also now work closely with social services departments. In England each group services about 100,000 patients and may have about 50 GPs, but this varies according to local circumstances. PCGs have replaced the former GP fundholding system that was introduced in the 1980s.

PCGs may do all or any of the following tasks (see Figure 1.9), although the majority of PCGs will initially operate at Level 2.

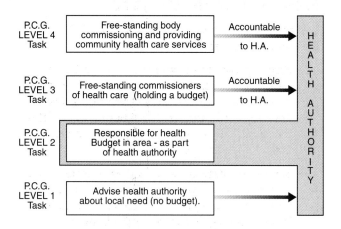

Figure 1.9 Primary Care Groups: levels of responsibility

- Become a free-standing body for providing community care services – again accountable to the HA.
- Become a free-standing body for commissioning health care – accountable to the HA.
- Take responsibility for managing the health budget in its area – as part of the HA.

⋄ Advise the health authority (HA) about needs of the local community.

In addition they are responsible for:

⋄ contributing to and implementing the government's Health Improvement Programme

⋄ promoting the health of the local population

⋄ developing primary care services in their areas

⋄ integrating primary and community health services

⋄ being involved in the development and monitoring of the quality of services.

This is the situation in England. In Scotland, primary care trusts oversee the delivery of services, and GPs are responsible only for primary care budgets. Wales has local health groups (equivalent to PCGs) but these have only an advisory role. At the time of writing it has yet to be decided whether Northern Ireland will have PCGs or primary care partnerships.

Provision of health care

The provision of health services is divided into these following areas:

1 **Primary care** is usually the first contact a person has with the health services and this is often provided in the community (GPs, dentists, opticians, etc.). Primary care is often preventative in nature (e.g. routine dental check-ups and eye tests).

2 **Secondary care** usually follows referral from a primary care worker (e.g. a GP may refer a patient to a hospital for tests and specialist investigations) Secondary care is often curative in nature (e.g. operations, setting broken bones, removing wisdom teeth etc.) and is given in hospitals, day surgeries and out-patient clinics.

Some services function as both primary and secondary care. A paramedic giving treatment at the scene of an accident is an example of primary care; a paramedic working in the ambulance service collecting a patient for treatment at a hospital is an example of secondary care.

3 **Tertiary care** may be provided by specialist units which are able to give longer-term, rehabilitative treatment – for example, a unit providing intensive physiotherapy following an accident where a patient suffered spinal injuries.

4 **Community services** provide care for people within the community, often in their own homes. Examples include district nurses, health visitors and chiropodists.

5 **Public health services** include health education and programmes and schemes to prevent illnesses and disease. Both the health services and Local Authorities have various roles in the promotion of better health.

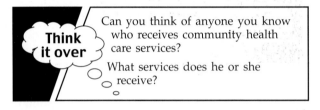

Think it over

Can you think of anyone you know who receives community health care services?

What services does he or she receive?

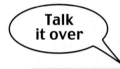

Talk it over

What is the difference between primary and secondary care?

The structure of the social services

The introduction of the National Health Service in 1948 also meant a range of health and social care services came under the direct control of the Minister of Health. It was hoped this direct control would result in a more unified and co-ordinated range of services. The responsibility for providing for old and disabled people and children by the Local Authorities was extended further. Also, services for people with mental health problems were strengthened through the setting up of the Provisional Council for Mental Health. However, until the 1960s these three areas of care were operated quite separately from one another. The publication of the **Seebohm Report**, in 1968, resulted in the amalgamation of the children's departments and the welfare services. Then, in 1970, the Local Authority Social Services Act set out a new framework for social care provision, which required the Local Authorities to set up Social Services Committees (see Figure 1.10).

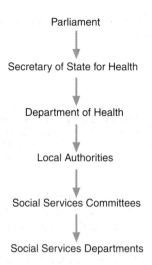

Figure 1.10   The structure of social care in England

Although the Secretary of State is responsible for the provision of social care, it is the Local Authorities who administer those services. In England and Wales, county councils, metropolitan councils and the London boroughs run the Local Authorities. In Northern Ireland there are four boards who administer the combined health and social services. In Scotland regional Local Authorities control social services departments.

However, the powers and responsibilities of Local Authorities are defined by parliament, which passes legislation outlining the Local Authorities' duties.

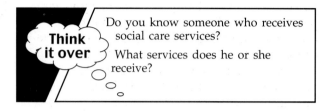

Local Authorities have the responsibility for the co-ordination of many aspects of social care in their communities, including services for children, for people with physical disabilities, people with learning disabilities and people with mental health problems, as well as responsibilities for housing, education, leisure facilities, refuse collection and highways.

Each Local Authority must appoint a Director of Social Services and must have a Social Services Committee. Some Local Authorities have separate directorates for each of their responsibilities (e.g. social services, housing, education, etc.). Others combine these departments at senior management level (e.g. housing with community care for adults – i.e. services for the elderly, people with

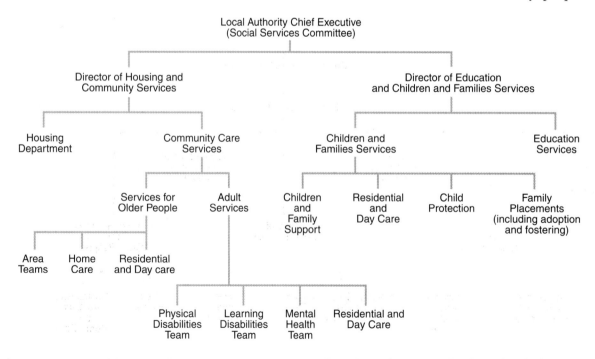

Figure 1.11   Combining different social care functions: an example

disabilities, people with health problems – and children and families with education) (see Figure 1.11).

The organisational structures of social services departments have changed considerably in the past few years. This has happened so that they can carry out their new roles and responsibilities as required by new legislation, particularly the NHS and Community Care Act 1990. As mentioned earlier, this Act made Local Authorities the purchasers of care, rather than the providers of care. Many social services departments reorganised their staffing structures to reflect these changes in responsibilities (see Figure 1.12).

The role of social service departments

The role of the social service departments has changed as their function as direct providers of services has decreased and their role as assessors of need and purchasers of services has increased. Their main role now is to offer advice and to provide access to services, such as residential care, for all client groups (e.g. children, people with physical or learning disabilities, people with mental health problems or older people). Previously, Local Authorities owned and managed a number of residential homes themselves. Today they are more likely to purchase residential care

for individuals in private or non-profit-making residential homes.

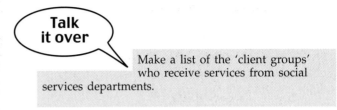

Make a list of the 'client groups' who receive services from social services departments.

Social workers are employed within the social services departments, and their role is to assess the needs of people requiring social care services. Social workers are often organised into teams that deal with a specific client group (e.g. children and families teams, teams for older people). Sometimes, teams consist of health and social care workers (for example, teams dealing with people with mental health problems may work side by side with social workers and community psychiatric nurses).

With their increased role in the purchasing of services, many social services departments have created special commissioning and **contracting** sections. (Contracting means employing someone who does not regularly work for your organisation to do a specific job for you – for

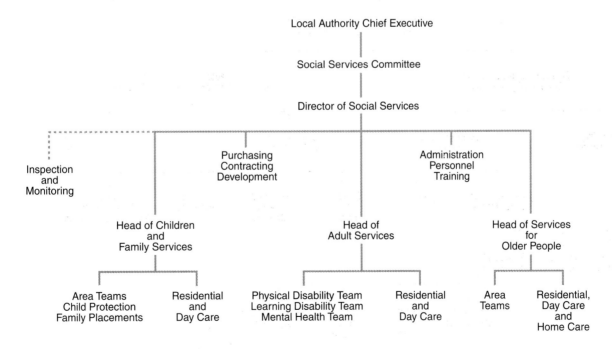

Figure 1.12 A Local Authority's social services department

example, employing cleaners through an agency). These new sections operate alongside divisions created as a result of the 1990 Act (e.g. complaints, inspection and registration units, quality monitoring and planning and development). Planning and development has become even more important as social services departments are required to work closely with health service colleagues, as well as with the private and voluntary sectors.

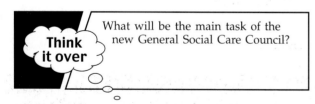

Talk it over

How could you find out if there are any services in your area where health and social services staff work together in teams to provide care?

The government has plans for modernising social services departments. These plans are set out in the white paper *Modernising Social Services*. Changes include new independent inspection units for care homes and other services and better support for adults – including the introduction of direct payment schemes to clients. Clients will then be able to spend their allowance on care providers of their own choice. There will also be Quality Projects to ensure children are properly protected against abuse; to raise standards of care in children's homes; and to give children better opportunities to receive a good education. Additionally, a new General Social Care Council will be formed. Its function will be to raise the standards of care given by social care staff. To achieve this there will be more emphasis on staff training and on monitoring the services provided.

Think it over

What will be the main task of the new General Social Care Council?

Joint work and planning

Health and social services must now work together to modernise the front-line care they provide for people. In September 1998, the targets set for achieving this were outlined in *Modernising Health and Social Services: National Priorities*

Guidance 1999–2002. The priorities contained in this document included the following:

- Cutting waiting lists and waiting times.

- Modernising mental health and primary care services.

- Reducing deaths from cancer and coronary heart disease, and improving the health of the most disadvantaged in society.

- Improving the quality and safety of children's services and providing better rehabilitation services for older people.

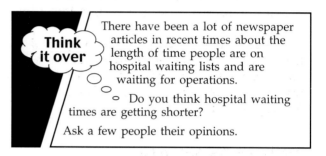

Think it over

There have been a lot of newspaper articles in recent times about the length of time people are on hospital waiting lists and are waiting for operations.

Do you think hospital waiting times are getting shorter?

Ask a few people their opinions.

Previous governments tried to encourage joint planning between the health and Local Authorities. However, this was difficult to achieve because of the different ways the authorities were structured. For example, in terms of health, the care of the elderly, mentally ill people was the responsibility of the mental health services, whereas, in terms of social care, the same people came under the remit of services for older people.

Other problems have arisen because Health Authorities and Local Authorities do not share the same geographical boundaries. For example,

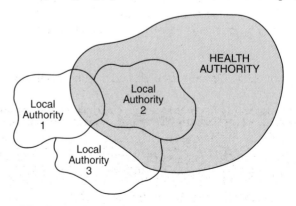

Figure 1.13 A Health Authority that covers more than one Local Authority area

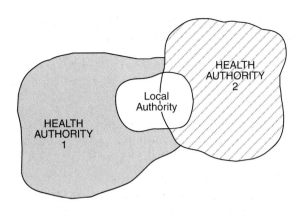

Figure 1.14   A Local Authority that comes under the control of more than one Health Authority

one Health Authority may cover all or part of a Local Authority's area (see Figure 1.13) or one Local Authority's area may come under the responsibility of a number of Health Authorities (see Figure 1.14).

Early years services

Structure

The early years services are those services that provide health, care and education services to children between the ages of 0 and 8, when not at school. As with the health and social services, the early years services involve both the statutory sector and voluntary and private groups

Statutory services

The government's role is to provide statutory services directly, or to supervise services through government departments. The four main government departments concerned with children are shown in Figure 1.15. Funding from these central government departments is passed on to Local Authorities in the form of grants. The authorities then use these grants to provide services for children and families in their areas. The three main services are health, education and social services.

Health services for children

In addition to the health care offered to all, there are special services for children:

1   *Health screening*   From the age of 10 weeks, all children are seen in their own homes by health visitors, who give children regular developmental tests. These tests are for growth and development, sight and hearing.

2   *Vaccinations and immunisations*   Children are given a programme of injections starting at the age of 8 weeks to protect them from whooping cough, polio, tetanus, measles and other infectious diseases.

3   *School health services*   Once they start school, children are seen by a school nurse and given health education.

4   *Dental services*   Dental check-ups and orthodontic treatment (straightening the teeth) are free to children up to the age of 16 years.

5   *Maternity services*   Before a baby is born and up to 10 weeks after the birth, the mother and child are looked after by a midwife.

6   *Community and hospital services*   If children need referral for specialist treatment, they may see a paediatrician (a doctor who treats sick children), audiologist, speech therapist, optician or dietician.

All these services are free to children under the age of 16 years.

Figure 1.15   Government departments concerned with children

Department	Responsible for
1 Department of Health (DOH)	Health services, including hospitals and local health care
2 Department for Education and Employment (DfEE)	All aspects of education and employment, including standards in schools and day nurseries
3 Department of Social Security (DSS)	Providing benefits for children and families
4 Department of the Environment, Transport and the Regions (DETR)	Local government, housing, planning and the countryside

Talk it over

Jake is 3½ years old. He is small for his age and doesn't want to eat.

Which health services might Jake's family make use of?

Education for children

Local Education Authorities are responsible for delivering nursery, primary and secondary education in their areas. Children are required to be in full-time education in the school term following their fifth birthday. However, many children start a year earlier (the 'reception year').

By law every 4-year-old is entitled to receive some nursery education. This may take place in private day nurseries or playgroups. Any nursery wanting to receive government funding for 4-year-olds must be inspected by Ofsted, the school inspection service. Nurseries must follow the Early Learning Goals, which is a special curriculum for children aged 3–5 years.

Social services for children

The Department of Social Security (**DSS**) is responsible for providing benefits for children and families, and it also runs the **Child Support Agency**. A number of benefits are available for children and families, and the main ones are as follows:

- *Child Benefit*   A fixed payment to all parents who have a child or children.

- *Maternity Benefit*   Money paid to working mothers while they are on leave from work to have a baby.

- *Family Credit*   Payments for families with a child or children where the family's income is low.

The benefits system is complex and changes frequently.

Local Authorities are responsible for a range of services, particularly for registering people who work with children in early years settings. These settings may be statutory, private or voluntary (see Figure 1.16).

Talk it over

The Rajiahs have two children aged 1 and 4 years. Both parents work full time and have well paid jobs. Their current nanny is leaving them after three years and they feel Manzoor, the 4-year-old, might be ready for a nursery or playgroup.

What care might suit the Rajiahs – a nanny, a day nursery or both? Discuss this in groups and give reasons for your recommendation.

The National Childcare Strategy

The government has recently made a decision to focus on the early years to ensure that preschool children are provided with good-quality care and education. There have been a number of key developments:

- A national framework of qualifications for people who work with children to ensure everyone understands the levels and achievements attained through the various training courses currently on offer.

- The preschool curriculum entitled 'Early Learning Goals'.

- Inspection by Ofsted of all preschool settings to ensure they are following a balanced programme of learning and play.

- Early Years Development Partnerships, where all Local Authorities have to produce a plan to show how the local health, social care and education services are working together for children.

Early Years Development Partnership and Plans

These plans are seen as the key to ensuring there is good quality local provision for all children. Some of the key aims of the plans are to:

- make sure every 4-year-old has three terms of good quality preschool education

- include children with special needs within the same care and education settings as other children

- show how the provisions of the Children Act 1989 and other laws relating to children are being fulfilled

Figure 1.16 Child care settings

Setting	Sector	Description
Childminders	Private; registered with Local Authority	A childminder looks after other people's children in the childminder's own home. This might include looking after other children after school as well as looking after children under 5 years of age during the day
Nannies	Private; no registration required	A nanny looks after children in the children's own home
Day nurseries	Statutory or private; inspected by Ofsted	A day nursery is open all year round and children under 5 years of age can stay all day
Workplace nurseries	Statutory or private; inspected by Ofsted	A workplace nursery is organised by an employer and the places are often subsidised. This means the employee does not pay the full cost
Créches	Private or Local Authority run	Créches look after children under 8 years of age for short periods of time. For example, they are found in new shopping centres, allowing parents to shop for a few hours
Playgroups	Voluntary or private	Playgroups are non-profit making groups designed to give children under 5 years of age an opportunity to play. Sessions are often two to three hours long
Nurseries or kindergartens	Statutory or private; inspected by Ofsted	Nurseries and kindergartens offer sessions in mornings and afternoons that allow children under 5 years of age to learn and play
Nurseries within schools	Run by Local Education Authority	Some infant or primary schools have a nursery attached. The nurseries take children from 3 to 4 years of age. No charge is made to the parents
Infant and primary schools	Run by Local Education Authority; inspected by Ofsted	Infant and primary schools take children from the age of 5 years. The normal school day is about six hours long
After-school clubs	Can be voluntary or private	After-school clubs look after children over the age of 5 years after school has finished during term time. They are often used by working parents
Holiday play schemes	Run by Local Authorities, and private and voluntary groups	Holiday play schemes look after children over the age of 5 years during school holidays. They are often used by working parents

- promote training for all early years workers (for example, NVQs in early years care)
- provide grants for training.

For example, a childminder might decide she would like to be NVQ trained so that she is better equipped to help the children she looks after. She could apply for a grant from her Local Authority to help her with her training to achieve this.

CASE STUDY — Michelle and her children

Michelle is a single mum with two children, Jade aged $4\frac{1}{2}$ years and Kai aged 2 years. She is living with her own mother at the moment, but wants to find her own home and to obtain a part-time job to help her support the children. Both the children are at home at present, but Jade is due to start school in 3 months. Michelle is anxious that Jade won't find it easy to be separated from her. Kai worries her too, because he is asthmatic and has had two recent serious asthma attacks. Michelle needs to find good-quality care and health support for him. Then there is the problem of finding a job. Michelle wants something that will fit in with her plans for the children and will pay enough to cover her child care costs. Her mum can help for a few hours a week, but no more.

Questions

1 What early years services will Michelle need for herself and her children? You could note them down under the headings: 'Health', 'Education' and 'Social care'.

2 How could Michelle find out about these services?

3 Imagine Michelle had moved into your local area. Where would she find the services she needs?

Voluntary and private organisations

Voluntary organisations

The UK has a long tradition of voluntary services, and this sector has always been involved in the provision of health and social care. For example, in the eighteenth and nineteenth centuries private benefactors established many hospitals which provided care free of charge. In 1866, Dr Barnardo's (now known simply as Barnardo's) was established to help orphaned and underprivileged children and, in 1889, the NSPCC (National Society for the Prevention of Cruelty to Children) was founded. By the middle of the nineteenth century there were so many voluntary organisations (many of them overlapping in the services they provided), that the Charity Organisation Society (COS) was set up to help co-ordinate these various organisations.

Today, the National Council for Voluntary Organisations (NCVO) is the main co-ordinating agency in England. Its main function is to provide links between voluntary organisations, official bodies and the private sector. Councils in Scotland, Wales and Northern Ireland have similar roles. There are over 200,000 voluntary organisations in the UK, and more than 170,000 of these are registered as charities. Throughout the UK, the Home Office is the government department with responsibility for co-ordinating government interests in the voluntary sector (see Figure 1.17).

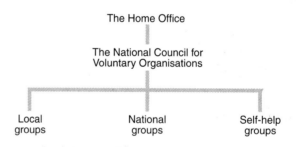

Figure 1.17 The structure of voluntary organisations in England

There are thousands of voluntary organisations involved in health and social care, ranging from national agencies (such as Age Concern) to local small groups. In recent years **self-help groups** have greatly increased in number. Self-help groups are usually set up by people who share a particular concern and who want to help other people in similar situations. For example, Compassionate Friends was set up to help the brothers and sisters of children who have died. Groups representing women's interests (e.g. the

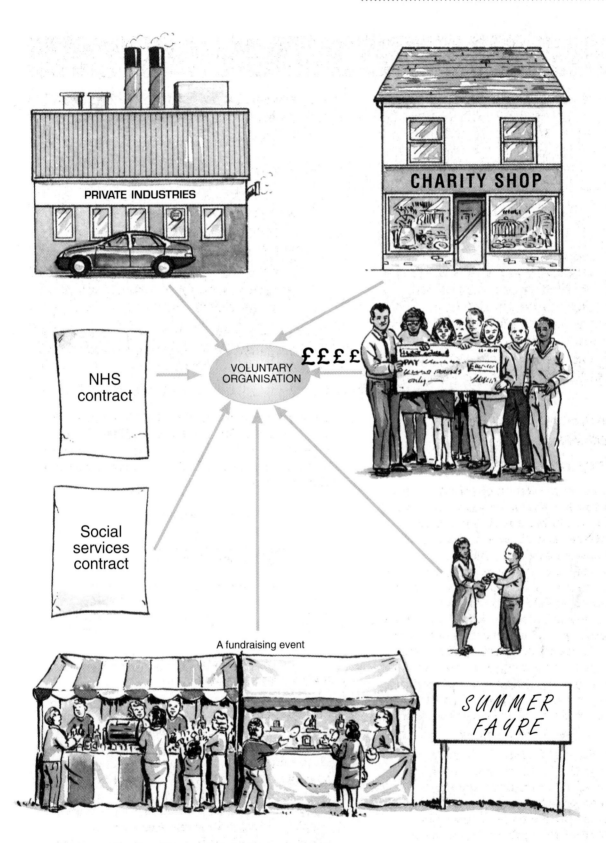

PRIVATE INDUSTRIES

CHARITY SHOP

NHS contract

VOLUNTARY ORGANISATION

£££££

Social services contract

A fundraising event

SUMMER FAYRE

Figure 1.18   The funding of voluntary organisations

Irish Women's Housing Action Group) and ethnic minority groups (e.g. the Cantonese Healthline) have also increased in number recently.

Funding for voluntary organisations comes from various sources. Some have contracts with Health Authorities or Local Authorities, who provide services for them. For example, some hospices (who provide specialist care for people with terminal illnesses) have contracts with Health Authorities and Local Authorities have contracts with local branches of Age Concern, through which they provide luncheon clubs for the more able older people in their areas. Other funds are obtained through fund-raising events, through charitable donations from individuals or groups of people, and through grants from grant-awarding bodies. Some larger companies donate money to charities for specific purposes (see Figure 1.18).

Voluntary organisations tend to focus on specific issues (see Figure 1.19).

Some examples of health, social care and early years voluntary agencies are given below.

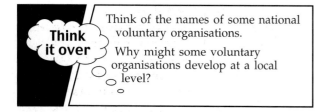

Think it over

Think of the names of some national voluntary organisations.

Why might some voluntary organisations develop at a local level?

Health: John Groomes Association for the Disabled

This charitable organisation was set up in 1866. It provides residential accommodation for people with severe disabilities, sheltered work and specialist housing throughout England and Wales. The association also provides holidays and short breaks for people with disabilities, their families and friends. It runs an information service about the problems and needs of people with disabilities.

Social care: Age Concern

Age Concern is a registered charity, which depends largely on public support for the financing of its activities. Although Age Concern provides services throughout the UK, it is divided into four regions: England, Scotland, Wales and Ireland. There is a network of over 1,400 local groups, with the support of around 250,000 volunteers plus some paid staff. The aim of Age Concern is to improve the quality of life for older people and to develop services appropriate to local needs. These services may include advice and information, day care, visiting services, transport schemes, clubs and specialist facilities for older people who have physical disabilities or who are mentally frail.

Early years: National Society for the Prevention of Cruelty to Children

The National Society for the Prevention of Cruelty to Children (NSPCC) was set up to protect

Figure 1.19 Voluntary organisations and their principal areas of concern

Area of concern	Organisation
Personal and family problems	Family Welfare Association; Child Poverty Action Group; Relate (formerly Marriage Guidance); Barnardo's; ChildLine; National Council for One-Parent Families; National Society for the Prevention of Cruelty to Children; Claimants' Union (advice on social security benefits); Samaritans (for lonely, depressed and suicidal people); Women's Aid
Health and disability	WRVS (Women's Royal Voluntary Service); MIND (National Association for Mental Health); Gamanon (for people with gambling problems); Help the Aged; Brook Advisory Centres; Institute for the Blind; National Institute for Deaf People; Alcoholics Anonymous; British Red Cross Society; Haemophilia Society
National organisations whose work is religious in inspiration	Salvation Army; Church Army; TocH; Church's Urban Fund; Church of England Children's Society; Young Men's Christian Association (YMCA); Catholic Marriage Advisory Council; Jewish Welfare Board

children from abuse. The organisation receives approximately 88% of its running costs from public donations. It operates throughout the UK and its workers are organised into area teams. These child protection teams assess and help abused children and their families. The work is carried out either in the family's home or in NSPPC centres. The teams also offer a 24-hour advice service and local education, training, consultation and advice for other professional and voluntary organisations.

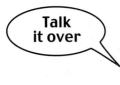

Talk it over

Do you know which voluntary organisation uses this symbol? Find out who founded it.

(The answer is given in the 'Answers to tests' section at the end of the book.)

Private health and social care organisations

The work of private organisations in the provision of health and social care has always been important. These organisations charge for their services with the intention of making a profit (i.e. they are run as businesses). Some of the services provided by the private sector are shown in Figure 1.20.

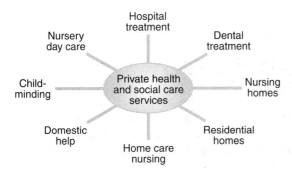

Figure 1.20 Health and social care services provided by the private sector

The range and extent of services available from private organisations have increased considerably in recent years. In particular, there was a rapid growth in private health care in the 1970s and 1980s when central government introduced the

Today, over three million people subscribe to private health care insurance schemes.

idea of a **mixed economy of care**. It is now government policy that NHS and private and voluntary health care provision should co-operate in meeting the nation's health needs. Private health care may be provided by NHS hospital trusts or in totally separate health care facilities. Similarly, the government expects Local Authorities to use private and voluntary agencies to provide them with social care, rather than own and manage these services themselves. Consequently, a number of small businesses have emerged in recent years, for example, ironing services, home-help services and private health clinics.

Services for older people

Local Authorities have the **duty** to assess the needs of older people and the power to provide services in order to meet those needs. However, they do not have to provide services themselves. For example, an older person may need assistance in getting up and washed each morning but this 'home care' service may be provided either by people employed directly by the authority or by people employed by a private agency. In the latter case, the Local Authority may have a contract with the agency to provide home care for such people. The range of services provided by a Local Authority can include:

- personal care (e.g. getting up, getting washed, dressing, going to bed and bathing)
- meals and light refreshments
- domestic help (e.g. shopping, housework, laundry and pension collecting)
- equipment (e.g. stair lifts and bath aids)
- personal alarm systems
- adaptations to the home (e.g. ramps, widening doorways, downstairs toilet)
- day care facilities
- residential homes
- nursing homes (although these may be funded by the health service).

Health Authorities also have a duty to assist older people who live at home. Community Health Services employ, for example, district nurses, occupational therapists, speech therapists, continence advisers, and chiropodists, etc., to provide these services. The help that may be offered includes:

◦ nursing care at home

◦ personal care – especially if the person has a terminal illness

◦ equipment (e.g. bath seats, hand-rails, walking frames, wheelchairs, commodes)

◦ aids to dressing, eating and carrying out everyday tasks

CASE STUDY – Mrs Low Ying

Mrs Low Ying is an 80-year-old Chinese lady. She was widowed seven years ago and lives alone in a two-bedroomed house. None of her family live nearby and Mrs Low Ying is very isolated and often lonely. About a month ago Mrs Low Ying's arthritis, which she has in her hands, legs and feet, became very bad and her mobility was greatly reduced. She also has angina and high blood pressure. Following a joint assessment visit by a district nurse and a social worker the following services were provided.

Local Authority

1   Every morning a home carer helps Mrs Low Ying with getting up, washing and dressing (the Local Authority has a contract with a private agency for home care services). In the evenings she can still manage to get herself back to bed.

2   Once a week the Local Authority provides help with her shopping, with the collection of her pension and with her household tasks (also provided through the private home care agency).

3   Meals-on-wheels are provided five days a week as she can no longer prepare her own food (the WRVS prepare and deliver meals on behalf of the Local Authority).

4   A stair-lift has been installed, as she can no longer get up the stairs by herself.

5   Ramps have been fitted from the front and back doors.

6   A disabled badge has been provided for her niece's car so that her niece can take her out and park close to shops, etc.

7   A personal alarm system has been installed so that she can call for help if she should have a fall.

8   Day care is provided at a local centre one day per week (Age Concern run the centre and arrange transport for Mrs Low Ying).

Health Authority

1   A district nurse helps Mrs Low Ying to have a bath once a week and also monitors her medication.

2   A bath seat, grab-rails and a raised toilet seat have been installed.

3   She has been supplied with a walking frame for use inside the home, and a wheelchair for going out.

Informal Carer

Mrs Low Ying's niece visits each Sunday and provides a meal that day. She also does her Aunt's laundry for her.

Questions

1   Does Mrs Low Ying receive a 'mixed economy of care' package?

2   What is meant by a 'mixed economy of care?'

3   What other care needs might Mrs Low Ying have in the future? Who might provide these?

- help with continence problems, including pads, pants and other aids
- help with speech and swallowing problems
- foot care and chiropody.

Informal carers

In recent years the term **carer** has been used to describe anyone, other than a paid worker, who is looking after someone who is ill or disabled. The carer may be a family member, friend or neighbour (for example, a wife looking after a disabled partner, a parent looking after a child with learning difficulties, an adult looking after a parent who has dementia or a friend looking after someone who has a long-term illness). It could even be a child who is looking after a sick or disabled parent.

Some people do not like the term 'carer' but it does at least acknowledge that the carer is doing a 'job' of work and one which can be very difficult and demanding. Informal carers may:

- help people to get from and return to bed
- help people to wash and dress
- help people to bathe or shower
- prepare refreshments and meals
- do domestic work and shopping
- monitor and dispense medicines
- provide transport.

Informal carers may also be people who belong to a local group, such as a church, or a group set up to help and advise other carers.

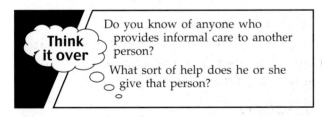

Think it over

Do you know of anyone who provides informal care to another person?

What sort of help does he or she give that person?

The main jobs in health, social care and early years services

People who work in health, social care and early years services may be involved in either **direct care** or **indirect care**. People who deliver *direct* care will meet clients face to face (for example,

occupational therapists, social workers and nursery nurses). However, there are jobs that are necessary to support those who deliver direct care but the people who perform these jobs may not come into face-to-face contact with the clients (for example, laboratory technicians, secretaries, catering staff and cleaners).

There are too many jobs in the fields of health, social care and early years services to include all of them in this book but the following pages describe a respresentative selection. You will be able to find out about the jobs not described here from careers guides (copies of these will be found in your local college or local library as well as at your local careers office).

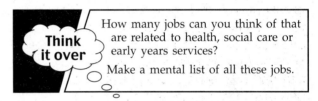

Think it over

How many jobs can you think of that are related to health, social care or early years services?

Make a mental list of all these jobs.

Jobs in the direct provision of health care

The NHS is the biggest employer of staff in Europe but not everyone who is involved in the provision of health care is employed by the NHS (see Figure 1.21). As we have already seen, some health care professionals are employed by voluntary organisations, by private companies, by government departments or are self-employed. While some health care jobs require basic training (such as nursing), others require more specialised training in addition to the basic training (such as midwifery).

Talk it over

What is the difference in the roles of a midwife and a health visitor?

You may need to talk to someone who is a midwife or health visitor to find out about this.

In the past ten years the use of **complementary therapies** (such as aromatherapy and homeopathy) has increased, and these therapies are rapidly becoming accepted and are now used alongside **conventional medicines and treatment**. This has resulted in yet a further increase in the

Figure 1.21   A few of the main jobs in health care

Doctors	Nurses	Therapists	Others	Support staff
Gynaecologist	District nurse	Physiotherapist	Chemist	Environmental health officer
Psychiatrist	Community psychiatric nurse	Aromatherapist*	Pharmacist	Administrator
Cardiologist	Ward co-ordinator or manager (sister)	Speech therapist	Chiropodist	Health service manager
Dermatologist	Health visitor	Art therapist*	Radiographer	Ambulance crew
Physician	Hospital nurse	Hypnotherapist*	Dietician	Catering officer
General practitioner	Midwife	Counsellor	Optician	Domestic supervisor
Surgeon	Nursing auxiliary	Drama therapist*	Pathologist	Laboratory technician
Geriatrician	Nurse for people with learning disabilities	Acupuncturist*	Anaesthetist	Medical records officer
Neurologist	Occupational health nurse	Homoeopath*	Dentist	Medical secretary
Paediatrician	Paediatric nurse	Osteopath*		Radiotherapist
Rheumatologist		Psychologist		Receptionist

Note: * **Complementary therapies.**

range of health care work currently available, although most complementary therapies are provided outside the NHS.

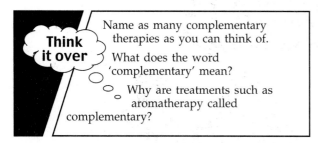

Think it over

Name as many complementary therapies as you can think of.

What does the word 'complementary' mean?

Why are treatments such as aromatherapy called complementary?

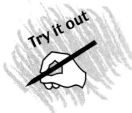

Try it out

Find out about how at least one complementary therapy works. For example, try using scented oils in your bath.

Hospital nurses

Hospital nurses are responsible for the nursing care of patients when they are in hospital. Nursing care involves such tasks as the following:

- Taking the patients' temperature, blood pressure and respiration rate.
- Giving patients injections.
- Administering medications.
- Cleaning and dressing wounds.
- Bandaging and splinting.
- Administering blood transfusions and drips.
- Routine tasks, such as bed-making, ensuring the patients are comfortable or escorting patients to other departments, such as X-ray or the operating theatre.

Nurses must familiarise themselves with the patients' medical history and circumstances; they must keep a careful record of the treatment that is given; and they must record the patients' progress. They must also take into account the patients' emotional and social needs, thus bringing a **'holistic' approach** to patient care (i.e. by addressing all these different needs, nurses provide an overall service to their patients that

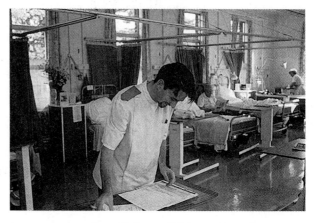

A nurse on a hospital ward

means more to the patients than if nurses simply performed practical tasks).

A nurse works as part of a *team* of nurses on the wards, or in other units within the hospital, such as the accident and emergency unit or out-patient clinics. A nurse also works as part of a multi-disciplinary team, which includes doctors, occupational therapists, physiotherapists and social workers. All the members of the multi-disciplinary team come together to ensure that patients receive as much help and support as they need so they can return to the community (see Figure 1.22).

There are many different types of ward on which nurses may work, including medical, surgical, orthopaedic (the correction of deformities in a patient's skeleton) and children's. There are also various units where they may be employed, such as operating theatre, out-patient clinics, maternity care units and intensive care units. There are areas of specialist work as well, for example, working with people who have neurological problems (such as people who have epileptic fits), or people who are receiving treatment for cancer.

The type of hospital a nurse might find him or herself working in can also vary enormously.

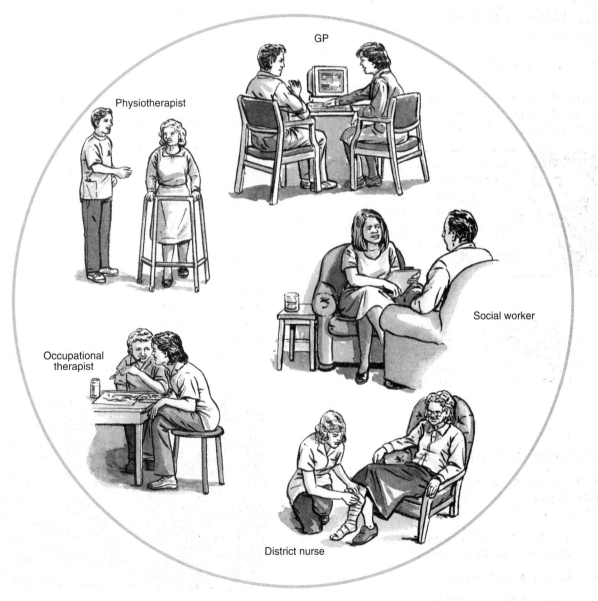

Figure 1.22   A multi-disciplinary team

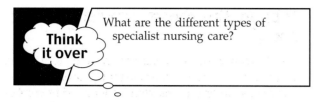

Some are very large and have a number of specialised wards and departments, out-patient clinics, an accident and emergency unit and operating theatres. Others may be much smaller and may specialise (for example in care for the elderly, for people with mental health problems or in health care specifically for children).

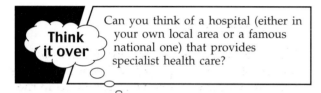

From the beginning of their training, nurses may choose to specialise in one form of nursing (see Figure 1.23). Nurses undertaking adult and general nursing training will spend time on many different wards and units during their training, but may still specialise in specific aspects of nursing.

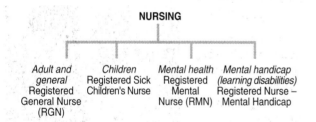

Figure 1.23   The specialised divisions of nursing

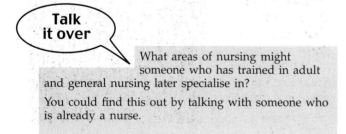

Skills and qualities
Nursing is physically, intellectually and emotionally demanding work. Trainee nurses are required to take in large quantities of knowledge, and the work itself can be very physically draining, as much time is spent walking from one location to another and can involve the trainees helping the patients move about the hospital. Being faced with illness or injury is always traumatic for both patients and their relatives, and the nurse will often be required to talk with patients about their situation, their problems and their fears, as well as having to deal with their worried relatives. Nurses need to be able to deal with difficult situations and distressed patients and families. They must remain calm and caring and must not become distressed themselves. They also need to be observant: they have to take in a lot of information and make sense of it. They must also be able to communicate clearly, both verbally and in writing.

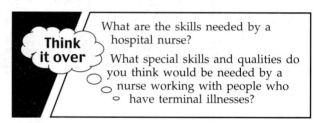

Nurses often have to work shifts, sometimes starting work early in the morning and finishing late in the evening. They may also be required to work at night, at weekends and on bank holidays. They therefore need to be adaptable in their working patterns (see Figure 1.24).

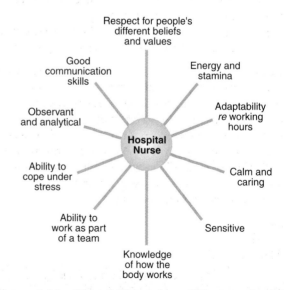

Figure 1.24   The skills and qualities required of a hospital nurse

General practitioners (GPs)

The GP, or family doctor, is very important in the provision of primary health care. The GP is often the first person to be consulted when someone is feeling unwell. It is the job of the GP to make any necessary examinations and, where possible, to make a diagnosis of the problem or illness and to prescribe appropriate medicines. GPs are now also increasingly performing minor operations.

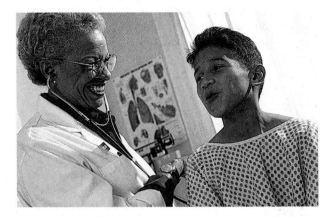

A general practitioner

GPs will advise people on how to manage an illness, disability or problem. They often become concerned with the patients' personal and social problems as well as their health problems. Where appropriate, GPs refer patients to hospitals or clinics, or other agencies, for specialist services.

General practice differs from other areas of medicine as GPs are not salaried. GPs receive a basic allowance plus additional payments depending on the number of patients registered with them and the types of service they offer.

Most GPs work as part of a team, the size of the team depending on the number of doctors working together and the variety of other professionals working with them (e.g. practice nurses, counsellors, receptionists, etc). However, much of their time is spent on a one-to-one basis with the patients. GPs often work long hours, seeing patients at their surgery or visiting them at home when necessary.

Talk it over

Do GPs and nurses need similar qualities for their work with people?

Jobs in the direct provision of social care

People who work in social care may be employed by public, private or voluntary organisations. They may undertake residential work, day care or 'fieldwork'. **Fieldwork** is the term used when a worker operates from a base (usually an office) but goes out to meet people, sometimes in their own homes ('working in the field'). As with health care, many other people are employed in jobs that support the direct provision of care (such as clerks and catering staff) but who may not come into direct contact with the clients.

Care assistants

Care assistants often provide **social care**. Most care assistants are employed by Local Authorities but they are increasingly being employed in the private sector as Local Authorities move away from the direct provision of services to the purchasing of private care services. Care assistants often work in residential homes, day centres, day nurseries or in people's own homes. Hence they work with people in a variety of ways and in various settings. Numerous other people are also employed in jobs that are concerned with people's social welfare (see Figure 1.25).

Care assistants assist people who require help with everyday tasks, such as getting up, washing, bathing, going to the toilet, dressing, shopping and housework. Obviously these tasks vary according to the individual client: care assistants can work with children and young people, people with

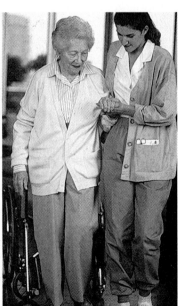

A care assistant who works with the elderly

CASE STUDY – Catherine

Catherine is a nurse on a hospital ward for elderly people. This is how she describes a typical day's work:

'I started work this morning at 7.00 am. When I came on to the ward many of the patients were already awake. This ward is for women only but in other hospitals the wards sometimes have both men and women. There are twenty beds on this ward grouped in bays of four. In some older hospitals the beds are just in lines down two sides of a long, narrow ward. The patients on this ward have a variety of problems: some are recovering from heart attacks or strokes, others have progressive illnesses such as motor neurone disease or Parkinson's disease, others have cancer.

My day begins with a "hand-over" from the night staff, who tell us how each patient has been during the night. It is then very hectic as the breakfast trolley arrives, and then we have to go round with the patients' medication. After this, the patients want to have a wash or bath. Later, various members of the multi-disciplinary team start arriving, such as the doctor, physiotherapist, social worker and occupational therapist. If we are beginning to plan a patient's discharge, there is often a meeting of the multi-disciplinary team to discuss how plans are going; often this also includes the patient and her relatives.

During the morning a patient may need to go to one of the other units for treatment, and I will often accompany her. Several of our patients have to have their blood pressure taken every 4 hours and those who are diabetic will need their blood sugar levels tested; others may need their dressings changed. Sometimes during the morning I will have a break for about 15 minutes but then it's back to the ward to help make beds, help the patients' get to

the toilet, answer patients' and relatives' queries about medication, etc. Patients are sometimes very anxious about what is happening to them and need a lot of reassurance and explanation from us. At the end of the shift, after the patients have all had their lunch and we've been round with the medication again, it's time to record what has been happening on each patient's file and to hand over to the afternoon shift. I love the work very much but it can be very tiring.'

Questions

1   What tasks might Catherine perform as part of her duties as a nurse?

2   What is meant by a multi-disciplinary team?

3   What skills does a ward nurse need in order to carry out his or her role?

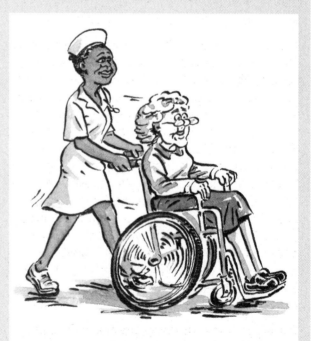

'I love the work very much ...'

Figure 1.25 A few of the main jobs in social care

Social workers	Care workers	Counsellers	Others
Children and families	Residential care	People with AIDS	Community workers
Older people	Day care	Bereavement	Housing officers
People with disabilities	Home care	Drugs and alcohol	Instructors
People with learning disabilities	People with disabilities	Family work	Liaison officers
People with mental health problems	People with learning disabilities	General counselling	Probation officers
Medical social workers	People with AIDS	Marital problems	Social work assistants
Palliative care social workers	Children and families	Students	Wardens
People with AIDS		Teenagers	

CASE STUDY – Pamela

Pamela is a care assistant in a residential home for older people. This is how she describes a typical day's work:

'Today I started work at 7.00 am. This means I was there when the residents began to wake up. The home I work in has forty residents and there are four units, so that 10 people live in each unit. There are six single bedrooms in each unit and two double rooms. One of the units, Snowdrop unit, is mainly for people with dementia.

Today I worked in Primrose unit where there are five women, three men and a married couple. My first task of the day was to help get people up, and to help them toilet, wash and dress. There are three assistants on the unit first thing in the morning, as this is a busy time. Once people are ready I help with the breakfasts. One of the three ladies I mainly work with is unable to feed herself, so I help her with this. Once breakfast is over the residents like to do various things. Some listen to the radio or watch TV, but when the weather is fine, like it was today, some like to go out into the garden. I took Joe out in his wheelchair this morning for a stroll around the grounds.

Throughout the morning people will need help with various things, such as going to the toilet or having a bath. Much of my time is taken up with toileting, washing and with meal times, but it's really nice when there is time to talk with a resident. They often have very interesting stories to tell.'

Questions

1 How might a care assistant help the residents who live in the home?

2 How could you find out about services for older people in your area?

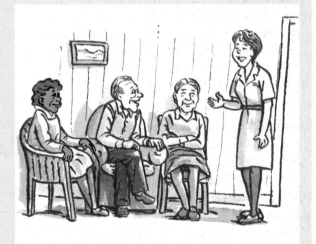

'The residents often have very interesting stories to tell'

physical or learning disabilities and with older people.

Some of the tasks include helping people with their personal hygiene (washing, bathing, cleaning their teeth, washing their hair, etc.). The tasks may also involve domestic duties (such as washing up, making beds, ironing, preparing and cooking meals, shopping, etc.). Sometimes care assistants will help people to learn new skills, including budgeting and cooking. They may also help set up activities for their clients that will help them improve or maintain their independence; they will also provide friendly support and a listening ear.

As already mentioned, care assistants can work in a variety of settings (nursing and residential homes, day centres, hostels and group homes or in the client's own home as a home carer). Hence a care assistant's working hours can vary greatly. Those working in a day centre will often work regular hours, Monday to Friday. However those working in a residential home, hostel or group home may be required to work shifts, sometimes starting early in the morning and finishing early in the afternoon, or starting in the afternoon and working through the evening. They may also have to work over weekends and at bank holidays. Care assistants working in the clients' own homes may work split shifts (i.e. a few hours in the morning and again in the evening). Many care assistants work part time.

Skills and qualities

Care assistants must be able to work with people from all sorts of backgrounds, religions, cultures and of different ages. They will need to be able to work alone and as part of a team. Maturity and common sense are very important. They must also have the right attitude and personality to be able to work with frail people, people with disabilities or with people who have difficulty doing everyday tasks. Patience, tolerance and the ability to encourage clients to do for themselves those things they are able to do are similarly very important.

Social workers

The majority of social workers are employed by Local Authorities although some may be employed by the health service or by voluntary organisations,

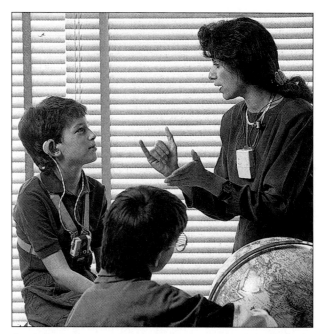

Social workers might work with people who have physical disabilities

such as the National Society for the Prevention of Cruelty to Children (NSPCC). The role of the social worker is to help people of all ages who need support with various aspects of their lives. These problems may be connected to low incomes, unemployment , poor housing, difficulties due to illness, disability, old age or relationship problems. As already noted, most social workers are employed by Local Authority social services departments (England and Wales), social work departments (Scotland) and area health and social services boards (Northern Ireland). They often work in teams that specialise in working with particular client groups, such as children and families, older people, people with physical disabilities, people with learning disabilities or people with mental health problems.

Social workers aim to assess the needs of individuals and families, then to set up and co-ordinate the services required to meet those needs. For example, a young adult who has had a road traffic accident, which results in him or her having to use a wheelchair, may need someone to help with personal care (getting up, washed, and dressed), someone to help with household tasks (cleaning, shopping, laundry) and may need special transport to get about. Sometimes the team includes other professionals, such as occupational therapists, home carers and clerks.

Social workers working with children and families might specialise in fostering and adoption work, in cases where child abuse or neglect is suspected or in cases where children have special needs (for example, when the child has a disability or behavioural problems). Social workers involved in child care may be required to attend juvenile courts.

When appropriate, social workers meet their clients and families to assess their needs and to determine the short and longer-term courses of action. Sometimes this can be done quickly and easily, but in other instances careful assessment and planning over a long period of time may be required. Social workers need to build up a relationship of trust with their clients so that they can help their clients explore the options open to them and to make informed choices about how their needs can best be met.

Social workers often work on a one to one basis with their clients, but at other times they will work with whole families or groups of people who have specific needs. They may also help clients to help themselves – in setting up support groups or self-help groups.

Some social workers specialise in other areas of work, for example:

- medical social work
- social work in palliative care
- work with people who have HIV and AIDS
- helping people who are drug or alcohol dependent
- work with people who have eating disorders
- helping women who have been abused.

These social workers often provide ongoing emotional support to the people they work with. Many social workers who choose to specialise work for voluntary organisations, but some might work for the NHS.

Most social workers work a 36-hour week, Monday to Friday. However, they are required to be flexible in their working hours, which can sometimes involve evening and, occasionally, weekend working.

Skills and qualities

Social workers deal with all sorts of people, from different backgrounds, religions, cultures and of different ages. They therefore need to respect

Talk it over

Do you know someone who has been assessed, or has received help from a social worker?

What sort of help did he or she need and how was this need met?

individuals' personal beliefs, identities and the choices they make. They also need to be very good communicators, both verbally and in writing. Although a great deal of time is spent in client contact, there is also a lot of paperwork and administration that must be attended to. Keeping records and writing reports is an important aspect of the social worker's role. To assess people's needs they must be able to:

- build up a rapport with people
- collect and analyse large amounts of complex information
- explain the options available to meet people's needs
- negotiate with others in order to obtain the services necessary to meet those needs.

There are often many conflicting demands on the social workers' time. Therefore they must be able to prioritise the tasks they need to do and to be capable of working under pressure. Much of the work can be emotionally demanding, but they must come to understand their clients' problems without getting involved at a personal level. Social workers must be strong enough to deal with a lack of co-operation from some of their clients while still trying to help them (see Figure 1.26).

Think it over

Do you know of anyone who has a learning disability?

What activities is he or she involved in during the week?

Does he or she go to work or attend a course at his or her local college?

Talk it over

What qualities and skills would a care assistant and a social worker have in common?

Make a list of them.

CASE STUDY – Justin

Justin is a social worker in a team which works with people who have learning disabilities. This is how he describes a typical day's work:

'I work in a team where there are four social workers, a social work assistant and three community nurses. Our team leader is also a social worker. This morning began with us all meeting together to talk about any problems we have had in helping the various people we work with and to agree who is to work with the new person who has just been referred to us. This is a 30-year-old woman with mild learning disabilities who has always lived with her parents. A few years ago her father died and now her mother is seriously ill. I have been asked to meet Pat and her mother to talk about how Pat will manage in the future and what sort of support she will need; whether she will be able to remain in the family home or whether she might need to move into a home with other people with learning disabilities.

I met them this afternoon. The meeting was a very emotional one, with Pat's mother having to face up to the fact that she will not be able to look after Pat any longer and Pat having to think about her mother's impending death. Having talked about some of the options, I agree to meet Pat and her mother again in a few days, when they will have had time to think things through.

During the morning I attended a review meeting at a day centre. This centre is for people with learning disabilities and clients got there once a week to meet one another and to have group discussions about any issues that are worrying them. Today we are reviewing the care plan and activity plan of a young man who I've been involved with for the past three years. At the moment he

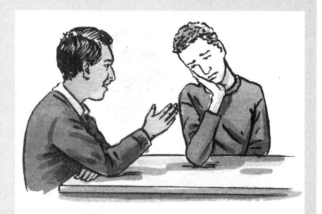

'The work can be emotionally draining, but it is also very rewarding'

is very unhappy about the computer course he has been attending at the local college and wants to talk about finding an alternative course. Also at the meeting are Ben's parents and his key worker from the day centre. After a lot of discussion Ben decides he would rather be doing an art course. I agree to find out more about these for him.

Sometimes the work can be very frustrating – there aren't enough funds to put in all the support services someone really needs. It can be emotionally draining, but it is also very rewarding!'

Questions

1   What social services might a person with learning difficulties need?

2   What social care services are available in your area for people with learning difficulties?

3   What skills would a social worker need when working with someone who has learning difficulties?

28

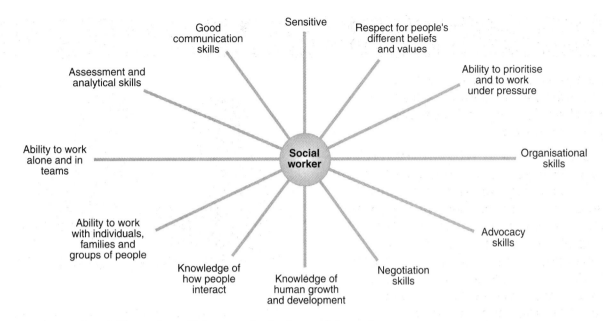

Figure 1.26   The skills and qualities required of a social worker

Jobs in the direct provision of early years services

Local Authorities, voluntary organisations and private agencies are involved in the provision of day care services and playgroups for children aged 5 years and under, and they may also provide out-of-school 'clubs' for children between the ages of 5 and 8 years. The main jobs in early years services include nursery nurses, childminders, and play and playgroup leaders. However, they also include 'nannies' and au pairs who are employed directly by parents, often through agencies. They similarly include other child care professionals, such as educational psychologists.

Other professionals involved in providing appropriate health care services for babies and young children include paediatricians, midwives, health visitors, nurses who specialise in working with ill children, speech therapists, physiotherapists and play therapists.

As in health and social care, there are also many people in jobs that provide support to those giving direct care but who may not come into direct contact with the clients. These include managers of services, secretaries, cooks and cleaners (see Figure 1.27).

Nursery nurses

Nursery nurses can work in a variety of settings, such as day nurseries, residential nurseries,

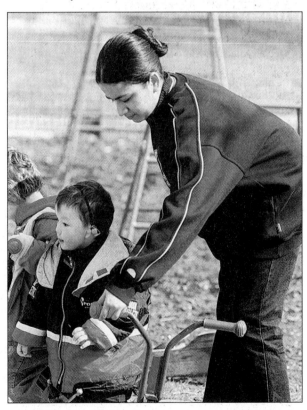

A nursery nurse

Figure 1.27 A few of the main jobs in early years services

Health care	Social care and early years education	Support staff
Midwives	Play leaders	Managers
Health visitors	Play therapists	Administrators
Paediatric nurses	Social workers	Secretaries
Nannies	Nannies	Cooks
Nursery nurses	Nursery nurses	Cleaners
Speech therapists	Au pairs	
Physiotherapists	Psychologists	
	Childminders	
	Specialist teacher assistants	

schools, crèches, hospitals or in the child's own home. They may work as part of a team (e.g. when working in a nursery) or they may work alone with one or two children or a group of children (i.e. when working privately for a family or when working in a crèche).

Nursery nurses can be involved in many care tasks – for instance, feeding, washing and toileting. They are also responsible for planning activities and play following the guidelines set out in the Early Learning Goals. The Early Learning Goals provide guidance on what children should be able to do at the ages of 3, 4 and 5 years. At the end of the reception year at school (when aged 5–6 years), that is, from school year 1 onwards, the children's learning is planned according to the requirements of the National Curriculum.

Nursery nurses take responsibility for the overall care of the children in their charge.

Skills and qualities

The children may come from all sorts of backgrounds and from different ethnic or religious groups. Nursery nurses therefore need to respect the different beliefs and values of the children's families. They also need good communication skills, especially with the children but also with the adults: they will often need to talk with the parents about their children. They similarly need good writing skills as they will be required to write reports on the children's development and achievements. Patience is a very necessary quality as children can be very demanding, and some may have emotional or

behavioural problems. Nursery nurses must have an understanding of child development and of the principles of preschool education. Sometimes they work alongside other professionals, such as social workers, speech therapists or physiotherapists, and so need to be able to work as part of a multi-disciplinary team. Nursery nurses also need a lot of energy, as children can be very active (see Figure 1.28).

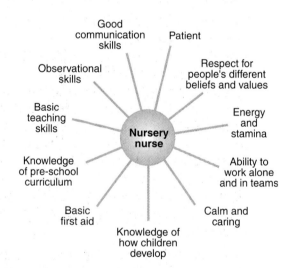

Figure 1.28   The skills and qualities required of a nursery nurse

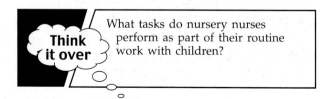

Think it over

What tasks do nursery nurses perform as part of their routine work with children?

Talk it over

Nursery nurses and social workers need similar skills and qualities. What are they? Make a list of them.

What are the different skills and qualities each need?

Jobs providing indirect care

To care for their clients effectively, those people who provide direct care often need the help of support services. In hospitals, clinics, social services departments and early years services, all sorts of administrative staff are needed. In

CASE STUDY – Lynn

Lynn is a nursery nurse in a private day care nursery. This is how she describes a typical day's work:

'The nursery opens at eight o'clock in the morning and closes at six o'clock at night. It is open from Monday to Friday every week of the year and only closes for bank holidays. All the children live in the local community and come from various ethnic backgrounds. Many come to the nursery because their parents are at work. About half come from one-parent families. The children are aged from 18 months to 5 years.

My day begins by greeting the children. Today, a new 3-year-old little boy came for the first time. He was very upset when his mother left and I stayed with him until he stopped crying and joined in with the other children. We give the children breakfast at about 9.00 am, dinner at 12.30 and afternoon tea at 4.00 pm. I sometimes help serve the food and I help the younger children to feed themselves. I am involved in all aspects of the children's routine care, including washing, dressing and toileting.

After breakfast I help set out the play equipment, such as colouring or picture books, jigsaws and puzzles, dressing-up clothes and toys. If the weather is good we go out into the garden where there are swings, slides, climbing frames and sand trays. After lunch we have 'quiet time'. I often read a story to the children before they have a rest. We have little beds where

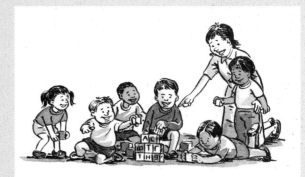

'I feel I am a friend to many of the children'

the children can have a nap. Later in the afternoon we often sing songs or play games. I also help the children to learn how to tie their shoe-laces and about table manners and other social skills.

It is a very demanding job. Sometimes the children can be quite naughty and will not listen to what is being said to them. You need a lot of patience. You also need a lot of energy to keep up with them. But it is also a very rewarding job and I feel I am a friend to many of the children.'

Questions

1   What qualifications does a nursery nurse have to have?

2   What skills does a nursery nurse need in order to work with small children?

3   What services are available in your area for pre-school age children?

residential and day care centres, whether run by Health Authorities or Local Authorities, catering services and possibly laundry services are required. As new technology is increasingly being employed in health care services, the equipment used for diagnosis and treatment is becoming ever more sophisticated. Similarly, information technology is now used for recording service users' records, which means that staff must be employed who have specialist technical skills (see Figure 1.29).

Receptionists

Receptionists are to be found working in many health and social care units, and their roles will vary according to the setting where they are employed. However, the receptionist's basic tasks remain the same and they usually involve operating the telephone switchboard and greeting people as they arrive at the unit. Sometimes they are also required to do general clerical tasks or to take on administrative or secretarial duties. They must also be able to use a computer for sending out letters and to keep the unit's information up to date.

Skills and qualities

Receptionists must be able to put people at their ease and to greet them with courtesy and warmth. They should be very sensitive to other people's feelings and be able to cope with people

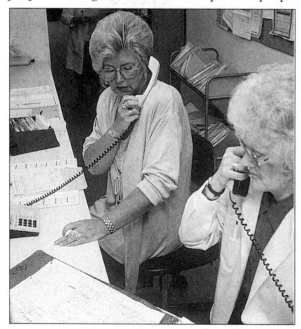

Receptionists in a GP's surgery

Figure 1.29 A few of the jobs indirectly involved in health, social and early years services

Job
Ambulance drivers
Porters
Catering assistants
Cooks
Domestic staff
Gardeners
Caretakers
Laboratory technicians
Radiographers
Drivers
Managers
Administrators
Secretaries
Clerks
Receptionists
Record keepers
IT officers
Finance officers
Supplies officers
Personnel officers

who are upset. They must be very clear in their communication, both verbally and written. Patience is also very important when dealing with people, and it often helps to have a good sense of humour. As already mentioned, the particular skills a receptionist will need will depend on the requirements of his or her job (see Figure 1.30)

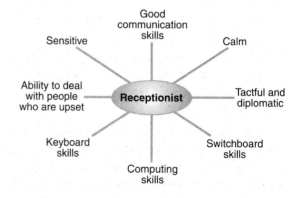

Figure 1.30   The skills and qualities required of a receptionist

Think it over

Make a list of the different offices or establishments you visit that employ a receptionist.

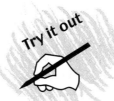

Try it out

Choose one of the job roles you have just read about or you know about and write a short description of the skills needed. Which skills do you think are the most important, and why? You could interview someone working in this sector and base your description on his or her job.

CASE STUDY – John

John is a receptionist in a hospice. This is how he describes his work:

'There are three receptionists at the hospice where I work, and I am the only man among them! One works on Saturdays and Sundays from 9.00 am to 5.00 pm. I work Monday to Friday from 8.00 am to 4.00 pm and the third works Monday to Friday from 4.00 pm until 9.00 pm.

A lot of my time is spent answering the telephone. Sometimes it is a relative who needs to speak to the nurses or a doctor. Sometimes it's another professional who needs to speak to one of the hospice staff. We have lots of different professionals working at the hospice. These include doctors, nurses, social workers, occupational therapists, physiotherapists and a chaplain. I often have to take messages when staff are not available.

The other main part of my job is greeting people when they come to the hospice. Often relatives who are visiting patients can be very upset, and I sometimes have to spend some time talking to them. I often make them a cup of tea.

Part of my role involves selling cards and small gift items to people. This is one way we help to raise money for the hospice. People often bring in donations as well. It is part of my job to receive these donations.

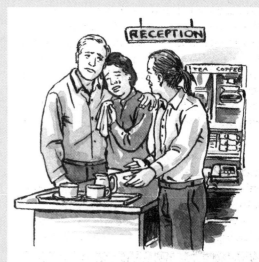

'I am often the first person in the hospice people have contact with'

Even small amounts of money help, so I like to make everyone who brings in a donation feel really special. I am also responsible for sending out "thank you" letters to these people.

I feel the work I do is very important, as I am often the first person in the hospice people have contact with.'

Questions

1   What skills are needed by someone working as a receptionist?

2   What tasks might a receptionist perform?

Effective communication skills

The main skill a care worker needs to work effectively is the availability to understand and communicate with others. Communication skills are vital in care work because they enable care workers to:

◦ understand the needs of others

◦ form relationships with clients

◦ show respect towards clients and other members of staff

◦ meet the clients' social, emotional and intellectual needs.

Some people might think that 'communicating with clients' involves nothing more than common sense. This is not true: care workers have to develop a range of skills (Figure 1.31).

Being an effective carer involves learning about the individual people you work with. Learning about other people involves listening to what they have to say and understanding the messages people send with their body language. It is not always easy to get to know people: we need the skills of being able to listen, of being capable of sustaining a conversation and of interpreting other people's body language correctly to help us understand each other and to build relationships.

Non-verbal communication

Immediately we meet someone we are usually able to tell what that person is feeling – whether that person is tired, happy, angry, sad, frightened – even before he or she has said anything. We can usually tell what people are feeling by noting their body language.

The proper term for body language is 'non-verbal communication'. Non-verbal means without words, so non-verbal communication is the messages we send out without putting them into words. We send out messages using our eyes, the tone of our voice, our facial expression, our hands and arms, by gestures with our hands and arms, through the angle of our head and by the way we sit or stand (the latter is known as body posture).

When people are sad they may signal this emotion with eyes that look down – there may

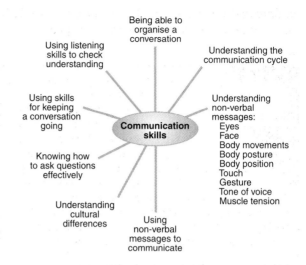

Figure 1.31   The communication skills needed for care work

also be tension in their faces, their mouths may be closed. The shoulder muscles are likely to be relaxed but the person's face and neck may show tension. A happy person will have 'wide eyes' that make contact with you – his or her face will 'smile'. When people are excited they move their arms and hands to signal their excitement (Figure 1.32).

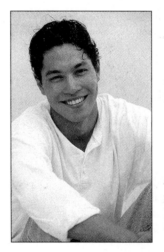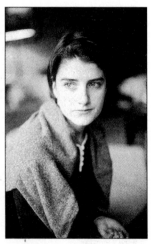

Figure 1.32   We signal our emotions through the expression on our faces

Most people are able to recognise such emotions but skilled carers must go one stage further than simply identifying emotions: they must understand the messages they send out with their *own* bodies when working with other people.

Non-verbal messages

Our bodies send out messages to other people – often without us consciously meaning to send these messages. Some of the most important body areas that send out messages are shown in Figure 1.33.

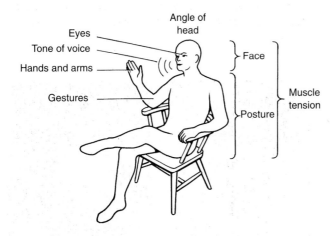

Figure 1.33   Areas of the human body that send out non-verbal messages

The eyes

We can often tell what other people's feelings and thoughts are by looking at their eyes. Our eyes get wider when we are excited, or when we are attracted or interested in someone else. A fixed stare may send the message that someone is angry. In European culture, to look away is often interpreted as being bored or not interested.

The face

Our face can send very complex messages and we can read these easily – even in diagrammatic form (see Figure 1.34).

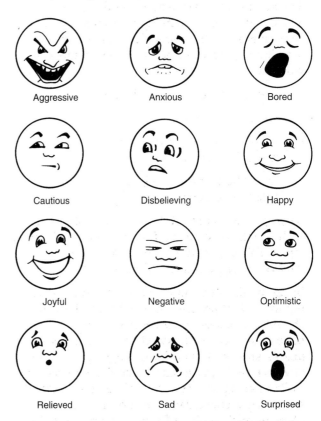

Figure 1.34   Facial expressions that send out messages

Tone of voice

It's not just *what* we say, but it's the *way* we say it. If we talk in a loud voice with a fixed voice tone, people think we are angry. A calm, slow voice with a varying tone may give out the message that we are being friendly.

Body movement

The way we walk, move our heads, sit, cross our legs and so on sends messages about whether we are tired, happy, sad or bored.

Posture

The way we sit or stand can send messages (Figure 1.35). Sitting with crossed arms can mean 'I'm not taking any notice'. Leaning can send the message you are relaxed or bored. Leaning forward can show you are interested.

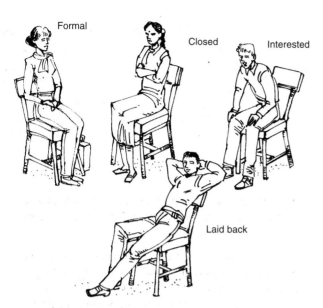

Figure 1.35   Our body posture can send out messages

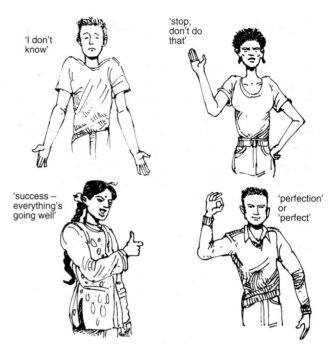

Figure 1.36   Some gestures commonly used in Britain

Muscle tension

The tension in our feet, hands and fingers can tell others how relaxed or tense we are. If people are very tense their shoulders might stiffen, their face muscles tighten and they might sit or stand rigidly. A tense face might have a firmly closed mouth, with lips and jaws clenched tight. A tense person might breathe quickly and become flushed.

Gestures

Gestures are hand and arm movements that can help us to understand what a person is trying to say. Some gestures carry a meaning of their own (see Figure 1.36).

Touch

Touching another person can send messages of care, affection, power over that person or sexual interest. The social setting and other body language usually help people to understand what a particular touch might mean. Carers should not make assumptions about touch: even holding someone's hand might be interpreted as an attempt to dominate them!

How close people are

The space between people can show us how friendly or 'intimate' the conversation is.

Different cultures have different codes of behaviour with respect to the space between people when they are talking.

Face-to-face positions

Standing or sitting eye to eye to someone else can send the message of formality or anger. A slight angle will create a more relaxed and friendly feeling (see Figure 1.37).

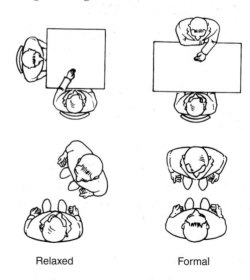

Relaxed   Formal

Figure 1.37   Face-to-face encounters

Organising a conversation

Skilled communication involves thinking about how we start and how we finish a conversation. Usually we start with a greeting or by asking how the other person is. As conversations have a beginning, a middle and an end, we must create the right kind of atmosphere for a conversation from the very start. We might need to help someone relax by showing we are friendly and relaxed. Next comes the conversation. When we end the conversation we usually say something like 'See you soon'. When we end a conversation we must leave the other person with the right feelings about what we have said (see Figure 1.38). A conversation is rather like a sandwich: the beginning and ends are the 'bread' and the conversation itself – the middle – is the 'filling'.

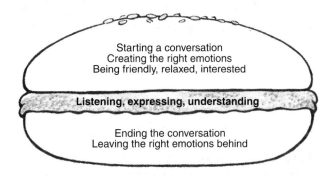

Figure 1.38   The conversation 'sandwich'

Starting a conversation
Creating the right emotions
Being friendly, relaxed, interested

Listening, expressing, understanding

Ending the conversation
Leaving the right emotions behind

The communication cycle

Communication is not just about giving people information. While we talk we go through a process or 'cycle' of:

- hearing what the other person says
- watching the other person's non-verbal messages
- having emotional feelings
- beginning to understand the other person
- sending a message back to the other person.

The communication cycle or process might look something like Figure 1.39.

Listening skills

We might be able to understand other people's emotions by observing their non-verbal

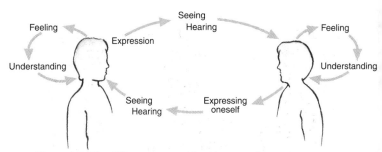

Figure 1.39   The communication cycle

communication but we can't usually understand what's on someone's mind without being a good listener.

Listening is not the same as hearing the sounds people make when they talk. Listening skills involve hearing another person's words – then thinking about what they mean – then thinking what to say back to the other person. Some people call this process 'active listening'. As well as thinking carefully and remembering what someone says, good listeners will also make sure their non-verbal communication demonstrates interest in the other person.

Skilled listening involves:

1 looking interested and ready to listen

2 hearing what is said

3 remembering what is said

4 checking understanding with the other person.

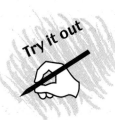

This is a practical exercise in listening: Take a piece of paper. Divide it into four areas and write four headings: 'Where I live', 'My last birthday', 'Something to look forward to' and 'My favourite lesson'. Any four titles will do as long as you have lots to say about the four areas. Think about what you can tell another person about yourself based on these four areas. Then get together with a partner who has also planned a talk about him or herself in this way. Describe the four areas to each other. See what you can remember about the other person from what he or she said and how detailed and how accurate this is!

How good are you at understanding and remembering?

Checking our understanding

It is usually easier to understand people who are similar to ourselves. We can learn about different people by checking our understanding of what we have heard.

Checking our understanding involves hearing what the other person says and asking the other person questions. Another way to check our understanding is to put what a person has just said into our own words and to say this back to them to see if we did understand what they said.

When we listen to complicated details of other people's lives, we often begin to form mental pictures based on what they are telling us. Listening skills involve checking these mental pictures to make sure we are understanding correctly. It can be very difficult to remember accurately what people tell us if we don't check how our ideas are developing.

Good listening involves thinking about what we hear while we are listening and checking our understanding as the conversation goes along. Sometimes this idea of checking our understanding is called 'reflection', because we reflect the other person's ideas (Figure 1.40).

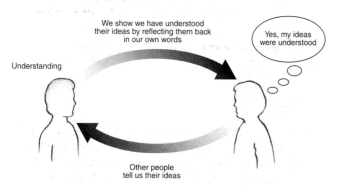

We show we have understood their ideas by reflecting them back in our own words

Yes, my ideas were understood

Understanding

Other people tell us their ideas

Figure 1.40   'Reflecting' back to the other person proves we have listened

Good listening is hard work. Instead of just being around when people speak, we must build up an understanding of the people around us. Although listening is difficult, people who are attracted to work in care usually enjoy learning about other people and their lives.

Cultural differences

Listening is one of the main ways we usually learn about other people, but skilled carers use a range of conversational techniques when working with clients. These techniques include being sensitive to cultural differences and social contexts, and getting a conversation going and keeping it going.

Culture means the history, customs and the ways people learn as they grow up. The expressions people use and the meanings non-verbal signs can have vary from one culture to another. For example, people from different regions of Britain use different expressions. In parts of the North of England, for example, the word 'canny' means a 'with it' and/or attractive person. In the South this word is unlikely to be understood and may be taken to mean something bad. In Ireland the term 'good crack' means 'good fun', but in England the term 'crack' refers to a very dangerous drug!

White middle-class people often expect other people to 'look them in the eye' while talking. If someone looks down or away a great deal, this is interpreted as a sign that they may be dishonest, or perhaps sad or depressed. In other cultures, for example, among some black communities, looking down or away when talking is a sign of respect – a way of showing you are using your listening skills! Care workers must be careful not to assume that statements and signs always mean the same thing – culture, race, class and geographical location can alter meaning.

There is a vast range of meanings that can be inferred from different types of eye contact, facial expression, posture or gesture and every culture develops its own special system of meanings. It may be impossible to learn about all these possible meanings but carers must be alert to them and must respect them.

Having said all this, it is possible to learn what your clients mean when they communicate with you. One way to do this is to remember what people say or do and try to understand what they really mean. However, this understanding needs to be checked. To do this it is usually possible to ask polite questions, or to work out what people mean over time by watching and listening to the other things they say or do.

The important thing to remember is that our own way of behaving and communicating is not the only way – or even the right way!

Keeping a conversation going

Once we have started a conversation we must keep it going long enough to meet our purpose and the emotional needs of others. Skills that help us achieve this are turn-taking, using non-verbal communication to show interest, the skilful use of questions and using silence at the appropriate moments.

If we are trying to get to know someone, we will probably listen more than we will talk: we must give the person we are talking to the opportunity to express him or herself. This involves taking turns. The person we are talking to will give us clues about this: people often slow down the rate at which they speak when they are reaching their last words, and they might change the tone of voice slightly, and look away from us. They might then stop speaking and look directly at us. If we are sensitive to these messages, we will be ready to ask a question or say something which keeps the conversation going.

We must also be interested in what the other person is saying. This demonstrates to the person we are talking to that we respect them – and carers must be interested in and respect what their clients say.

Showing interest means giving the other person your full attention and is the way you will keep the other person talking. Non-verbal messages we can employ to do this include:

- eye contact – looking at the other person's eyes

- smiling – looking friendly rather than 'cold' or 'frozen' in expression

- hand movements and gestures that show that we are interested

- slight head nods while talking to signal non-verbally, that we 'see', 'understand' or 'agree'.

Asking questions

Some of the questions we might ask will not encourage people to talk: these are closed questions. Questions such as 'How old are you?' are 'closed' because there is only one, right, simple answer the person can give: 'I'm 84'. Closed questions do not lead on to a discussion. 'Do you like butter?' is a closed question because the person replying can only say yes or no. 'Are you feeling well today?' is also closed – the person replying can again only say yes or no.

Open questions 'open' up the conversation. Instead of giving a yes/no answer, the person we are talking to is encouraged to consider his or her reply. A question such as 'How do you feel about the food here?' means the other person has to think about the food and then discuss it. Open questions keep a conversation going; closed questions can block a conversation and cause it to stop.

The more we know about someone, the more sensitive we will be about the questions we ask. For example, people often do not mind answering questions about their feelings or opinions, but dislike questions that ask for personal information. Getting to know people often takes time and will involve a number of short conversations rather than one long, single conversation.

Silence

Pauses in a conversation can be embarrassing – it can look as if we are not listening or interested in what is being said. However, sometimes a silent pause can mean 'let's think' or 'I need time to think'. Silent pauses do not always stop the conversation as long as our non-verbal messages demonstrate to the other people we respect them and are interested in them.

Misusing language

Think it over

Read the short conversation below. Using your knowledge of communication skills, work out what is wrong with them.

A young child is talking with a childminder:

Child: Why do people drive cars?

Childminder: Never mind that, you just keep playing – don't be a nuisance.

A young person with a learning disability is talking with a care worker:

Young person: I can help do it.

Care worker: No you can't help with this, go and help Fran lay the table.

Young person: But I want.

Care worker: No! You do what I tell you.

A care worker is helping an older person to get up in the morning:

Care worker: Come on – time to get up!

Older person: Who are you? Where am I?

Care worker: Come on, I'm in a hurry, your breakfast is waiting.

Older person: Where is my daughter?

Care worker: I don't know – just hurry up.

In these conversations the care workers are not listening. They are hearing what is said but are ignoring the client's feelings. There is no effective communication cycle or conversation. The conversations have no beginning, middle or end. There is no skilled questioning to try to understand what the clients are saying. In each situation people are told to do something with no respect being shown for their needs or feelings.

Barriers to communication

There are three main ways in which communication can become blocked:

1   If a person cannot see, hear or receive the message.

2   If a person cannot make sense of the messages.

Think it over

Children who are not encouraged to ask questions may learn 'not to bother'. This may limit their social and intellectual development. Children whose questions are often ignored may learn to do other things to get attention. Throwing toys, shouting or breaking things may result in getting attention if asking questions does not.

People who are ignored may feel they are of little value. A person who is never listened to may have a poor opinion of him or herself. People with learning difficulties treated this way will have unfulfilled social and emotional needs.

Older people may not be given the respect they deserve. If their questions are ignored they are likely to feel they are not worth much. Without purposeful conversation, they may feel life is not worth living.

Effective care hinges on good communication skills.

3   If a person misunderstands the message.

Apart from visual and hearing disabilities, the first kind of block can be created by environmental problems:

- poor lighting
- noise
- speaking from too far away (Figure 1.41).

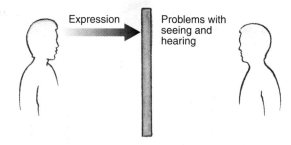
Expression

Problems with seeing and hearing

Figure 1.41   Environmental problems, such as noise and poor lighting, can create communication barriers

Occasions when people might not be able to make sense of messages include the following:

- Different languages are being used, including sign languages.

- People are using different terms, such as **jargon** (technical language), **slang** and **dialect**.

⬧ One of the speakers has a physical or intellectual disability, such as an illness, memory loss, or a learning dysfunction.

Examples of misunderstanding include the following:

⬧ *Cultural differences*: different cultures interpret non-verbal and verbal messages, and humour, in different ways.

⬧ *Assumptions about people*: assumptions about race, gender, disability, etc. can lead to stereotyping and misunderstanding.

⬧ *Emotional differences*: very angry or very happy people may misinterpret what is said.

⬧ *Social contact*: conversations and non-verbal messages understood by close friends may not be understood by strangers.

Supporting individuals

The care **value base** (see the next main section in this unit) requires care workers to value people's equality and diversity as well as their rights. People will feel valued and respected when they have been listened to, and when they feel their needs and wishes have been understood by the care worker. Good communication skills are vital for this, and care workers must find ways of overcoming the communication barriers that often arise between the client and worker (Figure 1.42).

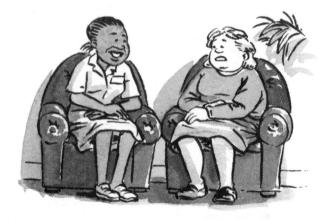

Figure 1.42 Care values are often expressed in our conversations with clients

Ways of overcoming barriers to communication

Visual disability

⬧ Use conversation to describe things.

⬧ Help people to touch things (e.g. touch your face so that the person can recognise you).

⬧ Explain the details sighted people take for granted.

⬧ Check what people *can* see (many registered blind people can see shapes or tell the difference between light and dark).

⬧ Check that spectacles are being worn, if necessary, and that they are clean.

Hearing disability

⬧ Do not shout: speak normally and make sure your face is visible so that those who can lip-read are able to do so.

⬧ Use pictures or write messages.

⬧ Learn to sign – for people who can use signed languages, such as Makaton or British Sign Language (BSL).

⬧ Use the services of a professional communicator or interpreter when sign languages are employed.

⬧ Check that hearing aids etc., are being used and are in working order.

Environmental barriers

⬧ Check and, if necessary, improve the lighting.

⬧ If possible, reduce the background noise.

Move to a quieter or better-lit room, if this will help.

⬧ Work in smaller groups if this will help you see and hear each other more easily.

Language differences

⬧ Use pictures, diagrams, and non-verbal signs and expressions.

- Use a translator or interpreter.

- Do not make assumptions or stereotype. Do not assume that people with physical or sensory disabilities have learning disabilities. Similarly, older people who have communication difficulties should not be labelled as 'confused'.

Jargon, slang and dialects

- Try different ways of saying things – try to make sense of sounds or words people do not seem to understand.

- Speak in short, clear sentences.

Physical and intellectual disabilities (such as learning or memory disability)

- Use pictures and signs as well as clear, simple speech.

  Be calm and patient.

- Set up group meetings where people can share their interests or where they can reminisce.

- Make sure that people do not become isolated

Misunderstandings

- Be alert to different cultural interpretations.

- Avoid making assumptions or discriminating against people who are different.

- Use your listening skills to check your understanding is correct.

- Stay calm and try to calm people who are angry or excited.

- Be clear about the context of your conversation. Is it formal or informal? Use the appropriate form of communication accordingly.

What if it is not possible to communicate with a client?

Sometimes, when people have a very serious learning disability or an illness (such as dementia), it is not possible to communicate with them. In such situations care services will often employ an **advocate**. An advocate is someone who speaks for someone else: a lawyer speaking for a client in a courtroom is working as an advocate for that person and will argue the client's case. In care work, a volunteer might try to get to know someone who has dementia or a learning disability. The volunteer tries to communicate the client's needs and wants – as the volunteer understands them. Advocates should be independent of the staff team and so can argue for the client's rights without being constrained by what the staff think is easiest or cheapest to do.

> **Think it over**
>
> Think about a care setting, hospital home or day centre you have visited. What barriers to communication have you noticed? Apart from people's disabilities and differences, what communication barriers were created by the environment or by the staff's communication skills and assumptions?

The care value base

All care work is about improving the client's quality of life – and improving the quality of life means meeting people's intellectual, emotional and social needs, as well as their physical needs.

If care is about making life better for clients, then clients should be:

- helped to take control or stay in control of their lives

- treated as valuable people

- given respect and dignity

- listened to.

Care values attempt to define the key principles that should guide how carers behave. These principles include the need to respect people and to listen to what people say – even though at times the language used in the principles may seem complex and daunting.

For example, the Care Sector Consortium was a group of people who devised the National Vocational Qualification (NVQ) training

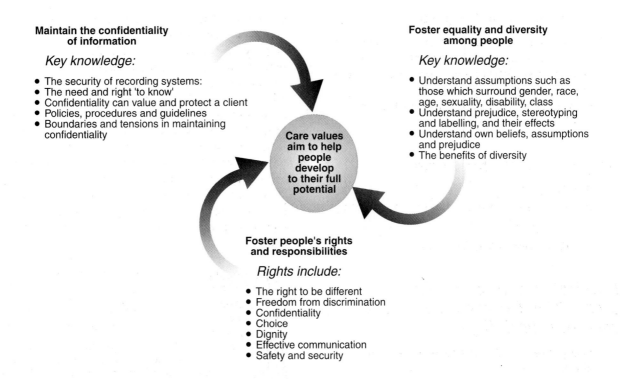

Maintain the confidentiality of information

Key knowledge:

● The security of recording systems:
● The need and right 'to know'
● Confidentiality can value and protect a client
● Policies, procedures and guidelines
● Boundaries and tensions in maintaining confidentiality

Foster equality and diversity among people

Key knowledge:

● Understand assumptions such as those which surround gender, race, age, sexuality, disability, class
● Understand prejudice, stereotyping and labelling, and their effects
● Understand own beliefs, assumptions and prejudice
● The benefits of diversity

Care values aim to help people develop to their full potential

Foster people's rights and responsibilities

Rights include:

● The right to be different
● Freedom from discrimination
● Confidentiality
● Choice
● Dignity
● Effective communication
● Safety and security

Figure 1.43   The care value base

standards for people who work in care. These standards define the values all care workers should follow. These standards are known as the care value base and this is set out in Figure 1.43.

Foster equality and diversity

Carers must value the ways people are different. They must understand the prejudices, stereotypes and assumptions that discriminate people on the grounds of gender, race, age, sexual orientation, disability or class. Carers must prevent such prejudices and assumptions damaging the quality of care provided to clients.

Foster people's rights and responsibilities

People have the right to their own beliefs and lifestyles, but no one has the right to damage the quality of other people's lives. This means that rights often come with responsibilities towards other people.

The easiest way to understand this is to think about the issue of smoking. Adults have a right to choose to smoke even though smoking usually damages health and often shortens a person's life. Smokers have a responsibility to make sure their smoke is not breathed in by other people. (See Figure 1.44.) This means that, in most places today, smoking is only allowed in specially designated areas.

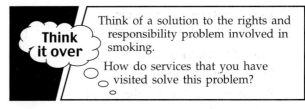

Think it over

Think of a solution to the rights and responsibility problem involved in smoking.

How do services that you have visited solve this problem?

Maintain the confidentiality of information

Confidentiality is an important right for all clients. It is important because of the following reasons:

⋄   Clients may not trust carers if the carers do not keep information confidential.

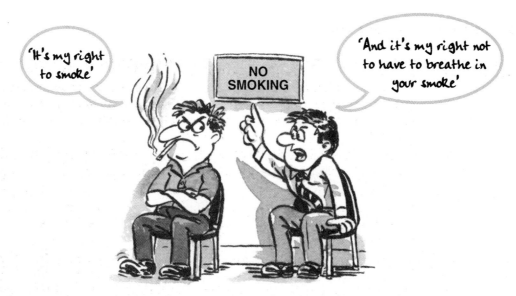

Figure 1.44 We all have rights, but we also have responsibilities to others

* Clients may not feel valued or may have feelings of low self-esteem if their private details are shared with others

* The client's safety may be put at risk if details of their property or their habits are widely known.

* A professional service that maintains respect for individuals must keep private information confidential.

* There are legal requirements to maintain the confidentiality of personal records.

Trust

Trust is very important. If you know your carer won't pass on things you have said to him or her, you will be more inclined to tell him or her what you really think and feel.

Self-esteem

If your carer promises to keep things confidential, this shows he or she respects and values you; it shows that you matter. Your self-esteem will therefore be higher than if the carer did not keep things confidential.

Safety

You may have to leave your home empty at times. If other people know where you keep your money and when you are out, someone may be tempted to break in. Hence carers must keep personal details confidential to protect their clients' property and personal safety.

Medical practitioners and lawyers have always strictly observed confidentiality as part of their professional code of conduct. If clients are to receive a professional service, care workers must follow this example.

Valuing diversity

No two people are the same and, because people are different, it can be easy to think that some people are better then others or that some views are right while others are wrong. Our individual cultures and life experiences may lead us to make assumptions about what is right or normal. When we meet people who are different from ourselves, it is all too easy to see them as 'not right' or 'not normal'. We must remember that different people see the world in different ways, and that our way of thinking may seem unusual to someone else.

Some of the ways in which people are different from one another are listed in Figure 1.45, which also lists the dangers of discrimination that might arise as a result of these differences.

Figure 1.45 The dangers of discrimination

Difference	Possible discrimination
Age	People may think of others as being children, teenagers, young adults, middle aged or old. Hence discrimination can creep into our thinking if we see some age groups as being 'the best' or if we make assumptions about the abilities of different age groups
Gender	In the past, men often had more rights than women and were seen as more important. Assumptions about gender still create discrimination problems
Race	People may understand themselves as being black or white, as European, African or Asian. People also have specific national identities, such as Polish, Nigerian, English or Welsh. Assumptions about racial or national characteristics lead to discrimination
Class	People differ in their upbringing, the kind of work they do and the money they earn. People also differ in the lifestyles they lead and the views and values that go with levels of income and spending habits. Discrimination against others can be based on their class or lifestyle
Religion	People grow up in different religious traditions. For some people, spiritual beliefs are at the centre of their understanding of life. For others, religion influences the cultural traditions they celebrate – for example, many Europeans celebrate Christmas even though they might not see themselves as practising Christians. Discrimination can take place when people assume that their customs or beliefs should apply to everyone else
Sexual orientation	Many people consider their sexual orientation as very important to understanding who they are. Gay and lesbian relationships are often discriminated against. Heterosexual people sometimes judge other relationships as 'wrong' or abnormal
Ability	People may make assumptions about what is 'normal'. Hence people with physical disabilities or learning disabilities may be labelled as 'not normal' or others may have stereotypical views about what they are capable of doing
Health	People who develop illnesses or mental health problems may feel they are valued less by others; they may feel discriminated against
Relationships	People choose many different lifestyles and have different emotional commitments, such as marriage, having children, living in a large family, living a single lifestyle but having sexual partners, or being single and not being sexually active. People live in different family and friendship groups. Discrimination can happen when people think that one lifestyle is 'right' or best
Presentation and dress	People express their individuality, lifestyle and social role through their clothes, hairstyles, make-up and jewellery. While it may be important to conform to dress codes at work, it is also important not to make stereotypical judgements about people because of the way they dress

Learning about diversity

To learn about other people's cultures and beliefs, we must take great care to listen to and observe what other people say and do. While learning about different cultures and beliefs can be very interesting and exciting, some people can find it stressful: we may feel our own culture and beliefs are being challenged when we realise there are so many different lifestyles. Such feelings may block our ability to learn about others.

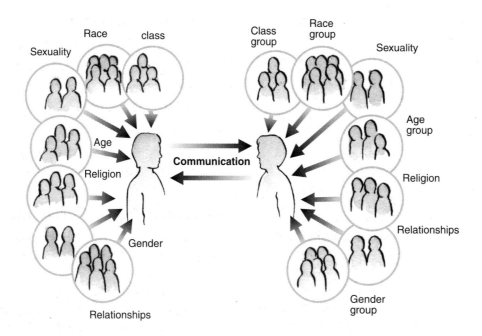

The groups a person belongs to will influence his or her beliefs and behaviour

Skilled carers must get to know the people they work with so that they will not make false assumptions about them. Carers must understand the ways that class, race, age, gender and so on influence individual people. Carers should also remember that a person's behaviour is not 'fixed': it will change as that person moves from one social group to another. For example, when we are at work we tend to take on the values of our workplace – we think and behave in the way our work demands and in the way our colleagues and those we come into contact with expect. In our private lives, however, we will take on other values: those of our friends when out for the evening or those of our family when at home or when we return for a family celebration.

Individuals may belong to the same ethnic group but they might have different religions or belong to different class groups. Simply knowing what someone's religion is will not necessarily tell you all about that person's beliefs or general culture. We can learn about different ethnic and religious customs but is impossible for us to know all the differences that might exist among individual clients. As mentioned earlier, the best way to learn about diversity is to listen to and communicate with people whose lives are different from our own.

Valuing diversity may make your own life better

Valuing diversity will enrich your life. If you are open to other people's life experience and differences, you will become more flexible and creative because you can imagine how other people see things. You will develop a wider range of social skills, and learning about other cultures will provide you with new experiences. Understanding other people's lives may also help you adapt your own lifestyle when you have to cope with change. For example, if you talk to people who are married or who have children, you will be better prepared if you choose these roles for yourself.

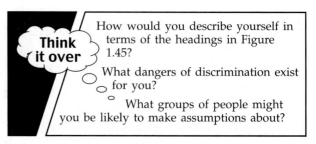

Think it over

How would you describe yourself in terms of the headings in Figure 1.45?

What dangers of discrimination exist for you?

What groups of people might you be likely to make assumptions about?

Employers are also likely to want to employ people who value diversity for the following reasons:

- Effective non-discriminatory care depends on all staff valuing diversity.

- People who value diversity are likely to be flexible and creative.

- People who value diversity will form good relationships with their colleagues and with the clients.

- Diverse teams often work together more effectively. If everyone has the same skills and interests, the team members may compete with each other. If people have different interests it is more likely the team will do all the work required and the people in the team will enjoy working together.

In care settings, everyone should receive a service of equal quality that meets their own personal needs. This is not, however, the same as everyone receiving the same service. Treating people as individuals, taking into account their different beliefs, abilities, likes and dislikes, is at the heart of caring for others.

If you encounter a situation where the services are not of equal quality, you should bring this to the attention of the management. In care settings there should be policies that have been designed to protect people from discrimination (see below).

Rights and responsibilities

Government legislation, codes of practice, employers' policies and national training standards outline the rights clients have when they are receiving health and social care services. These rights include:

- freedom from discrimination

- a right to independence and choice

- the right to be respected and to retain one's dignity

- safety and security

- confidentiality.

Figure 1.46 outlines some examples of these rights and responsibilities in more detail.

Freedom from discrimination

Discrimination means treating some groups of people less well than others and it may appear in the following ways:

- **Physical abuse** (hitting, pushing, kicking or otherwise assaulting a person). People may assault others because they hate certain groups or simply because they feel frustrated or annoyed at those who are different from themselves.

- **Verbal abuse** (insults, 'put downs' or damaging language). As with physical abuse, verbal abuse may make individuals feel more powerful if they think they can hurt other people with words.

- **Neglect** occurs when people are discriminated against by being ignored or by not being offered the help others might receive.

- **Exclusion** is a more subtle form of discrimination and may be hard to prove. Exclusion means stopping people from

Figure 1.46 The rights and responsibilities of people receiving care

Rights	Responsibilities
Not to be discriminated against	Not to discriminate against others
To have control and independence in their own lives	To help others to be independent and not try to control other people
To make choices and take some risks	Not to interfere with others, or put others at risk
To maintain their own beliefs and lifestyles	To respect the different beliefs and lifestyles of others
To be valued and respected	To value and respect others
A safe environment	To keep things safe for others
Confidentiality in personal matters	To respect confidentiality for others

getting services or jobs because they belong to a certain class, race or other group. Disabled people may be excluded from certain services because access is difficult – some buildings still do not have full disabled access. Some jobs may not be advertised in all areas, therefore excluding certain communities.

- **Avoidance** is where people try to avoid sitting next to people or working with people who are different from themselves. Such people are trying to avoid contact – perhaps because they do not want to learn about or rethink any of their prejudices.

- **Devaluing** means seeing some people as less valuable than others. Some people's self esteem is raised because they receive praise and their ideas are valued, but those who are 'different' may be criticised and their ideas ignored. People who are subjected to constant discrimination and prejudice may develop a very low sense of their own self-worth.

The effects of discrimination

Discrimination in all forms has permanent and extremely damaging effects (see Figure 1.47).

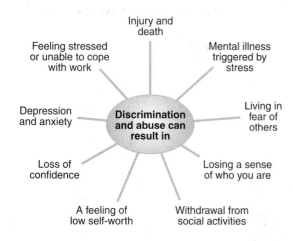

Figure 1.47   The effects of discrimination and abuse

Independence and choice

Although we all think of ourselves as being independent, there are times in our lives when we need another person's help. In care settings we can increase clients' independence by giving them control and choice over certain aspects of their care. To do this we must recognise the difference between doing things *to* or *for* clients and doing things *with* clients.

Wherever possible, clients should be helped to take control over their care. Even when people cannot do things for themselves, they can still be asked for their opinions about how they would like to be treated. This way we **empower** clients: feelings of independence increase a client's self-esteem. Feeling dependent on others may cause the opposite: clients will feel vulnerable and will have low self-esteem.

Talk it over

Discuss the difference between working *with* clients and working to do things *for* clients. Make a poster of *do's* and *don'ts* that shows how you could empower clients to be independent.

Dignity

Imagine you have been involved in an accident that puts you in hospital. Before this accident you were in control of yourself – you could do things for yourself – but now you need help with such basic things as washing and going to the toilet. How would you feel if someone had to help you to use the toilet? Perhaps if that person showed respect for your feelings and treated you with dignity, you might not feel so bad.

Clients must be treated with respect: when helping clients eat, wash, dress or use the toilet, it is vital we allow them to retain their sense of self-worth and dignity. We must show respect in the ways we give support. We must not have negative attitudes and we must provide the clients with the privacy and dignity they deserve.

Safety

All clients have the right to feel safe and secure when they are receiving care. They should not have to worry about themselves or their property; they must remain free of concern. The Health and Safety at Work Act 1974 makes it a duty of

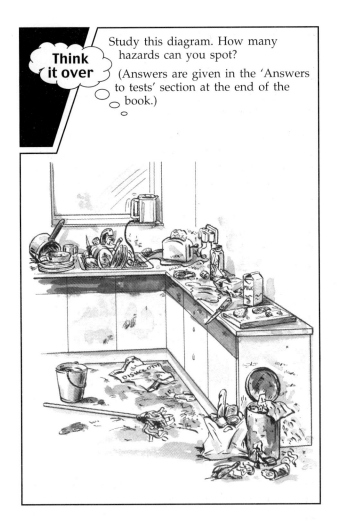

Study this diagram. How many hazards can you spot?

(Answers are given in the 'Answers to tests' section at the end of the book.)

Think it over

employers to ensure 'the health, safety and welfare at work of employees'. Equally, 'Employees have a duty to take reasonable care for the health and safety of themselves and others'.

When working in care it must be part of our daily routine to assess the safety of all situations. When working with clients who have impaired movement or poor sensory perception, it is doubly important to ensure there are no hazards.

Confidentiality

Confidentiality is a basic human right, but is so important that it has become a specific issue in the value base. The Data Protection Acts 1984 and 1998, the Access to Personal Files Act 1987 and the Access to Health Records Act 1990, make it a legal requirement that health and social care agencies keep client details confidential.

You will often be given personal information about the clients you are caring for, and this information must be kept confidential. Confidential personal information passed on to the wrong people might result in the client being discriminated against or put in danger. If care workers were to pass such information on to friends, neighbours or other members of the public, clients might feel they have lost control

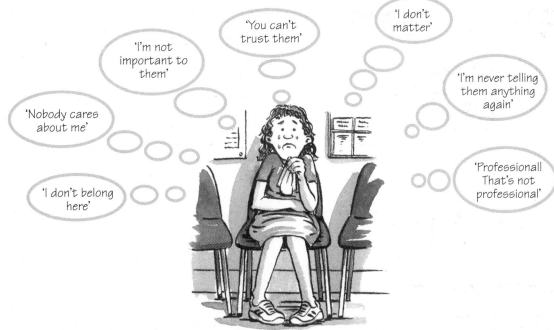

Figure 1.48   The confidentiality of the things clients tell you about is of vital importance

over their lives. For example, imagine your next-door neighbour starts to treat you as though you had a terminal illness when you thought that whatever was ailing you had been getting better. Or have you ever felt really good about yourself, but someone tells you that you look ill? How would you feel now about yourself?

And what of client's property and safety, if their personal details are common knowledge? What could be the consequences if someone says, 'Poor Mrs Jenkins at no. 27 is poorly again, but she leaves the key under the flowerpot by the front door so I can go in and make her a cup of tea'?

Sometimes it is important we tell a manager about a client's personal details, and this is known as 'keeping confidentiality within boundaries'. For example, we must inform managers if clients are at risk of damage to their physical or mental health. We must also tell senior staff of any risks a client may pose to other people, including ourselves. When serious risks are involved, confidentiality might be broken.

> **Think it over**
>
> If you go to see your doctor or go into hospital, you will expect to receive good quality care. What is good quality care?
>
> Different people have different ideas about what constitutes quality. Everyone will say he or she wants the right treatment, but some will also want:
>
> ⋄ a nicely decorated room
> ⋄ peace and quiet
> ⋄ no waiting.
>
> Others will want:
>
> ⋄ friendly conversations with those involved in their care
> ⋄ time to talk about their problems
> ⋄ respect.
>
> What do you think is most important?

Codes of practice and charters

Codes of practice and charters help to define the quality of care clients can expect if they receive care services and they can be used as a basis for measuring the quality of care provided.

Codes of practice

What constitutes good care is not a matter of individual debate. Codes of practice are needed to define what quality means. These codes can then be used to measure whether or not a particular service is providing good quality. For example, *Home Life: a Code of Practice for Residential Care*, first published in 1984, has a checklist of 218 recommendations for monitoring the quality of social care. Many of these recommendations have now been built into regulations inspectors check before a residential home can be registered or for a home to remain registered.

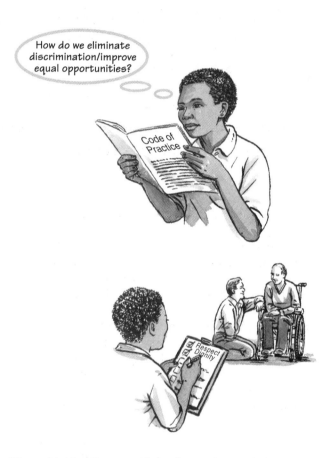

How do we eliminate discrimination/improve equal opportunities?

Figure 1.49   Some codes of practice mainly give advice and guidance; others can be used to measure the quality of care

The first ten recommendations, which concern staff qualities, are listed in Figure 1.50.

Codes of practice often advise workers on how to behave. For example the Equal Opportunities

STAFF

148 Staff qualities should include responsiveness to and respect for the needs of the individuals.

149 Staff skills should match the residents' needs as identified in the objectives of the home.

150 Staff should have the ability to give competent and tactful care, whilst enabling residents to retain dignity and self-determination.

151 In the selection of staff at least two references should be taken up, where possible from previous employers.

152 Applicants' curriculum vitae should be checked and for this purpose employers should give warning that convictions otherwise spent should be disclosed.

153 Proprietors should consider residents' needs in relation to all categories of staff when drawing up staffing proposals.

154 Job descriptions will be required for all posts and staff should be provided with relevant job descriptions on appointment.

155 In small homes where staff carry a range of responsibilities, these must be clearly understood by staff.

156 Any change of role or duty should be made clear to the member of staff in writing.

157 Minimum staff cover should be designed to cope with residents' anticipated problems at any time.

Figure 1.50 *Home Life*: **recommendations about staff quality**

Commission has published a code to help eliminate sexual discrimination, and the Commission for Racial Equality has issued a code that gives guidance on the elimination of racial discrimination. Similarly, the Department of Health has published a guide to the professional behaviour expected of social workers, doctors and the police when working with people who are mentally ill. These codes do not provide checklists to help in the assessment of qualities. Rather they provide guidelines for service managers when they are devising policies and procedures staff must follow.

1 Social workers will contribute to the formulation and implementation of policies for human welfare, and they will not permit their knowledge, skills or experience to be used to further dehumanising or discriminatory policies and will positively promote the use of their knowledge, skills and experience for the benefit of all sections of the community and individuals.

2 They will respect their clients as individuals and seek to ensure that their dignity, individuality, rights and responsibility shall be safeguarded.

3 They will not discriminate against clients, on the grounds of their origin, race, status, sex, sexual orientation, age, disability, beliefs, or contribution to society, they will not tolerate actions of colleagues or others which may be racist, sexist or otherwise discriminatory, nor will they deny those differences which will shape the nature of clients' needs and will ensure any personal help is offered within an acceptable personal and cultural context. They will draw to the attention of the Association any activity which is professionally unacceptable.

4 They will help their clients both individually and collectively to increase the range of choices open to them and their powers to make decisions, securing the participation, wherever possible, of clients in defining and obtaining services appropriate to their needs

5 They will not reject their clients or lose concern for their suffering, even if obliged to protect themselves or others against them or obliged to acknowledge an inability to help them.

6 They will give precedence to their professional responsibility over their own personal interests.

7 They accept that continuing professional education and training are basic to the practice of social work, and they hold themselves responsible for the standard of service they give.

8 They recognise the need to collaborate with others in the interest of their clients.

9 They will make clear in making any public statements or undertaking any public activities, whether they are acting in a personal capacity or on behalf of an organisation.

10 They will acknowledge a responsibility to help clients to obtain all those services and rights to which they are entitled; and will seek to ensure that these services are provided within a framework which will be both ethnically and culturally appropriate for all members of the community; and that an appropriate diversity will be promoted both in their own agency and other organisations in which they have influence.

11 They will recognise that information clearly entrusted for one purpose should not be used for another purpose without sanction. They will respect the privacy of clients and others with whom they come into contact and confidential information gained in their relationships with them. They will divulge such information only with the consent of the client (or informant) except where there is clear evidence of serious danger to the client, worker, other persons or the community or in other circumstances, judged exceptional, on the basis of professional consideration and consultation.

12 They will work for the creation and maintenance in employing agencies of conditions which will support and facilitate social workers' acceptance of the obligations of the Code.

Figure 1.51 The BASW principles for social work (taken from the BASW *Code of Ethics*, 1996)

Most professional bodies have a code of conduct or code of practice which explains the values that guide people who work in that profession. The

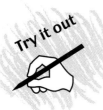

Try it out

When you visit a care setting, ask if you can have copies of the setting's policy documents on equal opportunities or confidentiality. How might these documents help to protect the rights of vulnerable people?

Think it over

Compare *Home Life*, the BASW code, and the UKCC code. There are similarities among all three 'codes', but there are also differences because social workers have slightly different responsibilities from nurses.

Pick out three points that are similar in all codes of practice. Why do you think they are there?

British Association for Social Work (BASW) has published 12 principles for social work that are contained within its code of ethics (see Figure 1.51). The UK Central Council for Nursing, Midwifery and Health Visiting (UKCC) has similarly published a 16-point code of professional conduct (see Figure 1.52).

As a registered nurse, midwife or health visitor, you are personally accountable for your practice and, in the exercise of your professional accountability, must:

1 Act always in such a manner as to promote and safeguard the interest and well-being of patients and clients.
2 Ensure that no action or omission on your part, or within your sphere of responsibility, is detrimental to the interests, condition or safety of patients and clients.
3 Maintain and improve your professional knowledge and competence.
4 Acknowledge any limitations in your knowledge and competence and decline any duties or responsibilities unless able to perform them in safe and skilled manner.
5 Work in an open and co-operative manner with patients, clients and their families, foster their independence and recognise and respect their involvement in the planning and delivery of care.
6 Work in a collaborative and co-operative manner with health care professionals and others involved in providing care, and recognise and respect their particular contributions within the care team.
7 Recognise and respect the uniqueness and dignity of each patient and client, and respond to their need for care, irrespective of their ethnic origin, religious beliefs, personal attributes, the nature of their health problems or any other factor.
8 Report to an appropriate person or authority, at least the earliest possible time, any conscientious objection which may be relevant to your professional practice.
9 Avoid any abuse of your privileged relationships with patients and clients and of the privileged access allowed to their person, property, residence or workplace.
10 Protect all confidential information concerning patients and clients obtained in the course of professional practice and make disclosures only with consent, where required by the order of a court or where you can justify disclosure in the wider public interest.
11 Report to an appropriate person or authority, having regard to the physical, psychological and social effects on patients and clients, any circumstances in the environment of care which could jeopardise standards of practice.
12 Report to an appropriate person or authority any circumstances in which safe and appropriate care for patients and clients cannot be provided.
13 Report to an appropriate person or authority where it appears that the health or safety of colleagues is at risk, as such circumstances may compromise standards of practice in care.
14 Assist professional colleagues, in the context of your own knowledge, experience and sphere of responsibility, to develop their professional competence and assist others in the care team, including informal carers, to contribute safely and to a degree appropriate to their roles.
15 Refuse any gift, favour or hospitality from patients or clients currently in your care which might be interpreted as seeking to expert influence to obtain preferential consideration and
16 Ensure that your registration status is not used in the promotion of commercial products or services, declare any financial or other interests in relevant organisations providing such goods or services and ensure that your professional judgement is not influenced by any commercial considerations.

Figure 1.52 The UKCC code of professional conduct

Codes of practice: summary

◊ All codes of practice enable both members of the public and professionals to measure whether quality care is being delivered or not.

◊ *Home Life* includes a checklist to help people assess the quality of care. Other codes are perhaps more abstract but they still help people to decide whether a service is good or not.

◊ Some codes provide professionals with advice and guidelines; others define the detailed values relevant to a specific service.

Talk it over

You are on a placement in a residential nursing home and have noticed that one of the care assistants is 'less than polite' to one of the residents, who speaks hesitantly because of a stammer. The care assistant interrupts the client and often makes choices for the client 'because we haven't got all day'. How would you handle this situation?

1 At coffee time, argue with the assistant about the rights and wrongs of the assistant's behaviour. Or

2 Talk with the client about how the client would like the situation to be handled, offering your support if wanted. Or

3 Go straight to the manager and tell him or her about the incident?

Discuss the pros and cons of each of these three approaches. Which is the best course of action? Is there anything else you could do? Is there a better way to deal with the situation?

Charters

Recent governments have produced a series of charters that outline the standards people can expect from a wide range of services. These charters are like codes of practice but they are designed by Government. The Citizen's Charter, in particular, sets out the quality we can expect from public services. The charter contains information about the services and gives advice about how we can seek redress (chase up our rights) if a service does not fulfil all the stipulated standards. An important section of the Citizen's Charter is the **Patient's Charter**. A new NHS Charter is expected which provides a statement of national standards and offers a localised approach to the services patients can expect.

The existing charter (which was produced in January 1995) set out the rights and standards people could expect of the services (for example, waiting times for out-patient appointments and for operations).

Many GPs are now producing practice charters that give information about the standards of service provided by their particular health centres. These cover such information as opening times, test results collection, how to get a repeat prescription, facilities for people with disabilities and out-of-hours treatment.

The Department of Health requires all Local Authority social services departments to publish **Community Care Charters**. These charters explain what users and carers can expect from the community care services provided in that area are they also set out their services' commitments and standards (see Figure 1.53).

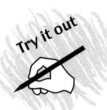

Obtain a copy of the charter your health centre has produced and find out the following information:

1 How could you contact the practice manager for information about his or her job?
2 If you rely on sign language, is there anyone at the surgery who can help you?
3 Suppose someone in your house is pregnant. Will she be able to give birth at home?
4 Is a social worker attached to the practice?

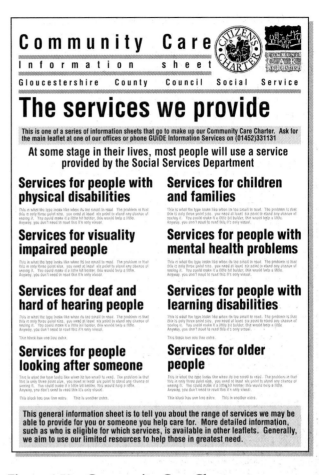

Figure 1.53   Community Care Charters

Unit I Assessment

Obtaining a Pass grade

To *pass* this unit you must produce a report based on two different health and/or social care settings. When writing your report you should use the records you have kept about your visits to or placements in two different settings. If you use your notes or logbook recordings, you should be able to do the following:

1 Describe the types of organisation you have worked in or visited and say whether it was in the statutory, voluntary or private sectors.

2 Describe the client group you have worked with or visited. What needs did the clients have, and why was a care service offered?

3 Describe the roles of two workers. What kind of work do they do? You could perhaps look at one worker in each care setting.

4 Explain how the care value base influences the way each of the two care workers does his or her job.

5 Describe any codes of practice or charters used in the organisation where the workers are based.

6 Demonstrate you have used the relevant communication skills (see below).

7 Explain the possible barriers to communication that might arise when dealing with clients (see below).

Ideas to help with these tasks:

1 You could find out which sector the organisation is in and the needs of its clients from either your tutor or from the senior staff you meet on your visits or placement. Write down the answers as soon as you are given them.

2 Talk to two different workers and make notes about the kind of work they do. If you take a copy of the care value base diagram on page 43 with you, you could show this to the workers and ask them how these values influence the way they do their jobs. Remember to make notes of what they tell you. Also remember to check your notes later that day to make sure you can read and understand them.

3 Ask a senior member of staff or your tutor about the codes of practice and charters that might be relevant to that particular service. You may be able to get a copy from the care setting, from a library or from the Internet. If you have your own copy of a charter or code of practice, this will help you to write about it.

4 Make notes of conversations you have had that demonstrate you have used the relevant communication skills. You could tape record a conversation you have had in college, or you could make notes about a conversation you have with someone in the setting as soon as the conversation has ended. Remember to make notes about your non-verbal behaviour as well as about the things you said. Look back at the communication section earlier in this unit and make a list of the non-verbal messages you used.

5 Ask the care workers in one setting about the barriers to communication they have encountered. Use the communication section given earlier in this unit to help you think about other barriers that might arise. Make a list of barriers that would cause you problems if you were to work with clients yourself.

Obtaining a Merit or Distinction grade.

To obtain a *Merit* or *Distinction* grade, you must analyse the way people do their jobs in the different settings so that you can compare the various ways in which the care value base is implemented.

First, to find out about the jobs people do, interview two different people in the two different settings. You will learn more about their jobs if you ask them about the types of client they mostly work with. The ask them: 'Do the clients you work with all have the same expectations of you?' You will probably discover that different clients have quite different expectations of staff members (see Figure 1.54). Part of the carer's role is to find a way of working that best meets his or her client's different needs. You could ask the workers how they organise their time so that they are able to do all the tasks they are required to perform.

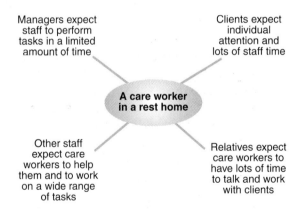

Figure 1.54   The expectations people have of a care worker who works in a rest home

You could then ask the workers to give you examples of how their settings foster diversity, protect the clients' rights and maintain confidentiality. You will probably be given different examples in each setting.

Obtaining a Distinction grade

To obtain a *Distinction*, you must write a detailed account of the care settings and of the work roles undertaken there, and you must explain how the work roles are influenced by the type of organisation the setting is and by the sector it belongs to (statutory, private or voluntary). Classify each of the two care settings you have visited accordingly. Remember to include the setting's size – it might be large (like the NHS or a large national company) or small (such as a voluntary organisation or a private rest home). It is also important to include a description of where the setting is located: in a town or city or in the country.

You will have to ask the staff about the ways the setting's size and nature influences their work with clients. You might also need to speak to a senior manager to learn about the advantages and disadvantages of different sectors and sizes. As well as asking questions, you will be able to learn a great deal just by observing!

Some general questions to consider that might help you prepare your report are as follows:

- How good is the transport to and from the home? Can relatives travel easily?

- How safe is the setting? What security measures are in place? Are crimes such as vandalism and burglary common in the area?

- How easy is it to get to community facilities, (e.g. shops, leisure facilities, temples, mosques, churches, clubs)?

- How easy is it to get staff? Do they have difficult journeys to work? Is it easy to get staff with the right qualifications?

- Look at the sort of resources the organisation can afford to buy. Consider the general condition of the furniture and decorations.

Skill area	Rating		
	Weakness I am not good at this	**In between** I can improve at this	**Strength** I am good at this
Using listening skills to ckeck I understand other people			
Using open questions			
Understanding the cultural differences in communication			
Being able to keep a conversation going			
Understanding other people's non-verbal messages			
Sending the right non-verbal messages to others			
Organising a conversation with an appropriate beginning, middle and end			

Figure 1.55   My strengths and weaknesses in the communication skills I use

⋄ What sort of staff training and supervision does the organisation provide?

⋄ What sort of equipment is provided for the clients? Are the staff trained to use any new equipment?

⋄ What type of management systems does the organisation have? Do people work in teams? How are duties shared and organised?

Communication
Obtaining a Pass grade

At *Pass* level, you will need to demonstrate relevant communication skills, either in real practical work with clients or in simulation exercises. As well as demonstrating listening, conversation and non-verbal communication skills, you must also explain what the barriers are that can block communication with clients.

Obtaining a Merit grade

To obtain a *Merit* grade, you must explain the communication methods you have chosen to use and must be able to identify your own strengths and weaknesses when communicating.

If you use simulated exercises you could tape record your performance and then analyse the skills you demonstrated. You could use a grid like the one shown in Figure 1.55 to help you assess your strengths and weaknesses. Your grid could be more detailed then the one shown here or it could include other skills than the ones listed in the figure.

When evaluating practical work you should similarly be able to assess your communication skills. For example, you might be able to say: 'Keeping a conversation going is one of my strengths because we talked for

Skill to develop	Action to improve these skill	The way to measure improvements in my skills
1 Listening	**(a)** Class exercises	Feedback from tutor
	(b) Listening to clients at a day centre	Recording their reaction: do I appear to be a good listener?
2 Understanding cultural differences	Talking to and listening to people from different cultural backgrounds	Listing the different gestures facial expressions and sayings they use
3 Understanding other people's non-verbal messages	Reading a book on body language - looking for real-life examples	Listing examples of non-verbal messages relevant to the clients
4 Sending the right non-verbal messages	Video conversation work with my friends	Listing ideas for changing the expression in my face and eyes so that I look more serious

Figure 1.56   Action plan: improving my communication skills

15 minutes and I kept the conversation going.' Or you might be able to say: 'Understanding other people's non-verbal messages is something I could improve on. I couldn't tell what the person I was talking to felt: her face and body movements didn't send a clear message.' When you have analysed your skills, try to record some evidence to support your evaluation.

Obtaining a Distinction grade

To obtain a *Distinction*, you must make realistic suggestions for improving your communication skills. One way to do this might be to design an action plan (see Figure 1.56).

Codes of practice and charters
Obtaining a Pass grade

To obtain a *Pass* grade, you must identify and describe codes of practice or charters used within the care settings you report on.

Obtaining a Merit grade

To obtain a *Merit* grade, you must explain how codes of practice and charters help to protect the users of services. You must explain that codes of practice and charters can provide definitions of good practice and can outline ways to protect people's rights. They are a measure of whether a service is providing good-quality care. If clients are not receiving a good-quality service, then charters and codes can help people to assert their rights and to make complaints.

You should obtain a full copy of the code of practice – perhaps from a library or from the organisation's web site. Pick out some examples in the code which you think provide clients with rights. Say what these rights are in your own words. How far does the code provide measurable standards or help people to understand their rights?

Codes of practice can also help managers to design policies and procedures that help staff provide a good service. If you interview senior care staff about the work people do in their organisations, you could also ask them if the value base, codes of practice or charters are used in staff training or staff supervision sessions. You could explain in your notes that, when staff work to improve the service they give, this will help to protect the clients. You could also explain that definitions of good practice can help professionals to think about the quality of their own personal practice. You could similarly ask staff about complaints procedures and about the ways the codes have influenced how these procedures are handled.

Obtaining a Distinction grade

To obtain a *Distinction*, you must evaluate the effectiveness of codes of practice and charters in upholding the broad principles of the care value base. This involves two tasks. First, you must show how different codes or charters include within their statements the principles of valuing diversity, clients' rights and confidentiality. You could discuss various codes with a friend and, together, try to work out what rights and what statements about confidentiality, equality and diversity the code includes. You will then have to write your own report on the code or charter. You could give your report the title: 'An analysis of the code (or charter) and its values'.

The second task is to find out just how seriously people use codes of practice or charters in real care settings. When you go on visits or on placements, ask the staff about values and codes of practice. You may find that some care settings give clients leaflets about their rights and offer training to their staff about rights and equality. They may also have complaints procedures that clearly explain these rights in relation to the codes or charters. If this is the case you can argue that codes and charters have a real effect on improving the quality of care services. On the other hand, you may come across care settings where values, codes and charters seem not to be understood. If you do, you could argue that theoretical ideas about rights do not always influence practice.

Try to work out why some care settings are better than others when it comes to rights and values. You could link this with the work you did on work roles and with the questions you asked staff for that task.

Unit I Test

1 What name is used to describe a service that has been set up because Parliament has passed a law requiring that service to be provided?

2 List three of the responsibilities of the new Health Authorities.

3 Which of the following definitions describes a 'mixed economy of care'?

   a People paying for their own care.
   b A mixture of provision through statutory, private and voluntary organisation.
   c People are means-tested before they can receive services from local social services departments or the NHS.

4 Describe briefly three different early years settings.

5 Describe the difference between the words 'direct' and 'indirect' when these words are used to describe jobs involved in the provision of care.

6 List three skills a nursery nurse should have.

7 At what ages can children receive early years services?

8 Explain what values are and why they are important in care work.

9 Explain two ideas for practical ways of valuing diversity in others.

10 Describe two general rights which clients might expect in a health or care setting.

11 Why are codes of practice and charters needed in care work?

12 Why are communication skills of great importance in care work?

13 What does 'non-verbal communication' mean?

14 How is listening different from just hearing what someone says?

Promoting health and well-being

This Unit covers the knowledge you will need in order to meet the assessment requirements for Unit 2. It is written in four sections:

Section one looks at definitions of health and well-being and how the health needs of different age groups differ. Section two explores the factors that affect health and well-being and the risks to health. Section three examines ways of providing health promotion information to support a health plan. Finally, section four explores indicators of good health. These are the actual physical measurements that can be done on the body.

Advice and ideas for meeting the assessment requirements for the unit and achieving Merit and Distinction grades are at the end of the Unit.

Also at the end of the Unit is a quick test to check your understanding.

Defining health and well-being

When we meet people we have not seen for some time, we usually ask how they are, and we would be quite surprised if they replied with full information about the state of their health – most of the responses we get are usually fairly simple and often inaccurate, such as 'fine' or 'not so bad'. Rarely do people tell us about details of their health or well-being.

Health and well-being are difficult things to understand or explain. Therefore the first part of this unit tries to provide clear explanations of the terms. It then goes on to explore the health and well-being of different groups of people. For example, to adolescents and young adults, being healthy might mean taking regular exercise by joining an aerobics group or playing football. However, this would not be a feature of the healthy lifestyle of an average 80-year-old person. To such a person, being healthy would more likely involve being able to do the tasks associated with independent daily living, such as shopping.

All people are unique and everyone has different health needs, but there are some things that affect everyone's health, such as what we eat and drink,

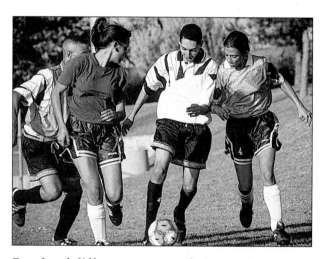

People of different ages get their exercise in different ways – young people often play sports such as football

where we live and the different incomes we have. These are the common factors that affect health, and these common factors are explored in greater detail later in this section.

Some people choose to do things that can be harmful to their health, such as smoking or taking too many legal or illegal drugs. Others choose not to do the things that are important to health, such as not wearing the correct protective clothing at work or not taking the right amount of exercise. This unit studies how these choices affect people's health and what people might be able to do to lessen their health risks.

This unit also explores ways to provide information to people to help them improve their general health, such as healthy eating leaflets and guidance on stopping smoking. Assessment tasks for this unit require you to investigate how to measure some aspects of people's physical health, to produce health targets for an individual (or group of people) and to understand how to involve them in improving their own health.

What is meant by health and well-being?

Health and well-being mean different things to different people; hence any definition has to involve everyone, which makes defining these terms difficult. The World Health Organisation has produced a definition of health which many people use: 'Health is a status of complete physical, mental, and social well-being and not merely the absence of disease and infirmity'. This definition was written in 1946 and has since been criticised on a number of points:

- The use of the word *complete* is seen by many people as being unrealistic (who can say he or she has 'complete mental well-being', for instance?).

- The use of the word *status* might imply that health does not change and that people do not change – that health is a level we reach and maintain. Clearly, this cannot be right: life is for ever changing.

- The definition implies that experts define our health but each individual may define his or her own health differently.

However, for all these criticisms, the World Health Organisation definition was a starting point to get people thinking about what health meant to them. Modern definitions of health emphasise health as the foundation from which people achieve all they are capable of – to enable them to satisfy their needs and realise their hopes; and to enable them to achieve quality in their lives. There is, and will continue to be, much discussion on the definition of health.

One thing most people agree with is that health is not just absence of illness or infirmity. It contains positive concepts about the physical, social, intellectual and emotional aspects of our lives (some might also include our spiritual needs).

Perhaps dividing the concept of health into these different aspects could be considered to be artificial, but it is useful for study purposes. However, it is important that we remember to consider people as whole human beings (this is called the holistic approach). The holistic approach is also known as PIES (and this might help us remember the four different aspects of health):

Physical
Intellectual
Emotional
Social

(see Figure 2.1).

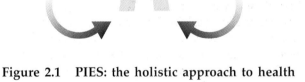

Figure 2.1 PIES: the holistic approach to health

Physical aspects of health

These aspects concern the physical functioning of the human body: sufficient food of the right types and proportions, clean drinking water, warmth provided by heating and clothing, having the right amount of sleep and rest and exercising regularly, etc. Illness and infirmity would also come in this category.

Social aspects of health

These include the ability to form good relationships with other people and the ability to maintain these relationships. Can people who live alone and avoid the company of others have good health? Using some definitions of health, the answer might be 'no'!

Intellectual aspects of health

These include the ability to think clearly and in an organised way. This does not mean that everyone should be trying to obtain academic qualifications although, for some people, this could be a feature of their health as they would be trying to achieve their own personal ambitions.

Emotional aspects of health

These include people's abilities to recognise emotions, such as grief, excitement, fear, joy etc., and to express these emotions appropriately. It also means being able to cope with stress, worry and depression (sadness) when these occur in our lives. Having emotional health does *not* mean *not* expressing your emotions!

Physical, social, intellectual and emotional are the aspects of health you need to consider in your health plan.

Different people and groups of people

For the purposes of study, people are often grouped into age ranges; they may also be grouped by other categories, such as vegetarians, smokers and people with learning disabilities.

The age ranges most commonly used are as follows:

- Infants (0–2 years, 11 months)
- Young children (3–9 years).
- Adolescents (10–18 years).
- Adults (19–65 years).
- Elderly people (over 65 years).

The physical, social, intellectual and emotional aspects of health we have just discussed will be very different for each of these age groups.

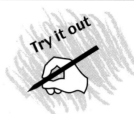

Jade is 2 years old. She goes to a morning playgroup three times a week. Sarah, her mother, is a single parent on benefit. They live on their own in a two-room flat on the fourth floor of an old house, which is difficult to heat. There is no garden and the house is situated on a busy road. After paying her rent and buying food, Sarah has not much money left, so she buys most of her clothing in charity shops.

Complete the chart in Figure 2.2. Try to imagine Jade's and Sarah's situations: you can be very imaginative about this. Examples are provided for each aspect to guide you.

Factors affecting health and well-being

Many factors affect our health and well-being. Some of these factors affect certain people only but some are common to us all. In this section we look at those factors that affect all of us.

Diet

Diet is our pattern of eating. Sometimes a person's diet may not be adequate to keep that person's body in a healthy condition. This is often known as malnutrition. Malnutrition may be caused by:

1   *Not having enough food.* We often see this in undeveloped countries when there is a drought or famine. But it can also happen in countries like the UK: for example, old people living alone who are unable to afford or to cook food.

2   *Eating the wrong types of food.* Some people may only eat one type of food, for example, chips and buns. This means the body is not getting all the nutrients it needs.

3   *Eating too much refined food.* Refined foods are ones that have been processed to remove texture or taste. Examples are white sugar and white sliced bread. Eating too much of

Different aspects of health	Aspects of Jade's health	Aspects of Sarah's health
Physical	Jade is vulnerable to colds and chest infections, probably as a result of the cold, slightly damp conditions in her home.	
Social		Sarah cannot afford to socialise; she would have to pay for a child minder. On the mornings when Jade is at playgroup Sarah does the washing, ironing and tidying up. Occasionally, she meets a friend while shopping, but doesn't stay long with her. Sarah is lonely for adult company.
Emotional		Sarah is afraid that Jade might be taken into care if she went to work. She suffers from low spirits most of the time. She is short of money and cannot afford treats. Her previous partner has no interest in Jade. He left her when Sarah became pregnant. She feels unable to trust anybody else.
Intellectual	Jade is getting the chance to play with water and sand at playgroup, but her vocabulary seems more limited than the other 3 year-olds. She will need more stimulation to be able to cope with school life in 18 months' time. She has some favourite soft toys from the charity shop.	

Figure 2.2 Jade and Sarah

these foods can cause digestive disorders, diabetes and tooth decay.

4 *Eating far too much food.* If a person eats more food than his or her body needs, then the excess is laid down as fat under the skin and around the internal organs. This puts a great strain on the whole body and can lead to heart disease and other serious illnesses.

Consuming the right diet for our lifestyles is important for our health, and this is often called eating a **balanced diet**. A balanced diet is one that contains the correct nutrients in the correct proportions for healthy living. So how do we know what is appropriate for us?

The nutrients our bodies need fall into five main groups, with two additional requirements. These are carbohydrates (starches and sugars), proteins, fats, vitamins and mineral salts (and the additional requirements are water and fibre) (see Figure 2.3).

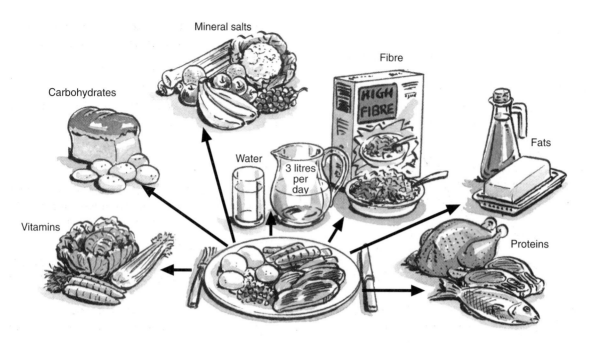

Figure 2.3 The nutrients our bodies need

Carbohydrates

Carbohydrates are the body's main source of energy. Complex carbohydrates, such as the starch in bread, rice and pasta, have to be broken down by enzymes in the digestive system; these are better for health than the refined sugars in sweets, soft drinks or sugar-containing foods. This is because sugar gives our bodies a quick boost of energy that falls rapidly, whereas complex carbohydrates provide our bodies with a slow build-up of energy that is sustained over a longer period.

Refined sugar also increases our chances of tooth decay and may play a part in causing diabetes. As complex carbohydrates usually contain fibre and certain vitamins and mineral salts, they can also help provide us with these nutrients.

Our diet should consist of 60% carbohydrates, mostly in the complex forms described above. From every gramme of carbohydrate we absorb into our bodies, we obtain 17 kJ (kilojoules) of energy.

Fat

Energy is also supplied by fat, but there is a danger here. Every gramme of fat we absorb gives our bodies 35 kJ of energy – twice as much as carbohydrates, but with more dangers attached to it, so only 20% of our diet should be composed of fats and less if possible.

As well as giving us energy, fat also helps to:

- store the fat-soluble vitamins A, D, E and K
- protect the body's vital organs
- provide us with a long-term energy store
- provide us with the raw materials we need for making certain hormones
- provide us with the raw materials we need to make new cell membranes.

Hence some fat is essential if the body is to function properly. In Western societies, far too much fat is consumed and this can lead to heart and circulatory problems, such as heart attacks and strokes and also to muscular and joint disorders through carrying too much weight.

Proteins

Our diet should contain 20% protein as our bodies need this for the formation, growth and repair of cell structures. Some of the essential chemicals in our bodies are also proteins, such as enzymes, some hormones, haemoglobin (which is present in red blood cells and which carries oxygen), and blood-clotting substances and so on.

Vitamins

Vitamins act on the body in complex ways, and it is sufficient for our purposes just to be aware that they are essential to a healthy diet. They are only required in very small amounts and, if a person eats plenty of fresh fruit and vegetables, wholemeal bread, dairy products and cereals, he or she will take in sufficient quantities of these essential materials. An individual who eats only burgers and chips, chocolate bars and other manufactured products may have vitamin deficiencies.

Mineral salts

Again these act in complex ways and are required in only small amounts. They are supplied by fresh fruits and vegetables, red meat and dairy products. The two main mineral salts (which are required in larger quantities but still relatively small quantities when compared with proteins, fats and carbohydrates) are calcium for bone and teeth formation and iron – an essential component of haemoglobin.

Fibre

Fibre is the collective word for all the plant cell-walls we eat in our diet. Some people call fibre roughage, bran or cellulose but it is still the same material. Although it does not provide us with raw materials or energy, fibre has several important roles:

◇   It provides bulk in our food. It fills us up and makes us feel less hungry. Therefore in one sense it can be said to slim the body.

◇   It stimulates the muscular control of our bowels, thus preventing constipation.

◇   It helps to prevent diseases of the bowel, such as bowel cancer.

Fruit, vegetables, cereals and wholemeal products provide us with enough daily fibre.

Water

Tea, coffee and soft drinks can all be thought of as water because water is the main ingredient of all drinks. Even milk is mainly water.

Water is essential for life: it is the main component of our bodies – it makes our blood flow, gets rid of waste substances in urine, keeps our body cells moist, cools our bodies and dissolves oxygen and carbon dioxide and so on. We should drink around 3 litres of water every day.

Healthy eating

Once we know which foods provide each of the essential nutrients, we can plan a healthy diet.

In 1983 the National Advisory Committee for Nutrition Education (NACNE) produced five dietary goals to follow when planning meals. These goals were also recommended by the Committee on Medical Aspects of Food Policy (COMA):

1   Reduce our overall fat intake, but when we do eat fat make sure it is polyunsaturated, not saturated.

Figure 2.4 Dietary goals and health risks

Goal	Health risk	Change from	To
Eat less fat	High cholesterol Heart disease Obesity	Animal fats e.g. lard	Vegetable oil, e.g. corn
Eat less sugar	Tooth decay Obesity	Sweet puddings	Fresh fruit
Eat less salt	High blood pressure	Seasoning with salt	Using herbs or spices
Eat more fibre	Constipation Bowel cancer	White bread	Wholegrain bread
Drink less alcohol	Liver damage Stomach disorders	Alcoholic drinks	Low-alcohol drinks

2   Eat less salt.
3   Reduce our intake of sugar.
4   Eat more fibre.
5   Drink less alcohol.

Figure 2.4 shows the health risks if we do not follow these goals. The table also makes some suggestions about changing to a healthier diet.

Energy needs

The amount of energy needed by individuals is linked to their levels of activity: although each of us requires a different amount, there are general recommendations for every age group. It is important to balance our food intake to match our energy needs. Otherwise:

1   too little exercise + too much food = weight gain

2   too much exercise + too little food = weight loss.

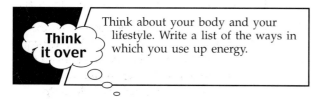

Think it over

Think about your body and your lifestyle. Write a list of the ways in which you use up energy.

1   **Basal metabolic rate** is the amount of energy required for your body to function when lying down, still and warm. It is lower for women than men because women tend to have smaller body masses. Any movement increases the number of kilojoules needed.

2   **Occupation** – different jobs require different levels of energy output and therefore different amounts of kilojoules are needed to sustain the people who do these jobs. Occupations are classified into groups:

   a   Sedentary – office workers, teachers, pilots, shop workers.
   b   Moderately active – postmen/women, nursery assistants, care assistants, hospital porters.
   c   Very active – miners, farm labourers, builders.

3   **Activity outside work** – the amount of exercise you take affects energy needs. Here are some examples of the energy use of different types of exercise:

	Average estimated kJ per hour
Sitting (watching TV)	400
Standing	425
Tennis	1645
Cycling	1900
Swimming	2500
Household tasks	950

4   **State of the body** – certain conditions, such as pregnancy and breast feeding (lactation), require an increase in energy intake to cope with the extra demands placed on the body.

5   **Age** – young children require more energy for their body size than adults as they are growing rapidly and also tend to be active all the time. On the other hand, ageing people require less energy as activity levels often slow down along with the general slowing down of the body processes.

Which foods provide energy?

All food provides some energy, but the amount per 100 g depends on the nutrient content of the food. Energy comes from four sources:

⋄   protein – 17 kJ/g
⋄   fat – 35 kJ/g
⋄   carbohydrate – 17 kJ/g
⋄   alcohol – 30 kJ/g.

Most foods are a combination of nutrients. The energy values of common foods are shown in Figure 2.5.

Figure 2.5 Some common foods and their energy values

Food	kJ per 100 g
Whole milk	274
White bread	1068
Butter	3006
Sugar	1680
Roast beef	950
Cod (steamed)	321
Apples	197
Cabbage	66
Crisps	2222
Chips	1028
Boiled potatoes	339
Sweet biscuits	1819

As can be seen from this table, a balance of input and output is complicated by the kilojoule values of food. A person's choice of foods can affect whether he or she achieves the right balance. An inactive person on a high-fat diet of chips, fried food, cakes, etc., would soon eat more than his or her energy needs. Excess calories taken into the body are stored as fat in the adipose layer under the skin which can lead to obesity.

Do all people need the same nutrients?

Everyone needs a balanced diet which contains all the nutrients. However, some groups have particular needs because of their life stage.

Children

Here are some tips for feeding children:

- This is a time of rapid growth so they need plenty of protein, vitamin D and calcium to develop strong bones.

- They also need fluoride to ensure strong enamel on their teeth to protect from decay, and iron for red blood cells.

- Milk is important, so if children do not like to drink it, give them plenty of milk in food.

- Children have small appetites, so give small portions and think about different ways to serve food attractively, for example, making faces in food might encourage a child to eat.

- Do not encourage children to eat sweets and snacks between meals as they will fill up on these and lose their appetite at meal times, which results in an unbalanced diet.

- Do not encourage the eating of sweet food between meals as this can contribute to tooth decay and obesity.

This advice continues right through until adolescence.

Pregnancy: 'eating for two'

It is essential that a pregnant woman eats a healthy balanced diet to ensure the health of both herself and her baby. Research has shown that a healthy diet is also vital before conception to help prevent foetal disorders and to ensure the woman's body is in the best condition to cope with the demands of pregnancy.

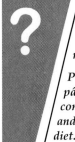

> *Vitamin A appears to be the only vitamin that is dangerous if taken in excess. In pregnancy, birth defects can result.*
>
> *Pregnant women are advised not to eat pâté during pregnancy, as it usually contains liver (and therefore Vitamin A) and might be too much on top of a normal diet.*

It is a myth that a pregnant woman should eat for two; this only leads to extra weight gain which may be difficult to lose after the birth. However, the intake of some nutrients does need to increase to meet the needs of the growing foetus. If the diet is lacking in any required nutrient, the body adjusts to ensure the baby has priority and the woman may hence suffer.

During pregnancy energy requirements increase as do the needs for certain minerals and proteins.

Calcium is required for the development of the foetus's skeleton. If there is not enough calcium to meet this demand, this will be removed from the mother's bones, which will then soften and bend (a condition known as osteomalacia). To help absorb the calcium, a greater quantity of vitamin D is also needed.

Iron is essential to the foetus as it develops its own blood supply. The baby also needs to build up a store of iron for its first three months of life as milk, either breast or formula, contains little iron.

It is also important that the mother's haemoglobin levels remain high as blood can be lost in delivery and a good iron level can help speed recovery. Iron tablets are often prescribed to pregnant women as iron in the diet is not always readily absorbed. One traditional source of iron, liver, should be avoided as the high amounts of vitamin A in liver have been linked to spina bifida. However, iron tablets tend to cause constipation and so an increase in fibre in the diet to prevent this is also needed.

Increases in energy requirements should come from healthy sources, such as pasta and bread, not sugar and fats.

The dietary goals outlined above should be followed throughout pregnancy and, in particular, alcohol consumption should be reduced. This is because alcohol crosses the placenta and can be harmful to the baby. Often, however, when pregnant, a woman finds she no longer likes certain foods such as tea, coffee and alcohol (all foods which could damage the foetus), but has cravings for other foods such as red meat and tomatoes. It is often suggested that these cravings are a result of deficiencies in the diet and are the body's way of getting the nutrients needed.

Older people

- As activity slows, the amount of calories eaten should be reduced to prevent obesity.

- The digestive system often slows, so the food chosen needs to be easily digested (such as fish).

- Poor teeth may cause problems with eating, so softer, well cooked foods should be chosen.

- It is wrong to say that older people do not like, or need to avoid, spicy foods. Ageing can dull the taste buds so some older people may like spicy foods for their flavour.

- Diets should be high in calcium and vitamin D to help prevent decalcification – removal of calcium from the bones and teeth. A loss of calcium can also lead to osteoporosis, which results in weaker bones more prone to fractures and breaks.

- Protein is important to maintain and renew cells.

- Fibre levels need to be increased as the slowing of the digestive system, along with reduced mobility, may cause constipation.

- Iron is needed to prevent anaemia.

- The NACNE food goal recommendations (see pages 65–66) should be followed.

Social factors also play a part in an older person's quality of diet, especially if living alone. Research has shown that older people living on their own often do not eat properly because it is 'not worth the bother of cooking for one'. In cases where a partner has died, the remaining person may become disorientated while grieving, and so miss meals and not eat properly. This can also happen if a person begins to suffer memory loss.

Physical difficulties may affect diet. For example, lack of mobility may mean it is difficult for an older person to go to a supermarket where there is more choice of healthy foods and food is cheaper. Older people may be restricted to shopping close to home in a corner shop. Level of mobility may also affect an older person's ability to cook, and this can also affect the quality of diet. A person with arthritis may have difficulty preparing fresh vegetables and so may rely on frozen varieties, which may contain fewer nutrients.

Work, rest and play

A **healthy lifestyle** may be thought of as a **balanced lifestyle**, one which includes the right amounts of activity – work and recreation – and rest – inactivity and sleep. Each person is different and we all live happily on differing amounts of work and rest. As life changes a person's work and rest patterns change. Take for example, the lifestyle of many young students. Their course may be considered their 'work'; but they may also have a part-time job.

Work may take up five days per week and they possibly work some evenings at their jobs. Younger students may spend much of their time working. They relax by going out in the evenings after work and may survive on five hours' sleep a night. The younger student may be able to cope with this balance.

Another type of lifestyle is that of an older care assistant who may work an eight-hour shift each day for five days of the week, with the remainder of the time spent on leisure activities, sleep and socialising. This may represent a balance that meets the needs of the older person.

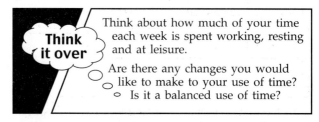

Think it over

Think about how much of your time each week is spent working, resting and at leisure.

Are there any changes you would like to make to your use of time? Is it a balanced use of time?

Why are sleep and rest important?

The human body is like a rechargeable battery. It cannot keep going without recharging itself. The body does this through sleep. During sleep the body is in a state of unconsciousness which allows the individual to cope with the activity of the day. If a person is not getting enough sleep, he or she is less able to cope with day-to-day life and is more prone to accidents and psychological problems, such as stress.

Non-physical activities

A large number of people enjoy non-physical activities that provide for their emotional, social and intellectual needs. For example, reading helps people unwind, particularly reading in bed before sleeping. It also provides intellectual stimulation and talking points when in the company of friends.

Sewing and knitting can be creative, useful and emotionally satisfying. Board games and quiz games are socially and intellectually enjoyable, while collecting stamps, coins, miniature cars, electric trains and other similar 'collectables' satisfies our emotional, and often intellectual, needs.

Many people with fairly ordinary jobs are amateur star performers in music making, singing and amateur dramatics!

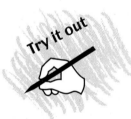

Try it out

With a partner, make a four-column chart like the one below. Write down in the first column all the leisure and recreational activities you can both think of (take 10 minutes to do this). Tick the appropriate columns for each activity, saying which need is satisfied by the activity. 'Reading' has been entered for you.

Activity	Emotional satisfaction	Intellectual satisfaction	Social satisfaction
Reading	✓	✓	✓

Another way the body recharges itself is through rest or inactivity. Doing very little physically, such as watching the television or reading, can also promote health for people who lead physically active lives.

Exercise and health

Taking exercise is an important part of keeping healthy, and there are many different and enjoyable ways to do so. A person can become fit by exercising about three times a week for 20 minutes. Exercise can range from walking to water-skiing, or from a gentle game of badminton to a hard workout in a gym.

Exercise should make use of the muscles but you should always warm up before any exercise, no matter how fit you are. You should also cool down as part of the routine.

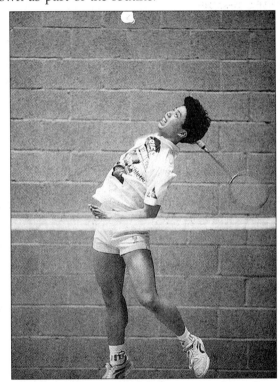

Vigorous exercise can be fun!

Most forms of exercise can be taken at different paces and levels. It is important to make sure the pace and level are chosen to suit the fitness of the individual.

Most exercise is a combination of **anaerobic** exercise, which stretches muscles, and aerobic exercise, which works the heart and lungs.

The benefits of exercise

Apart from the effects it has on our physical health, regular exercise has many other benefits. It helps us feel good and can also make us more relaxed, confident and able to cope with the strains of life (see Figure 2.7).

Figure 2.6 The effectiveness of different forms of exercise

Exercise	Strength	Stamina	Suppleness	Kcal/min
Badminton	**	**	***	5–7
Cycling (hard)	***	****	**	7–10
Golf	*	*	**	2–5
Dancing (disco)	*	***	****	5–7
Ballroom dancing	*	*	***	2–5
Swimming (hard)	****	****	****	7–10
Walking briskly	*	**	*	5–7
Climbing stairs	**	***	*	7–10

*Fair **Good ***Very good ****Excellent

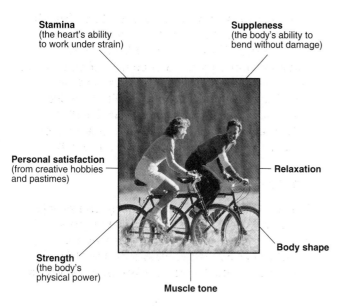

Stamina
(the heart's ability to work under strain)

Suppleness
(the body's ability to bend without damage)

Personal satisfaction
(from creative hobbies and pastimes)

Relaxation

Strength
(the body's physical power)

Body shape

Muscle tone

Figure 2.7 The benefits of exercise

Exercise can be a way for people to make new friends. It can also play a role in developing co-operative skills, especially in children.

The benefits of each form of exercise are often rated according to how much the exercise improves strength, stamina and suppleness (see Figure 2.6).

Environment

Environment includes an individual's immediate environment (such as his or her home, flat or place of residence), the individual's locality (such as an inner city, a leafy suburb or a rural community) or much wider regional, national or international environments. We must also include the environments of people who are homeless, of those in work and the play environments of children. The concept of 'environment' is hence very complex (see Figure 2.8).

The ideal environment for everyone would be in a land where there was no unemployment, no ill-health, no crime, no pollution, no poverty, the best housing, the best diet, the best education and total support for each other socially and emotionally. In reality, this is unlikely ever to happen.

Our environment can affect our growth and development, and it can afffect our potential. If we all lived in exactly the same environment, had the same illnesses and accidents, and ate the same diet, we would be likely to develop in a much more similar way than we really do. Our environment affects the opportunities we have in life, the attitudes we hold and the way we feel

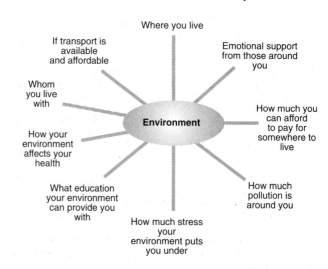

Where you live

If transport is available and affordable

Emotional support from those around you

Whom you live with

Environment

How much you can afford to pay for somewhere to live

How your environment affects your health

What education your environment can provide you with

How much stress your environment puts you under

How much pollution is around you

Figure 2.8 How our environment can affect us

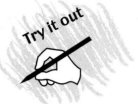

Try it out

Using flip charts and in small groups, brainstorm the possible ways in which an individual's health might be affected by his or her home environment. Here are some key words to get you started (you will be able to think of more):

location	overcrowding	solitary living
stairs	lighting	ventilation
damp	cooking facilities	sleeping arrangements
level (basement, high rise)	dirt	cleaning
noise	vulnerability	safety
sanitation	living accommodation	pets
garden/no garden	neighbours	heating

When you have exhausted your key words, put the charts up for the whole group to view and discuss. Next, take three 'post-its' each and, using three key words, write a sentence on each saying how the key word might affect someone's health.

For example: 'Vulnerability: an old person living in an inner-city flat might be very frightened of violent intruders – this would seriously affect his or her emotional and social health.'

about ourselves. We all have different experiences of life, partly because of where we live and whom we live with, and partly because of the situations we experience.

Look at the 'Try it out' above. You could repeat the same task for your own locality. Study the annual reports published by your local Health Authority or public health or social services departments. These reports will give you valuable information. For example, if you live in an area that has certain industries, such as chemical works, steel plants or oil refineries, there may be health risks associated with these industries. The reports may contain advice or guidance about these risks (see Figure 2.9).

Social class

The term 'class' is one way to categorise people, depending on their income. For many years people's income and jobs were used by the Registrar General when measuring the UK's population in the ten-yearly Census. However, in

---

Serious chemical incidents, like major outbreaks, are rare but the concentration of chemical sites in the area means that co-ordinated planning to deal with spillages are vital...

The Health Authority's role is perhaps not as well known as the role of other agencies (Police, Fire and Ambulance, Health and Safety Executive, Environmental Health). However, as part of its remit to protect the health of the population in the area it does have important responsibilities. These are:

- to ensure that there are hospital facilities to treat people affected by toxic chemicals

- to provide medical advice to the public and to other health professionals, in liaison with the emergency services. In the event of a serious incident to ensure collection of appropriate samples from people affected in an incident and

- to determine the need for long term surveillance of those affected and if this is necessary, to ensure that appropriate surveillance is carried out.

The local hospital has recently reviewed the facilities in the Accident and Emergency Department for dealing with chemically contaminated people and new decontamination facilities are being designed as a result of this review.

This report also mentions an outbreak of gastro-intestinal disease which affected 50 people. It was thought to have been associated with drinking water – another environmental factor that affects people's health.

Figure 2.9   Extract from the Wirral Public Health Report 1998, *Building Partnerships for Better Health*

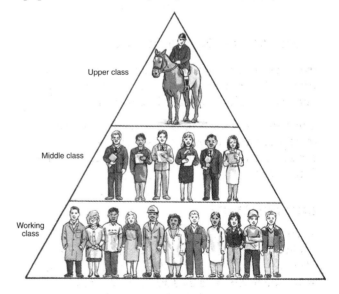

Figure 2.10   Social class

Figure 2.11

Social classifications expected to be used in the 2001 census	
1.1	Employers and managers in larger organisations, for example company directors.
1.2	Higher professionals, for example doctors, solicitors, teachers.
2	Lower managerial and professional occupations, for example nurses, journalists.
3	Intermediate occupations, for example clerks, secretaries.
4	Small employers and own account workers, for example taxi drivers, painters and decorators.
5	Lower supervisory, craft and related occupations, for example plumbers, train drivers.
6	Semi-routine occupations, for example shop assistants, hairdressers.
7	Routine occupations, for example cleaners, refuse collectors.

Those who are long-term unemployed form a final, eighth group.

December 1998, the National Statistics Office drew up a new method of classifying the population, and six **socioeconomic** classes first drawn up in 1911 were replaced by seven others (see Figure 2.11). People's socioeconomic status is now not just based on people's earnings but on the conditions of their employment (such things as job security, sick pay, pensions and the amount of control individuals have over their workloads). (See Unit 3 for details about income and wealth.)

Why should people's social class affect their health and well-being? Why should it matter how we measure social class? From the discussion of social class we have just had, these questions might come into our minds. But when we look at the population when it is categorised like this we find differences in the statistics about the amount of disease (morbidity) and early death (mortality) among the classes. For both males and females we find that, in over 80% of diseases, there is a steady rise in disease from social class 1 to the lower classes (see Figure 2.11). People at the bottom of the table and those who have been unemployed for a long time have higher amounts of heart and circulation problems, ulcers, mental illnesses, certain cancers, arthritis and many more illnesses. Such people also have a worse

likelihood of survival of certain cancers than people in the top classes.

It may also be the case that working-class areas of the country tend to have fewer (and worse) facilities for health care than other areas. People in the lower classes also tend to smoke and drink more than people in class 1 and, consequently, suffer more from smoking-related illnesses and alcohol problems. We could also perhaps assume that people from class 1 can afford leaner cuts of meat than people in other classes, and that they can easily afford balanced diets. Similarly, people with a good income may also have the money, time and education to take advantage of health clubs, exercise, sport and health information.

We could perhaps conclude from all this that social class has a serious effect on people's health and well-being.

Employment

A government health policy document called *Health of the Nation* states that 'people in manual groups are, for example, more likely to smoke and eat diets containing less Vitamin C and beta-carotene [a substance the body can convert to vitamin A]. There is also a higher proportion of heavy drinkers in manual than non-manual groups (though on the other hand there is also a higher proportion of people who never drink or who drink only lightly and infrequently). There is also evidence of lower take-up of preventive health services (e.g. immunisation, child health surveillance) in the most vulnerable groups.

Think it over

Why do you suppose the information in this document could be true? Try to give reasons for the three main points (smoking, diet and drinking) mentioned in the document. Could these be linked to the pressures and restrictions people in manual work suffer from?

Our work has a profound effect on our health and well-being: it provides our income, which, in turn, influences our standard of living. It also has far-reaching effects on us emotionally and mentally and can affect the 'speed' at which we live.

A person in a high-powered job will usually receive a salary that reflects the pressure he or she is under. However, such a person may find that, although he or she can afford a magnificent home, he or she never has the time to be there. His or her health and mental state may similarly be threatened because of the pressure he or she is under.

People in very low-paid jobs are equally under pressure though for different reasons. Trying to make ends meet and juggling the household bills are extremely stressful when someone is on a limited income. To have no employment at all has similar effects. No work means very little money coming in and a restricted lifestyle. In some areas of the UK unemployment figures are so high that it is very difficult for people to get jobs. Unemployment has a profound effect on self-esteem and motivation: what is the point of trying to get GCSEs if there are no jobs to go after?

Unemployment affects the way we treat other people. We may think that we cannot, or have no right to, approach others for help. It also affects the treatment that we receive from others, the services we are entitled to, and our attitudes to life. Finally, many people work simply for the money rather than for the satisfaction they get from their jobs. However, it could be argued that the more satisfaction a job gives us, the less stress we will be under. On the other hand, work itself is not without its problems, as we all know. And it perhaps comes as no surprise that there are far more employment-related accidents among the working classes than among the middle and professional classes. Many people are at risk of falls, cave-ins, 'dust' that can affect the respiratory system, injury to the eyes, etc., as a consequence of the work they do. The people who work in the emergency services (for example, the police, ambulance staff and firemen and women) have jobs that are dangerous in themselves but they must also deal with stressful incidents that may leave them depressed and anxiety-ridden. Research suggests that teachers, nurses and doctors also have very stressful occupations and that these people can be subjected to violent attacks from the people they come into contact with.

People who work in offices can develop repetitive strain injury, neck and back problems from poorly designed furniture, and depression and anxiety as a result of work overload and pressure. Similarly, we all might suffer emotional, social or physical problems that arise from racial, sexual, cultural or age discrimination.

Housing

Our income inevitably affects where we are able to live, and how we can afford to live there. For example, people on low incomes are more likely to rent rather than to buy and if we do not have regular work or a regular income, it is unlikely that banks or building societies will lend us the money for a mortgage.

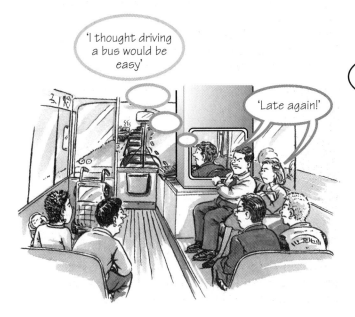

'I thought driving a bus would be easy'

'Late again!'

All types of work can put people under stress

Talk it over

With your friends, discuss which parts of the area you live in are most expensive and which the least. What are the reasons for this?

You could consider the facilities within each area, the amount of space between dwellings and the proximity of busy roads or heavy traffic.

Where we live and the type of dwelling we live in affect our health. If our home is in a badly maintained high rise in the inner city, with no access to safe play for our children, we are going to be under greater stress than someone living in more open conditions. Everyone lives with some stress but not everyone has the option or the money to escape for a while to relax. Stress can lead to ill health as a result of low income or poor housing; on the other hand, if we have a regular income and a secure job, we are more likely to be able to afford a better standard of living and the good health that accompanies this.

Income

Income is not just the amount of money we earn; it also has a great effect on our lives. If we have a high income we are less likely to worry about being able to pay the rent or feed our children. If we have a low income, we are less likely to worry about keeping up with the latest fashions or buying a new sports car. According to our incomes, different things become more or less important to us.

Education

Learning is something we do from birth, yet we only gain formal qualifications via the education we receive at school or college. The opportunities for education are not the same for everyone. By law, a child is entitled to education between the ages of 5 and 16 years but some children start and leave school earlier than others. All sorts of factors influence the amount of education a person receives (see Figure 2.12).

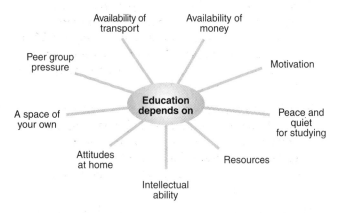

Figure 2.12   The factors that affect our education

Education can affect people in different ways. Sometimes our education turns us against those

things our upbringing told us were right and proper – be it our political views, our tastes for music, or simply those things that constitute 'a good square meal'. Although diet may seem trivial when put alongside politics, culture etc., if we think about what we eat it is very difficult to divorce our eating habits from our other attitudes about life – and it is our education (or lack of education) that has guided us in our eating habits. What we learn (or fail to learn) tells us what constitutes 'proper' food.

To confuse things even further, health messages have changed over the years. Dairy products were once considered to be very good for us but now the experts are saying that it is better to drink semi-skimmed milk. Potatoes and bread were once considered fattening, but now we are told to eat them – and to cut down on the butter instead! Red meat (i.e. beef, lamb and pork) was also considered to be an essential part of weekend meals, provided people could afford to buy it, but now healthy eating advice is not to eat too much red meat, but to eat more white meat – chicken and fish.

So how do we find out what is *supposed* to be good for us? One way is to read leaflets.

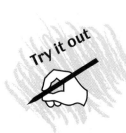

Carry out a survey, with permission, of shoppers in a local supermarket which supplies free information on healthy eating. Count the number of shoppers emerging from the cash tills and those who pick up or even look at the free information provided.

You could further extend this activity, with a simple questionnaire to shoppers asking them when they last looked at or picked up leaflets, then whether they read them.

How individuals can control the factors that affect their health and well-being

Many of the factors we have studied cannot be easily altered: issues such as income, employment, housing and social class. However, we can change some of the factors that affect our health and well-being, such as lack of exercise, diet, smoking, alcohol consumption, sexual behaviour and unsafe practices in the workplace.

It is not possible, however, in some situations to tell whether an individual has control or not and, in some instances, the individual may not want to believe he or she has control. A good example is education. There are many people who have not achieved their full potential educationally, but who were quite capable of doing so: they just did not want to challenge themselves.

Life choices and life chances

Some people say that everyone has a choice about his or her lifestyle. We can choose to exercise or be lazy; we can choose to follow a healthy diet or not; we can choose to practise safe sex; and we can choose not to take drugs. This all seems fine until we think about the ways poverty and stress can influence people.

If we live in a stressful neighbourhood or are under stress because we are unemployed we might not be able to choose our lifestyles as easily as someone who has a more comfortable life. Similarly, if we have to work long hours we may not easily be able to find the time to exercise. If we are depressed we may not care about the rules of safe sex, or we may feel the urge to take drugs. Hence people may *not* all have the same life chances.

Talk it over

In a group, discuss how you think young people's life chances are affected in the area where you live.

Is everyone able to shop easily, can everyone use the area's public and private facilities, and is everyone able to go out in the evenings?

In 1995, about a fifth of Britain's population and a quarter of Britain's children were considered to be living in poverty and, as we have already noted, poverty is one of the main influences on our life choices and life chances. There are different ways of measuring what it is to be poor. One measure is to use the amount of money paid to people receiving Income Support. This level of income is often called the poverty line.

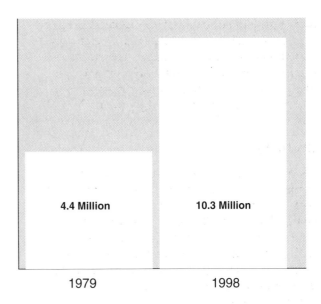

4.4 Million **10.3 Million**

1979 1998

Figure 2.13 Poverty in Britain

The key groups of people who have to live on or below the poverty line include:

◦ one-parent families

◦ elderly people

◦ single-earner, unskilled couples (where only one person works in an unskilled job)

◦ people who are unemployed

◦ people who are sick or disabled.

In 1998 an estimated 10.3 million people in Britain lived on or below this poverty line; in 1979, however, only 4.4 million people were estimated to be living in poverty (see Figure 2.13). The number of people who can be considered to be poor increased during the 1990s and may continue to increase in the future.

People who are poor may have enough money for food, for some clothes and for heating, but poverty means there is little money for the interesting purchases that make for exciting lifestyles: people who depend on benefits have limited life choices.

The latest clothes, comfortable and reliable cars, the latest electronic equipment, digital TV and so on may not be possible for people on a low income. People with little money have to restrict what they can buy when they visit a supermarket or shopping centre.

Many lifestyles are not possible for people in poverty. Belonging to a sports club is not possible if you can't afford the membership fees, the equipment and so on. Even jogging isn't possible if you feel your neighbourhood isn't safe to go out in.

Children living in poverty may have limited life choices and limited life chances to develop their full social, emotional and intellectual potential.

Risks to health
Substance abuse

People may use drugs or other substances in a way that feels pleasurable but that may be harmful to their health. For example glue is meant to stick things together, not to be inhaled. Many substances can be misused and these range from, for example, too much coffee causing nervous tension, to an individual who is addicted to 'crack' cocaine (see Figure 2.14). The word 'drug' also covers nicotine and alcohol, both of which are legal in the UK. Choosing to use any drug has an effect on our bodily functions.

Misuse of drugs
All kinds of drugs are available and they may be obtained in three main ways:

* The first way is from a doctor, via a prescription made up by the chemist. These are known as **prescribed drugs** and are part of a treatment given to combat an illness. Prescribed drugs are supplied with instructions and a list of side-effects you should be aware of.

* Some drugs are sold to the public by chemists or supermarkets. These are known as **over-the-counter drugs**. Supermarkets and other shops only sell paracetamol and similar drugs in small quantities in order to try and limit their misuse.

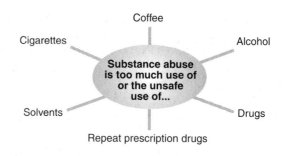

Figure 2.14   Substance abuse can take many forms

* It is illegal to possess **controlled drugs** except in certain special circumstances. These are often the types of drugs that can lead to addiction or that have dangerous side-effects if misused. Examples of controlled drugs are cannabis or cocaine.

Drugs misuse can have profound effects on us (see Figure 2.16). And the effects listed in the table are only the tip of the iceberg. Figure 2.17 analyses some of the most commonly misused drugs.

Solvent abuse
Solvents are substances used in the manufacture

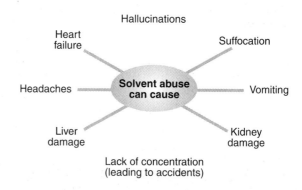

Figure 2.15   The effects of solvent abuse

Figure 2.16 The effects of misusing drugs

Psychological	Physical	Social
Depression	Heart problems	Crime
Paranoia (thinking people are against you)	Risk of HIV	Homelessness
Psychosis (total mental confusion)	Risk of hepatitis B/C	Employment problems

Figure 2.17 Chart to show effects and risks of some commonly misused drugs

Misused drug	Appearance and use	Effects of use	Possible risks to health
Cannabis or hash, grass, marijuana, Black Leb, rocky, weed	Like dried herbs, a dark brown block or sticky and treacle-like Usually smoked but sometimes eaten	Feeling of sickness, hunger or worry More alert and talkative Imagines things (hallucinations)	Bronchitis and damage to lungs Raised pulse rate and blood pressure Inactivity and loss of memory Mental illness
LSD or acid, trips, tabs	Blotters and micro-dots that are swallowed	Greater self-awareness Disorientated in time and place Altered hearing, panic Depression and feeling that everyone and everything is against them (paranoia)	Never quite returning to previous normal state and needing more and more to achieve the same effects (tolerance) Flashbacks Anxiety Disorientation and depression
Heroin or H, Henry, smack	White or brown powder that is injected, sniffed up the nose or smoked	Feeling sleepy and coddled	HIV/AIDS and Hepatitis B when it is injected Thrombosis of veins or abscess at the injection sites Blood infection (septicaemia) Heart and lung disorders Can be fatal if impure
Ecstasy or E, xtc, M25s, lovedoves, Adam	Flat, round tablets that are swallowed	Confidence, calmness and alertness Thirst, anxiety Symptoms of heat stroke Sexual feelings	Nausea, headache and giddiness Raised body temperature with no sweating Muscular cramps Collapse Mental illness including paranoia
Cocaine, coke, snow or Charlie	White powder that is injected or sniffed	Anxiety, thirst and heat stroke symptoms	HIV/AIDS and Hepatitis B when it is injected Thrombosis of veins or abscess at the injection sites Blood infection (septicaemia) Heart and lung disorders Addictive Raised body temperature with no sweating, muscular cramps Lack of appetite (anorexia)
Crack	Crystals that are smoked	Feel on top of the world, could do anything Panic, worry or hostility	
Amphetamines or speed, sulph, whizz	White powder in tablets or screws of paper that is swallowed, sniffed or injected	Palpitations (increased force and rate of heart beat), weakness, hunger Lots of energy and confidence Depression and worry	HIV/AIDS and Hepatitis B when it is injected Raised blood pressure and risk of stroke Mental illness Tolerance develops
Solvents or glue, Evo, aerosols, petrol, lighter fluid	Various fluids or sprays that are sniffed	Heightened imagination, depression, happiness or sadness, hostility Fatigue, confusion Liver and kidney damage	Liver and kidney damage Increased risk of accidents during the abuse Heart failure, suffocation, vomiting/choking, death

of glue, lighter fuel, petrol and aerosols. People sniff or inhale these products to get 'high' on the solvents they contain. For some people the effect is rather like being drunk: it makes them feel sad, happy, sleepy or wobbly on their feet. For others the reaction may be different. They may lose their appetites, have headaches or feel sick, or feel confused or hallucinate. Solvent misuse can cause convulsions, coma or death, even the first time a person tries it. It is against the law in the UK for children to buy items that may be misused, for example, lighter fuel and certain glues.

CASE STUDY – Cassie and Mick

Cassie and Mick are both aged 15 years and have been friends for about three months. They spend their Friday and Saturday evenings at raves where Mick often supplies Cassie with an ecstasy tablet. Recently they are both finding that school is even more tiring and boring than usual, but the weekends are much better: the ecstasy they take gives them more energy and life seems to be much more fun.

Jen, Cassie's friend, is worried about the ecstasy Cassie takes. She is for ever nagging Cassie about the dangers of heat stroke and dehydration: apparently, you can drink too much liquid and flood your brain. Cassie thinks this is funny. She knows that if you drink just *one* pint of water an hour you're usually OK. Jen thinks Cassie will become addicted, but Cassie knows she won't. This is just a way of relaxing at the weekend. Anyway, it's not as if she buys drugs from some shady looking character lurking in a doorway somewhere – Mick gets them from his mate – and your friends wouldn't mess you up.

Sometimes it is difficult to 'come down' after a rave. Cassie finds she can't get to sleep, and she always wakes up feeling tired and depressed that she has to go back to school on Monday. One of Mick's friends has offered to get them some 'brown', which he says makes you sleep like a baby and wake up feeling great. Neither Mick nor Cassie are aware that 'brown' is one of the names used for heroin.

Questions

Discuss the above case study:

1 What short-term benefits are Mick and Cassie getting?

2 How dangerous do you think their habit is?

3 Should Jen interfere further?

4 What longer-term effects are in danger of arising?

5 Could Mick be charged with supplying Cassie with drugs?

6 Where do you think they are getting their money to support their recreational habits?

7 What could the effects be if 'brown' was to replace ecstasy?

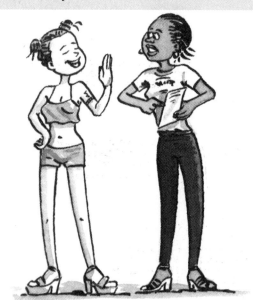

We do not always listen to good advice

As using solvents can cause dizziness or make someone pass out, misusing them by a busy road, by water, near a railway line or on top of high buildings adds to the chance of serious injury (see Figure 2.15).

The misuse of drugs and solvents: overview

Developing a tolerance to any drug can mean that more is needed each time to get the same effect. This means increased costs and increased risks. Also, most drugs that are misused are not made under safe laboratory conditions. Some drugs are contaminated with other dangerous substances, and so the effects are unpredictable. Some drugs may be deliberately mixed with other substances and some could be far weaker or stronger than those previously experienced.

Alcohol

Any decisions we make that affect our health have both short and long-term effects. Deciding to drink alcohol can, in the short term, make us feel good. In the slightly longer term it could mean loss of self-control. In the even longer term constant overuse of alcohol could mean alcoholism or cirrhosis of the liver. Cirrhosis is the condition where the liver enlarges in an attempt to cope with the excess amounts of alcohol: it becomes inflamed and hardens. It consequently stops working and the body is poisoned.

Some of the effects of alcohol are as follows:

- Alcohol slows down sections of the brain – abuse of alcohol can actually make your brain shrink!
- It causes weight gain – alcohol is very high in kilojoules.
- Alcohol weakens the immune system.
- Heavy drinking can affect sexual performance.
- Alcohol can give an initial 'high', followed by depression.
- It can become habit forming, and people can become dependent on it.

Tobacco

You will have noticed significant changes in social attitudes to smoking in the past few years. A very large number of workplaces and public places are now totally non-smoking areas or only permit smoking in certain restricted places. The hazards of smoking are now fairly well known as they have been well documented in the media and are printed on cigarette and other smoking material packaging. If you need to refresh your memory about these hazards, study Figure 2.18.

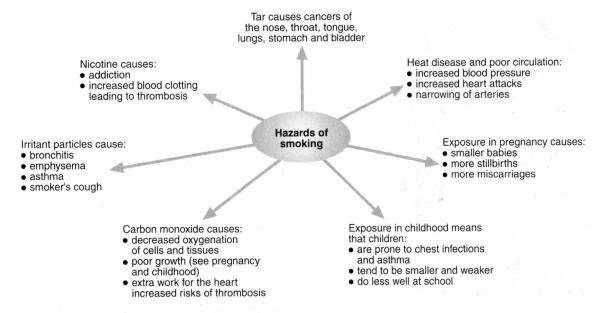

Figure 2.18   The hazards of smoking

Under the Health and Safety at Work Act 1974, employers have a duty to ensure the health, safety and welfare of their employees. More recently, European legislation has made it a requirement of employers that they must provide smoke-free rest areas and rest rooms. This requirement has been reinforced lately by reports about the risks to health from passive smoking. Passive smoking occurs when non-smokers inhale unfiltered smoke from the smokers around them. Such smoke has larger amounts of tar, nicotine and other irritants than that inhaled by the smoker.

Some non-smoking, well-known entertainers have died as a consequence of working for many years in smoky night-clubs and similar places. The foetuses of pregnant women are also passive smokers.

The following statistics about smoking have been compiled by the Royal College of Physicians:

◊ Smoking-induced illness accounts for 50 million lost working days each year.

◊ In England, 16 million working days are lost due to bronchitis, emphysema and asthma alone.

◊ Some 28% of people in paid employment would prefer it if their employers banned smoking altogether in their workplace.

Massive extra costs are incurred as a result of fire, refurbishment and redecoration, cleaning, drains on funds, health insurance, early retirement,

smoking breaks – the list could go on and on! (See Figure 2.19 for advice on how to assist smokers to stop smoking.)

Diet

'You are what you eat'. Although this is an old saying, it is largely true. Our health is greatly affected by our diet and the way we use the energy food gives us. There are many benefits from eating the right sorts of food in the correct quantities. If you eat too much once in a while, it is unlikely you will come to harm, apart from feeling a little bloated. If you constantly over-eat, your body will start to store fat under your skin in a thick layer. More importantly, it will store the excess fat on your organs and inside your arteries. Both of these are dangerous to our health and could lead to possible heart disease in later life.

When people put on weight, they do so gradually and usually do not notice it happening. Suppose over a few years you put on six kilogrammes. Carrying that extra weight is the same as carrying a vacuum cleaner around with you wherever you go. Imagine how tiring that would be. If you are overweight the same strain is put on your heart, muscles and back.

Under-eating is also unhealthy. A common condition induced by under-eating is anaemia, which is caused by a lack of iron in the diet. Anaemia occurs when the concentration of

The following is a list of traditional ways to stop smoking. There are also many new therapies, which can be found from web sites about the risks of smoking.

● Change the habits you have acquired that encourage you to smoke (for example if you usually smoke after lunch, take a short walk instead).

● Cut down on the number of cigarettes smoked over a period of time rather than trying to stop suddenly.

● Use substitute nicotine gum or patches (with counselling support).

● Ask friends and family for their support.

● Use the money saved to buy a longed-for treat.

● Restrict your opportunities for smoking, such as one cigarette only in the evening.

● Change your brand of cigarettes to one which has a very low tar content.

You will find several leaflets about stopping or reducing smoking at your local health education unit, or from the Health Education Authority and the anti-smoking organisation, ASH.

Figure 2.19   Advice on how to stop smoking

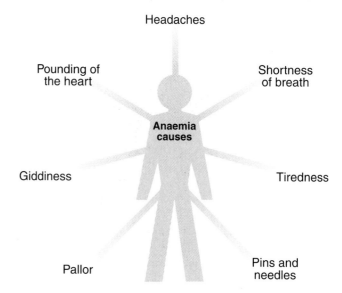

Figure 2.20   The effects of anaemia

haemoglobin in the blood falls and this prevents the oxygen in your blood from being carried around your body efficiently (see Figure 2.20).

People, who change their diet, for example, by becoming a vegetarian could be prone to anaemia. Another group who are susceptible to anaemia are teenage girls and young women, who are trying to alter or achieve their desired body shape. Because they cut down on iron-rich foods and generally eat less, they do not get the nutrients they need.

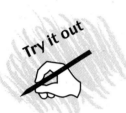

Weigh and measure yourself, and then see where you are on a standard height/weight chart. You will notice that the bands for each particular measurement are quite wide.

Why do you think this is?

Are you in the band you expected to be in?

Poverty and diet

Eating the right foods in the correct quantities is rather like putting petrol, oil and water in a car: it keeps you running and ensures all your parts are maintained in working order (see Figure 2.21). Poverty has a huge effect on the health choices

people are able to make. If you do not have enough money to buy the leanest cuts of meat, or the freshest fruit and vegetables, your diet is going to be less healthy than someone who can afford to buy these. The diets of people living 'on the breadline' are much worse than those with a higher income.

Suppose you have less than £50 a week to feed five of you: your main purpose in buying food would be to stop people from feeling hungry, rather than meeting all their nutritional needs. The easiest, fastest way to stop hunger is to eat

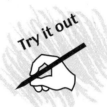

Try to work out a week's *healthy* menus for five people with only £50 to spend. Remember, that's only £10 per person for the whole week. You may have to undertake some research to do this realistically. Work out main meals for each day and then draw up a list of the things you need (you can exclude those things most people have in their 'larders' – things like salt, flour, sugar, jam, oil, margarine etc.). Go to a supermarket and check prices against those items on your list.

Can you afford to buy all the things you have planned to eat? Are you tempted to 'cut corners' and dive into the freezer compartment for that cheap bumper pack of burgers? How frustrating do you find the whole experience?

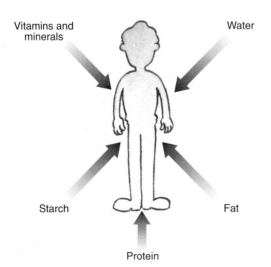

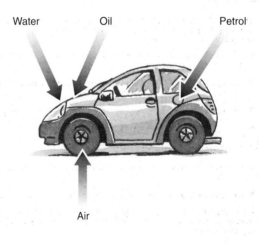

Figure 2.21   Just as a car needs petrol, we all need the correct food to keep our bodies in working order

high-fat carbohydrate foods: chip butties, tinned spaghetti on toast, deep-fried anything. Advice from the exerts about improving our diets by eating five helpings of fruit and vegetables a day is less easy to follow when you are living on a limited income. Alternatives have to be found.

Poverty can spiral people into ill-health. And once we enter this spiral, it is very difficult to break free of an inevitable descent into being unable to cope with the pressures of life (see Figure 2.22).

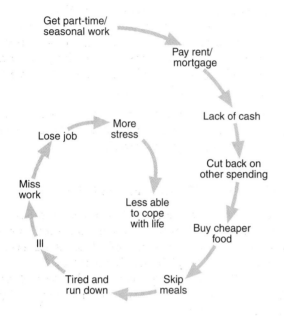

Figure 2.22   Poverty and diet: the vicious circle

Stress

Most people suffer from stress at some time in their lives, and a small amount of stress can be good for us: it makes our bodies respond more vigorously to meet the challenges of life. It is the grind of continual stress that is so harmful to us.

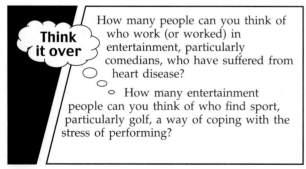

Think it over

How many people can you think of who work (or worked) in entertainment, particularly comedians, who have suffered from heart disease?

How many entertainment people can you think of who find sport, particularly golf, a way of coping with the stress of performing?

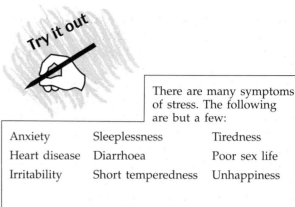

Try it out

There are many symptoms of stress. The following are but a few:

Anxiety	Sleeplessness	Tiredness
Heart disease	Diarrhoea	Poor sex life
Irritability	Short temperedness	Unhappiness

Try to add to this list.

Individuals or groups who suffer from stress will find that, eventually, their relationships will break down, they will become depressed and they may develop mental illnesses. They may even become violent or suicidal. Alternatively they may withdraw from the world and become anti-social. Either way people's health will suffer and this is why stress management training is now accepted as necessary to prevent people who suffer from stress from becoming ill. Stress management training helps find ways of minimising stress or ways to cope with stress.

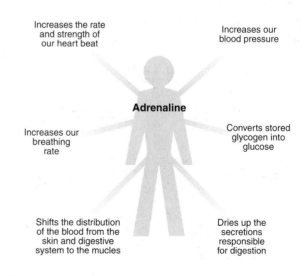

Figure 2.23   The effects of adrenaline

The way our bodies respond to stress is age-old: it evolved so that people could cope with predators, hunger and extremes of temperature, etc. These were things prehistoric people encountered regularly in their lives. However, such stress reactions are often not appropriate in modern society, and stress can now induce illness in people instead. Stress causes the body to secrete the hormone adrenaline. The effects of adrenaline are shown in Figure 2.23. Anyone who is stressed every day for a period of time is likely to develop heart and breathing problems.

Personal hygiene

Good personal hygiene is essential to us all: our skin, hair, and teeth soon start to lose their sparkle if not maintained properly (see Figure 2.24). When working in the field of health and social care, you will have to work closely with other people. Poor personal hygiene is very noticeable if in a combined space and can cause embarrassment and discomfort for everyone.

Poor personal hygiene isn't just unpleasant, it can affect our health in a negative way. Human beings are an ideal medium for bacteria to grow in. We are the right sort of temperature, we produce moisture in the form of sweat, and we produce food for bacteria in the form of dead skin cells, and in the chemicals in our sweat. Bacteria can be passed from one person to another and also on to food, so it's important to try to reduce the number of bacteria that are using us as host.

Watch the people in the room with you. See how often they touch their faces, scratch itches, play

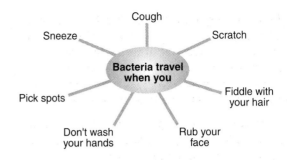

Figure 2.25   How we pass on bacteria

with their hair and rub their noses. Every time they do this they are transferring bacteria from one place to another (see Figure 2.25). Not only are they increasing the risk of spreading bacteria to themselves, they are also increasing the chances of spreading bacteria to others.

Examples of infections that can be passed on as a result of poor hygiene are headlice, threadworms, ringworm, impetigo and scabies.

Lack of physical exercise

A lack of physical exercise has many effects on our bodies (see Figure 2.26). Our lungs are never fully inflated and deposits collect at their bases. The bowel is sluggish and this leads to constipation. Our weight is not under control and, frequently, as middle age sets in, our body weight increases steadily.

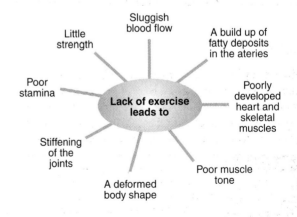

Figure 2.26   The effects of lack of exercise

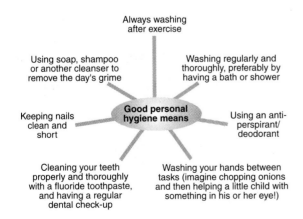

Figure 2.24   Good personal hygiene is essential

Sexual behaviour

The continuation of the human race depends upon males and females having sex, and sex is therefore a natural part of human life. Because people are actively engaging in sex at younger and younger ages, they are often not aware of the consequences of unwanted pregnancies, and of the possibilities of contracting diseases that are transmitted through the act of sexual intercourse.

Sex is exciting and pleasurable to both partners, and is a way of demonstrating love and affection for each other. Sex can occur between males and females or between two people of the same gender. The latter cannot result in pregnancy, but still carries a serious risk of disease. It doesn't matter whether the relationship is for one night or many nights, the risk of disease is still there. However, the greater the number of sexual partners a person has, the greater the risk of being infected with disease and the greater the risk of passing it on.

HIV (human inmmunodeficiency virus) and AIDS (acquired immune deficiency syndrome)

AIDS is caused by the HIV virus and, although only first reported as recently as 1981, AIDS is now a major worldwide epidemic. AIDS is the term used to describe the condition people who have advanced HIV infection suffer from. There is no cure for AIDS (although several therapies are now known to prolong the life expectancy of AIDS sufferers and some vaccines are now being tested on people). Therefore the only way to avoid HIV infection is to avoid behaviours that put a person at risk of contracting the virus. This means we should not have unprotected sex and drug users should not share needles.

HIV damages the human immune system by killing or injuring the immune cells such that the person's body is unable to fight off certain infections and cancers (see Figure 2.27). Generally, the AIDS victim is prone to **opportunistic infections** and cancers that do not usually cause illness in healthy people.

HIV/AIDS statistics

You will find the latest statistics on the Internet (www.avert.org/wwstatsy.htm). Statistics for the UK are given in Figure 2.28.

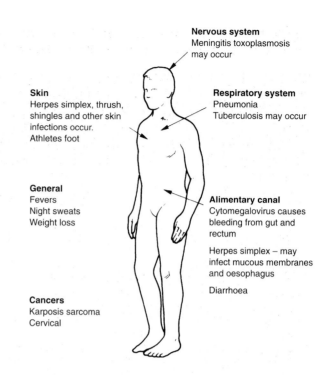

Skin
Herpes simplex, thrush, shingles and other skin infections occur. Athletes foot

General
Fevers
Night sweats
Weight loss

Cancers
Karposis sarcoma
Cervical

Nervous system
Meningitis toxoplasmosis may occur

Respiratory system
Pneumonia
Tuberculosis may occur

Alimentary canal
Cytomegalovirus causes bleeding from gut and rectum

Herpes simplex – may infect mucous membranes and oesophagus

Diarrhoea

Figure 2.27   AIDS-related illnesses

The figures in Figure 2.28 show only reported cases. As many people are unaware they are infected with the HIV virus, real figures will be much higher (it can take several months for HIV antibodies to develop and show up in tests). Clients and care-workers who have HIV infection, and those people who work with clients who have HIV infection, require information, tact, full treatment and support.

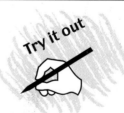

Examine Figure 2.28.

1   Calculate the percentage increase or decrease in cases of HIV and AIDS in each country between the years 1995 and 1998.

2   Comment on each country's apparent success in the promotion of health in relation to HIV and AIDS as suggested by these figures.

Examples of a calculation

Percentage increase of HIV cases between 1990 and 1991 in England = 2250 – 1969 × 100 = 37.8% increase in cases of HIV.

Figure 2.28 Table to show HIV and AIDS statistics in the different countries of the United Kingdom by year by kind permission of the Public Health Laboratory Service AIDS Centre

Year	Country							
	England		Wales		Scotland		N. Ireland	
	HIV-infected persons	AIDS cases	HIV-infected persons	AIDS cases	HIV-infected persons	AIDS cases	HIV-infected persons	AIDS cases
All to 1984	87	100	0	3	213	3	0	0
1985	2224	151	13	2	249	4	20	1
1986	2226	285	27	4	334	7	12	1
1987	2024	602	27	9	259	25	8	2
1988	1429	699	44	16	140	34	8	5
1989	1531	766	29	14	130	57	12	5
1990	1969	1177	67	16	130	62	12	8
1991	2250	1246	31	14	159	86	15	4
1992	2192	1370	46	17	135	77	16	7
1993	2153	1457	38	21	147	111	11	9
1994	2168	1622	45	23	137	121	7	7
1995	2432	1409	43	20	158	130	15	13
1996	2606	1738	38	12	159	94	10	10
1997	2331	1275	32	35	170	68	14	0
1998	2599	882	37	22	160	56	11	4
1999*	1320	368	27	10	71	33	4	1
Total	31541	15147	544	238	2751	968	175	77

* Only half-year figures for 1999 are available

Think it over

Look again at the trends and patterns of HIV and AIDS in the UK. Compile graphs or pie charts from the data provided. You could also write a short report that identifies the main trends of HIV and AIDS infection.

Transmission

Main ways in which the virus is passed on to others are as follows (see Figure 2.29):

- Unprotected sexual contact with an infected partner.

- The sharing of blood-contaminated needles or syringes between injecting drug users when one or more of the individuals is infected with the virus.

- An infected mother can pass the infection on to her baby during pregnancy or at birth.

Although rare, HIV can also arise from:

- Contact with infected blood. Blood donations are now screened and treated to destroy the virus (but this was not the case before 1985).

- Accidental jabs or cuts with needles, sharps and medical instruments when passed between an infected client and health care worker (and vice versa).

To date, scientists have found no evidence of transmission through:

- saliva, sweat, tears, urine or faeces

- towels, bedding, toilet seats, swimming pools, telephones or food utensils

- mosquitoes, bed bugs, or other biting insects.

Figure 2.29   Analysis of routes of HIV and AIDS infection for the United Kingdom for all cases between 1984 and 1998

Routes for infection	AIDS cases	HIV cases
Sex between men (homosexual route)	10771	23226
Sex between men and women (heterosexual route)	2715	8568
Injecting drug users	1030	3489
Exchanging blood or tissue	764	1622
Unknown	457	1672

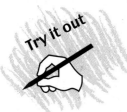

Look at Figure 2.29. Find the percentage of HIV-imfected persons who were injecting drug users. Calculate the percentage of people with AIDS infected by the heterosexual route.

Note: Having other sexually transmitted diseases, such as herpes, syphilis and gonorrhoea, seems to make sufferers more susceptible to HIV infection if they have intercourse with an HIV-infected person.

To protect yourself from HIV infection you should:

1   Practise safe sex (using kite marked condoms) or celibacy.

2   Limit the number of partners you have or wait until you are in a permanent relationship before having sex.

3   Wipe surfaces with good disinfectant after cleaning up spills of any body fluids.

4   Wear disposable gloves when dealing with blood, body fluids or wounds.

?   *The number of people who become infected by the heterosexual route each year is rapidly overtaking the number of people infected by the homosexual route. HIV infection can no longer be considered a disease of 'gays'. Overall figures for HIV infection suggest a further increase in 1999. The health promotion message for safe sex – use a condom – is not getting through to a large number of the population.*

Unsafe practices in the workplace

Workplaces are subject to various inspection systems and must comply with the Health and Safety at Work Act 1974 and the 1988 Control of Substances Hazardous to Health Regulations. The key features of the Health and Safety at Work Act (HASAW) are given in Figure 2.30. What HASAW basically means is that both the employer and the

- *employers must make all reasonable efforts to ensure the health, safety and welfare of all their employees by informing you:*

  –how to carry out your job safely without risk to yourself and others

  –of risks identified with the job that may affect you

  –what measures have been taken to protect you from the identified risks

  –and how to use these measures

  –how to get first aid treatment

  –what to do in an emergency

  –by leaflet or poster about the Health and Safety at Work Act and the local Health and Safety Executive's address

- *employers must provide free of charge:*

  –adequate safety training

  –clothing or equipment required to protect you while at work

- *as an employee, your responsibilities are:*

  –to take reasonable care of yourself and others (including the general public) who may be affected by your work

  –use any equipment provided for you for its intended purpose and in a proper manner

  –not to carry out tasks that you do not know how to do safely

  –let your manager know if you witness anything that is not safe and could place yourself or others at risk

  –to co-operate with employers on health and safety matters

  –inform the appropriate person in the organisation if you have an accident or witness a near miss

Figure 2.30   Key features of the Health and Safety at Work Act 1974

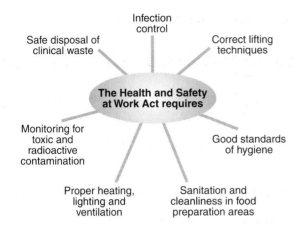

Figure 2.31 How the Health and Safety at Work Act affects care settings

employee share extra responsibilities for health and safety and that any organisation employing more than five people must have a written policy statement on health and safety. Figure 2.31 outlines the ways HASAW affects care settings.

The main requirements of the Control of Substances Hazardous to Health (COSHH) Regulations are that employers must:

⋄ complete risk assessments on all hazardous substances used in the workplace

⋄ keep records of risk assessments and review them regularly

⋄ inform employees about any substance hazardous to their health

⋄ provide appropriate training in the use of hazardous substances.

Hazardous substances include correction fluid used in offices, disinfectants used for cleaning,

drugs used in medical treatment and radioactive chemicals used in care settings.

Workplaces contain people, and people often take shortcuts to save themselves time or consider certain things they must do in the course of the jobs irrelevant or a waste of time. As a result, people often don't wear their protective clothing properly, they don't wear ear protectors against noise and fail to wear safety helmets and shoes and other safety clothing. Circuit breakers (designed to protect equipment) could be jammed open, the wrong fuses might be installed in plugs, incorrect waste disposal methods might be practised – a host of unsafe working methods could be mentioned. We must all be aware of hazards and unsafe practices in the workplace. We must investigate these and, if necessary, report them. Remember the responsibility for health and safety rests with all of us.

Health promotion

One way to promote people's health is to produce leaflets and brochures (Figure 2.32). Your tutor may have collected samples of these for you to study. Other good sources of such literature include:

⋄ doctors' surgeries

⋄ dentists' surgeries

⋄ health centres

⋄ health visitors

⋄ health promotion units

⋄ supermarkets

⋄ health food shops

⋄ specialist support agencies.

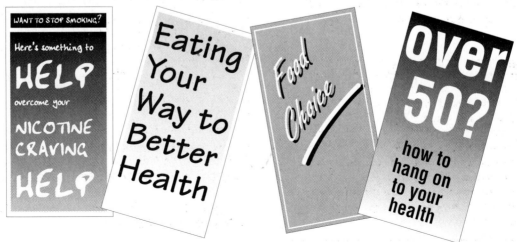

Figure 2.32 Some examples of health promotion literature

When collecting leaflets for use in your assignments, think carefully about what kind of information you need and who you intend to read it. For example, a child will not want to be told about kilojoule values or the risks of eating too much saturated fat. Similarly, a well-educated adult will not appreciate leaflets that contain lots of smiley faces faces eating high-fibre bread and fresh vegetables. You should also avoid those leaflets food manufacturers publish simply to promote their own products.

Not everything we read is 100% accurate. You will have to study the information carefully to assess whether it reflects the particular points you wish to make (see Figure 2.33). If you do not care for published material, you could make leaflets or posters of your own.

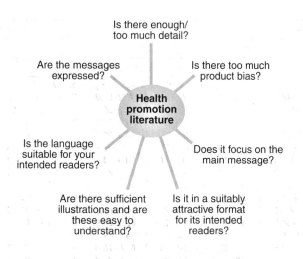

Figure 2.33   Assessing health promotion literature

Indicators of physical good health

There are a number of different physical (body) measurements that can be taken to assess a person's state of health. These include:

◦   height and weight

◦   peak flow

◦   body mass index (BMI)

◦   resting pulse rate and recovery after exercise.

Height and weight

There are standard ways of measuring a person's weight against that person's height. To do this, standard charts or tables are used that are available in three different forms. These different forms take into account the person's frame size. Frame size is a person's bone size and build. If you find it difficult to judge a person's frame size, ask him or her: most people know whether standard clothing and shoe sizes fit them and will be able to guide you as to their frame. Different tables are also used for men and women (see Figures 2.35 and 2.36).

If someone falls into the severely overweight range, he or she is at risk of cardiovascular disease, high blood pressure, diabetes, arthritis and other conditions. Such people should be advised to seek help from their family doctor.

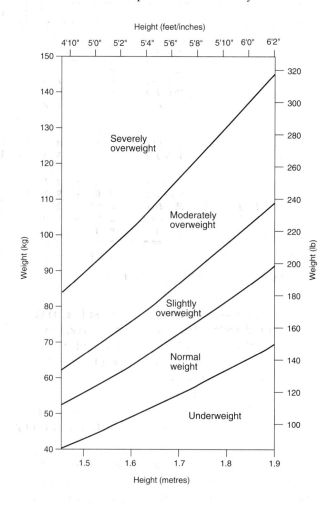

Figure 2.34   Example of a height/weight chart

Men																
Weight																
Height (in shoes)			Small frame						Medium frame						Large frame	
m	ft	in	kg kg	st	lb		st	lb	kg kg	st	lb		st	lb	kg kg	st	lb		st	lb
1.575	5	2	50.8–54.4	8	0	–	8	8	53.5–58.5	8	6	–	9	3	57.2–64.0	9	0	–	10	1
1.6	5	3	52.2–55.8	8	3	–	8	11	54.9–60.3	8	9	–	9	7	58.5–65.3	9	3	–	10	4
1.626	5	4	53.5–57.2	8	6	–	9	0	56.2–64.7	8	12	–	9	10	59.9–67.1	9	6	–	10	8
1.651	5	5	54.9–58.5	8	9	–	9	3	57.6–63.0	9	1	–	9	13	61.2–68.9	9	9	–	10	12
1.676	5	6	56.2–60.3	9	12	–	9	7	59.0–64.9	9	4	–	10	3	62.6–70.8	10	12	–	11	2
1.702	5	7	58.1–62.1	9	2	–	9	11	60.8–66.7	9	8	–	10	7	64.4–73.0	10	2	–	11	7
1.727	5	8	59.9–64.0	9	6	–	10	1	62.6–68.9	9	12	–	10	12	66.7–75.3	10	7	–	11	12
1.753	5	9	61.7–65.8	9	10	–	10	5	64.4–70.8	10	2	–	11	2	68.5–77.1	10	11	–	12	2
1.778	5	10	63.5–68.0	10	0	–	10	10	66.2–72.6	10	6	–	11	6	70.3–78.9	11	1	–	12	6
1.803	5	11	65.2–69.9	10	4	–	11	0	68.0–74.8	10	10	–	11	11	72.1–81.2	11	5	–	12	11
1.829	6	0	67.1–71.7	10	8	–	11	4	69.9–77.1	11	0	–	12	2	74.4–83.5	11	10	–	13	2
1.854	6	1	68.9–73.5	10	12	–	11	8	71.7–79.4	11	4	–	12	7	76.2–85.7	12	0	–	13	7
1.88	6	2	70.8–75.7	11	0	–	11	13	73.5–81.6	11	8	–	12	12	78.5–88.0	12	5	–	13	12
1.905	6	3	72.6–77.6	11	4	–	12	3	75.7–83.5	11	13	–	13	3	80.7–90.3	12	10	–	14	3
1.93	6	4	74.4–79.4	11	8	–	12	7	78.1–86.2	12	4	–	13	8	82.7–92.5	13	0	–	14	8

Figure 2.35 Weight/height chart for men

Women																
Weight																
Height (in shoes)			Small frame						Medium frame						Large frame	
m	ft	in	kg kg	st	lb		st	lb	kg kg	st	lb		st	lb	kg kg	st	lb		st	lb
1.473	4	10	41.7–44.5	6	8	–	7	0	43.5–48.5	6	12	–	7	9	47.2–54.0	7	6	–	8	7
1.499	4	11	42.6–45.8	6	10	–	7	3	44.5–49.9	7	0	–	7	12	48.1–55.3	7	8	–	8	10
1.524	5	0	43.5–47.2	6	12	–	7	6	45.8–51.3	7	3	–	8	1	49.4–56.7	7	11	–	8	13
1.549	5	1	44.9–48.5	7	1	–	7	9	47.2–52.6	7	6	–	8	4	50.8–58.1	8	0	–	9	2
1.575	5	2	46.3–49.9	7	4	–	7	12	48.5–54.0	7	9	–	8	7	52.2–59.4	8	3	–	9	5
1.6	5	3	47.6–51.3	7	7	–	8	1	49.9–55.3	7	12	–	8	10	53.5–60.8	8	6	–	9	8
1.626	5	4	49.0–52.6	7	10	–	8	4	51.3–57.2	8	1	–	9	0	54.9–62.6	8	10	–	9	12
1.651	5	5	50.3–54.0	7	13	–	8	7	52.7–59.0	8	4	–	9	4	56.8–64.4	8	13	–	10	2
1.676	5	6	51.7–55.8	8	2	–	8	11	54.4–61.2	8	8	–	9	9	58.5–66.2	9	3	–	10	6
1.702	5	7	53.5–57.6	8	6	–	9	1	56.2–63.0	8	12	–	9	13	60.3–68.0	9	7	–	10	10
1.727	5	8	55.3–59.4	8	10	–	9	5	58.1–64.9	9	2	–	10	3	62.1–69.9	9	11	–	11	0
1.753	5	9	57.2–61.2	9	0	–	9	9	59.9–66.7	9	6	–	10	7	64.0–71.7	10	1	–	11	4
1.778	5	10	59.0–63.5	9	4	–	10	0	61.7–68.5	9	10	–	10	11	65.8–73.9	10	5	–	11	9
1.803	5	11	60.8–65.3	9	8	–	10	4	63.5–70.3	10	0	–	11	1	67.6–76.2	10	9	–	12	0
1.829	6	0	62.6–67.1	9	12	–	10	8	65.3–72.1	10	4	–	11	5	69.4–78.5	10	13	–	12	5

Figure 2.36 Weight/height chart for women

Moderately overweight people are still at risk and should follow the same plan as severely overweight people. Slightly overweight people are still at greater risk than those of normal weight, but should follow a sensible weight-reducing plan and take more exercise. Anyone with health problems should be advised to consult his or her family doctor before beginning a new regime.

Being slightly underweight is not a problem but being very underweight *is* a problem. If someone has recently started to lose weight for no reason he or she may have an undiagnosed illness. Such people should be advised to consult a medical practitioner.

Some people (and not just overweight people) are very sensitive about other knowing their weight. When working with people you will have to anticipate such sensitivity. People might be able to weigh themselves and be able to find their position on the weight/height charts themselves. Do not tell other people about someone's weight without first asking the person for his or her permission to do so. If you are taking measurements from children, ask for the child's permission as well as asking his or her parents or guardians.

Peak flow

To measure peak flow you need a meter which records the maximum speed at which air can flow out of the lungs. This measurement is used to assess the width of the air passages (bronchi). The most common use of peak flow measurement is to monitor the degree of bronchospasm (narrowing of the air passages) in people who suffer from asthma, and their response to the drugs they take for the condition. It is also a useful measurement in people who have respiratory problems, such as intermittent coughing or difficulty with breathing. It can help to asses whether they have developed asthma (see Figure 2.37).

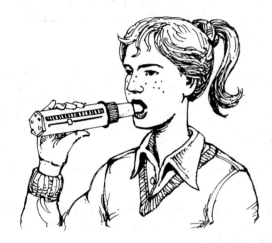

Figure 2.37   A peak flow meter

After first taking a deep breath, an individual blows through the mouthpiece with maximum effort. Fitness suites in gyms and sports centres often employ peak flow measuring equipment.

Body mass index

The body mass index (BMI) also uses weight in kilograms and height in metres to assess people's general state of health. BMI is worked out using the following calculation:

$$\frac{\text{weight (kg)}}{\text{height (m)}^2} = \text{BMI}$$

For example, if your height is 1.82 m, then you will divide your weight by 1.82 x 1.82. If your weight is 70.5 kg then:

$$\frac{70.5}{1.82 \times 1.82} = 21.3$$

People with BMIs between 19 and 22 appear to live the longest; death rates appear to be the highest in people with BMIs of 25 and over. BMIs are different for males and females (see Figure 2.38).

Figure 2.38   Body mass indexes

Female	Significance	Male	Significance
Less than 18	Underweight	Less than 18	Underweight
18–20	Lean	18–20	Lean
21–22	Average	21–23	Average
23–28	Plump	24–32	Plump
29–36	Moderately obese	32–40	Moderately obese
37+	Severely obese	40+	Severely obese

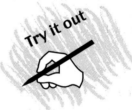

Try it out

You will find lots of useful references to BMIs and other physical measurements if you 'surf the web'. Some Internet health sites can be found in the 'Further reading' section at the end of the book.

Resting pulse rate and recovery after exercise

You can count someone's pulse rate where an artery crosses a bone. Pulse rates are usually taken either below the base of the thumb or on one side of the windpipe in the neck. It should be counted by lightly pressing two figures over the site until you feel the throbbing. Count the beats over 10 or 15 second intervals and multiply by 6 or 4, accordingly, to obtain the number of beats over one minute.

To take people's resting pulse, make sure they are calm and have been sitting quietly for 5–10 minutes. Take at least three recordings and calculate the average pulse rate. (To work out the average, add all the readings together and divide by the number you obtain by the number of readings you have taken).

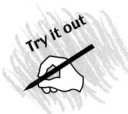

Zola had the following counts for her resting pulse rate:

65 68 72 74 68 65

The average would be 65 + 68 + 72 + 74 + 68 + 65 divided by 6. This works out at 69 beats per minute.

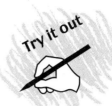

Working in pairs, take physical measurements of members of your group. Record your results in a table.

Discuss what the results suggest about each individual's level of fitness.

It is generally accepted that the lower the pulse rate in a healthy individual, the fitter he or she is. After exercise, when the pulse rate has increased, the same principle still applies.

To measure someone's 'recovery after exercise' pulse rate, you will need to provide your subject with some form of mild exercise, such as running on the spot or walking up and down stairs. Take readings immediately after the exercise and every minute until the pulse rate is back to resting level. You could draw up a graph of pulse rate against time to display your readings, and mark the point at which the resting pulse rate is regained. Note the time it took for this to occur.

To obtain valid results repeat this over three or four exercises and work out the average.

Safety note: When devising the exercise, bear in mind your subject's state of health and fitness! You could not ask an elderly lady to jog around

the block! Walking up a flight of stairs might similarly be too much, so stepping up and down one step a few times might be sufficient.

The shorter the recovery time, the fitter the individual. Pulse rates should generally recover within 2 or 3 minutes but, again, bear in mind the severity of the exercise you have asked someone to do.

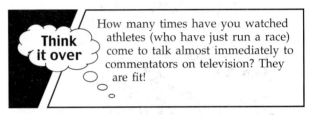

Think it over
How many times have you watched athletes (who have just run a race) come to talk almost immediately to commentators on television? They are fit!

To find out about negotiating health improvement plans with clients, see the assessment activities section, which follows.

Unit 2 Assessment

Obtaining a Pass grade

To obtain a *Pass*, you need to produce a plan to promote the health and well-being of at least one person whose health is at risk. This plan must include:

- information about the health risks
- an explanation of which risks the person can control
- at least two measures of health
- timescales and targets for improving the person's health

- supplementary health promotion material.

1   Study the outline profiles of the pretend family members shown in Figure 2.39 below. All these people have health risks. If you had to construct a health plan for one of these people, which one would you choose? At first sight June's may seem the easiest to work out, Julie's perhaps the hardest.

   June may appear to be a good choice, but a successful plan would depend on her desire for change. Jason may think a health plan is a big joke and may not take it seriously.

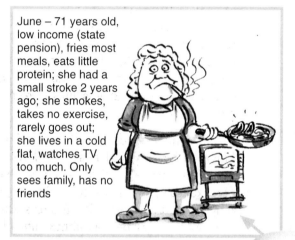

June – 71 years old, low income (state pension), fries most meals, eats little protein; she had a small stroke 2 years ago; she smokes, takes no exercise, rarely goes out; she lives in a cold flat, watches TV too much. Only sees family, has no friends

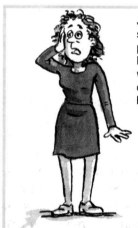

Julie, 42 years old, single parent, has two part-time jobs; works hard to make ends meet; worries about her children; had lump in breast removed last year

Health plan

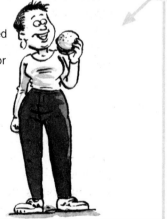

Jill, 18-years old, engaged to Jason, may have unprotected sex, eats mostly burgers and chips for main meals

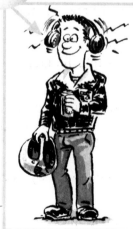

18-year-old Jason rides a motorbike, drinks a lot of alcohol, smokes, takes ecstasy occasionally, has unsafe sex; well paid assembly line work; listens to loud music through ear phones

Figure 2.39   Possible subjects for a health plan

It is hence important to give serious thought to whom you choose for your health plan, and the reasons why, before starting to collect your assignment evidence. Try not to choose the easiest person you can think of as this might limit your opportunities. In real life, the best advice is to talk to the person first about what you need to do to get his or her support for a health improvement plan. You *must* be tactful: think how you would feel if one of your friends or family decided you were 'unhealthy' and tried to change your lifestyle! It might be best to explain your task to more than one person to see what their reactions are before making your final decision. Having made your choice, discuss this with your tutor. He or she will be able to guide you.

2   Having identified the person you will provide the health plan for, you must now give some thought to the format in which you will present the plan. The most obvious way to present it is probably in table form. However, is your person a good reader and will he or she be able to understand tables? A child, an older person or an adult with learning disabilities will prefer larger, clear typing and lots of illustrations. A friend who is a student at college or university may be used to reading tables, but a person with a visual impairment might appreciate an audiotape. Many educational establishments also have the facilities for converting written notes into Braille.

3   You could produce a booklet or a large poster that could be put on display on the person's kitchen wall. Whatever form your plan takes, you must have valid reasons for the design you have chosen, and it must be easily understood by your subject.

You are required to consider both short and long-term targets for improving a person's health. Wherever possible, these targets should be measurable.

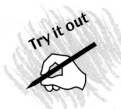

Try it out

Study the family members shown in Figure 2.39 once more.

How could members of the family control some of the health risks they face?

How could you measure their weight and overall fitness? How would you go about assessing their diets?

Obtaining a Merit grade:

1   Read the case study about Vikram. To obtain a *Merit*, you will have to relate the physical measurements you have taken from Vikram to his personal circumstances (i.e. explain how the results you have obtained in the height/weight tables, in measurements of his resting and recovery pulse rates and of his BMI, relate to Vikram's current diet and level of exercise).

2   You will also need to explain the links between his physical health and his emotional, social and intellectual health. For example, his inability to find a job may relate to his emotional stress and to the low feelings he has about himself.

3   You also need to explain why you have chosen the specific health promotion materials you have provided (e.g. lots of attractive illustrations, non-technical language, targeting people in Vikram's age range, not tied to commercial interests – particularly the healthy eating literature).

4   When you have constructed your plan, you will have to talk it through with your subject. Although you will have given a great deal of thought to your plan and will have chosen your subject carefully, when it comes to implementing it you may well find your subject is not so keen! No one likes to be dictated to, and people often dig their heels in and refuse to listen to advice.

UNIT 2 ASSESSMENT

CASE STUDY – Vikram

Vikram is 16 years old, is moderately overweight, smokes but doesn't drink alcohol, takes no exercise, and suffers from moderate stress due to a lack of money and because of criticism at home as he is unemployed. He has no important qualifications from school, but he has some Amateur Swimming Association certificates, including a 400-metre award.

The possible health targets you could produce for Vikram are outlined below:

Overweight Provide a sensible eating plan and expect (with the exercise plan) Vikram to lose 7 kg in four to six weeks (short term) and 15 kg in the next 12 months (long term).

Smoking Reduce from 40 cigarettes a day to 20 cigarettes in one month and none in 12 months.

Exercise The chosen exercise (negotiated with Vikram) is swimming – 10 lengths of the baths, three times per week for one month stepped up to 25 lengths, three times per week in six months. In one year's time, to have improved his swimming techniques and to have joined a water polo training club. Swimming to be funded by savings on cigarettes consumed. Consider lifesaving training when his swimming skills are improved.

Stress Provide social and physical targets that will help him alleviate his stress. Vikram will have a focus for his daily activities. While he still has time for job-searching, he might also have, in due course, a job possibility as a pool attendant if he manages to succeed on the lifesaving course. His self-esteem should rise and he

should become more confident as his skills improve.

You would need to explain these targets clearly to Vikram, and provide him with some health promotional literature to support your plan. These would need to be in a language he will understand and not too technical.

You might visit your local health education unit to find leaflets on:

* reducing smoking
* healthy eating
* the benefits of exercise
* coping with stress.

In addition, Vikram would probably find it helpful if you supplied him with information appropriate to his exercise targets (swimming pool costs, opening times, etc.) and about the skills required to join a water polo team.

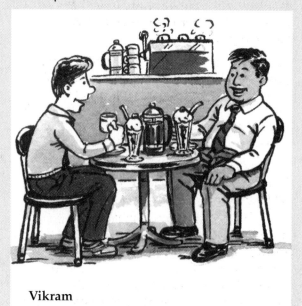

Vikram

5   When people understand the reasons for doing or not doing things they are more likely to listen – so explain your reasons carefully. Do not expect people to change their habits or lifestyle overnight: be prepared to change your timings and

be open to compromise. If someone smokes 40 cigarettes a day, you will get a better response if you gradually lower his or her habit to 30, then 20, 10 and finally single figures than if you suggest he or she stops smoking immediately. And you must also give him or her plenty of encouragement.

6 Discussing the health improvements you wish to achieve with your subject will make your plan much more effective. Give the person time to think about what you have said, and bring the issues up at appropriate, quieter moments. Don't 'nag' or get irritated or become

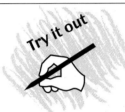

Try it out

Study the following people who might have been chosen to follow a health plan:

1 A busy, working mother who has a job that means sitting at a desk all day. Your plan suggests she exercises twice a week. However, your subject complains that she never has time for exercise and doesn't like it anyway.

2 Your friend's good-looking brother is very proud of his large number of 'girlfriends' – mostly single-night relationships. He does not practise safe sex and considers himself to be immune to sexually transmitted diseases.

3 Your subject is a 55-year-old relative who lives alone and exists mainly on fried foods (because he or she is not a good cook, and frying is quick and easy).

In pairs, take it in turns to role play, first, the subject and, secondly, the person who has devised the plan. When role playing the person who has devised the plan, be particularly careful to *negotiate*. Remember, people are much more likely to accept your plans if they feel they have been involved in devising them and if they feel they have been consulted first.

discouraged. Quiet encouragement and praise are far more likely to be effective.

Obtaining a Distinction grade

1 You will need to predict the physical, social and emotional effects on Vikram if he followed your plan. Discussing these effects with him might be a prime motivator for Vikram following your plan. You will need to be aware of Vikram's responses when he seems to have reached a limit or plateau, or even if he fails. Will this leave him with less self-esteem than before? When he 'plateaus' out, you might be able to suggest some workouts in a fitness suite so that he can develop more physical strength.

2 You will also need to anticipate difficulties and suggest ways to overcome them. For instance, Vikram will not be able to afford the swimming sessions if he cannot reduce his tobacco consumption. You might question him about his smoking habits and suggest ways to avoid temptation. If he smokes more when he is at home because other people at home smoke, then he should get away from home for longer periods. If he smokes with his friends, then perhaps he can suggest ways to involve his friends in more active pursuits, such as badminton, football or basketball.

3 If Vikram eats out at snack and coffee bars, he will have difficulty keeping to a healthy eating diet, but he might improve relationships at home by volunteering to prepare some meals – which will help to improve his diet at the same time. This will also save money.

4 To obtain a distinction, your plan must be detailed and it must address all relevant areas using the appropriate technical language.

UNIT 2 ASSESSMENT

Unit 2 Test

1   Which of the following diseases have been identified as risks associated with smoking?

   a Heart disease.
   b Diabetes.
   c Arthritis.
   d Tuberculosis.

2   Stress can produce:

   a lowered immunity to disease
   b heart disease
   c anaemia
   d vitamin deficiency.

3   Which of the following is an example of unsafe practices in the workplace?

   a Unhealthy diet.
   b Being overweight.
   c Not wearing ear protectors.
   d Not taking exercise.

4   Which of these is known as the body mass index?

   a Height divided by weight.
   b Height divided by weight squared.
   c Weight divided by height.
   d Weight divided by height squared.

5   A peak flow meter is used to measure:

   a maximum speed of heart rate
   b maximum speed of expired air
   c maximum speed of inhaled air
   d breathing rate.

6   Janis has difficulty forming relationships with colleagues. This is an aspect of his:

   a physical health
   b emotional health
   c social health
   d intellectual health.

7   The normal recovery rate of the pulse to its resting state is in the range of:

   a 6–8 minutes
   b 6–8 seconds

   c 2–4 seconds
   d 2–4 minutes.

8   Which of the following diseases are associated with being overweight?

   a Tuberculosis.
   b Heart disease.
   c Lung cancer.
   d Arthritis.

9   Professional people, such as doctors and lawyers, are in social class:

   a I
   b V
   c IV
   d II.

10   Which of the following deficiencies is most likely to give rise to anaemia?

   a Lack of calcium.
   b Lack of Vitamin D.
   c Lack of iron.
   d Lack of protein.

11   Modern definitions of health focus on:

   a experts defining health
   b complete physical and emotional well-being
   c absence of illness and infirmity
   d people's aspirations and their quality of life.

12   Define a balanced diet.

13   Provide three recommendations for people who want to follow a healthy diet.

14   Explain the benefits of a diet that contains the recommended amount of fibre.

15   Describe the uses of protein, fat and carbohydrate within the human body.

16   Explain why older people require fewer energy-containing foods than adolescents.

17 Write a few paragraphs about health needs and relate these to one social class.

18 Explain why fresh fruit and vegetables are recommended in balanced diets.

19 Describe four sources of health promotion literature.

20 List four potential difficulties people might encounter in keeping to a health plan.

Understanding personal development

This Unit covers the knowledge you will need in order to meet the assessment requirements for Unit 3. It is written in five sections.

Section one looks at human growth and development and the five main stages of human life. Section two considers how social and economic factors affect human development. Section three explores the idea of self-concept and analyses those factors that influence the self-concepts we hold about ourselves. Section four looks at the changes we all experience during the course of our lives. Finally, section five considers the support carers can give people when they have to cope with change in their lives.

Further information and advice for meeting the assessment requirements for the Unit (in particular, for Merit and Distinction level work) are at the end of the Unit.

Also at the end of the Unit is a test to check your understanding: this includes two scenarios for you to analyse and discuss.

Human growth and development

Life is about change: each year we live we notice changes in our body. As we live our lives we learn new skills and knowledge – we develop intellectually. As we develop we experience changes in the way we feel about ourselves and others; our emotions develop and change. Throughout life we find ourselves in different social situations and relationships – we develop socially.

One way of looking at the human life-span is to study the way we develop physically, intellectually, emotionally and socially. The first letters of these words spell **PIES**. Unit 2 explains that PIES is a way of thinking about human development.

This section explores physical, intellectual, emotional and social development at five **life stages**: infancy, early childhood, puberty/adolescence, adulthood and old age.

At one time life was considered to be a simple set of stages. During infancy, childhood and adolescence, a person would grow physically and learn the knowledge and skills he or she needed for work. Adulthood was a time when people worked and/or brought up their own family. Old age was when people retired and children would usually be grown up by the time their parents reached retirement.

At the beginning of the twenty-first century people's lives are much more complex. People now need constantly to relearn skills and to increase their knowledge because they are often required to change the kind of work they do. Some people have children late in life; some choose not to have children. Science now makes it possible for a woman to give birth in her 50s. Some people may 'retire' in their 30s or 40s – perhaps for a while before taking up employment again! Life stages are no longer as clear as they once were, and some writers now prefer to see life as a continuous process of change rather than a series of distinct stages. However, this section explores the five stages people still commonly use to categorise human development.

Infancy

Physical development

Growth is defined biologically by three stages:

- increase in the number of body cells

- increase in the size of individual cells as they carry more material

- body cells becoming more specialised in both structure and function.

All three stages are very important in a foetus's growth and development. However, after birth, it is the increases in the number of body cells and in the size of cells that are the most important factors in the infant's development.

At birth, on average, babies have a 'length' (later called 'height') of 50 cm and a weight of 3.5 kg. For a few days, babies lose weight as they learn to feed, but rapidly regain their birth weight. A baby's head circumference is also measured at birth and for a short while afterwards. This measurement is used to assess brain growth.

New-born babies are often known as **neonates**. Although they are helpless and would die if they were not cared for, human neonates show a surprising number of inborn physical reflexes. A reflex is an automatic response. Most of these fade away as babies become more mature, and other reflexes take their place.

Neonate reflexes

- *Suckling reflex*: Babies automatically suck on anything placed in their mouths.

- *Rooting reflex*: babies turn their heads when their faces are touched. They are trying to find their mother's nipple.

- *Stepping or walking reflex*: when the babies are supported and their feet are allowed to touch a solid surface, their legs move in an action resembling stepping or walking.

- *Startle reflex*: if babies are surprised by a loud noise, they pull up their arms and legs and ball their fists. (This is very similar to the Moro reflex, but in the Moro reflex the arms are extended and the hands are open.)

- *Plantar reflex*: when the sole of a baby's foot is stroked, the big toe curls upwards. (Plantar means referring to the sole of the foot.)

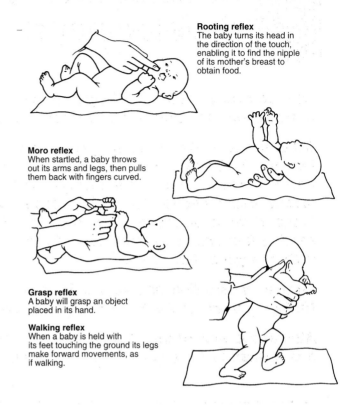

Rooting reflex
The baby turns its head in the direction of the touch, enabling it to find the nipple of its mother's breast to obtain food.

Moro reflex
When startled, a baby throws out its arms and legs, then pulls them back with fingers curved.

Grasp reflex
A baby will grasp an object placed in its hand.

Walking reflex
When a baby is held with its feet touching the ground its legs make forward movements, as if walking.

Figure 3.1 The primitive reflexes of a new-born baby

- *Grasping reflex*: babies hold on tightly to any objects placed in their hands.

In addition to these primitive reflexes, new-born babies will be able to recognise different colours and tastes, and be able to smell, and to hear and to blink their eyes. Babies have to learn to control their bodies. Learning to control the use of large muscles is called learning to use our gross **motor skills**.

Gross motor skills
Head control

Until they reach the age of about 4 months, when babies are pulled to sit from a lying position, their heads will fall back. Gradually they increase their control of their heads and, during the fifth and sixth months, they will have learnt to lift their heads when being pulled to a sitting position. When held in a sitting position, their heads fall forward until they are 1 month old, when babies begin to lift their heads for a few seconds. After a further four weeks, they can hold their heads up.

Sitting

At 4 months of age, when held while sitting, a baby's back is nearly straight. By 6 months, infants can sit by themselves with support from their arms held out in front of them. Two months later, infants can sit easily with no support and, close to their first birthday, they can turn sideways while sitting without toppling over.

Crawling and walking

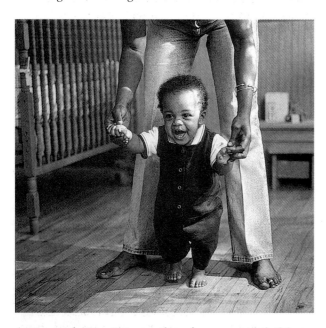

At around 11 or 12 months of age, many babies can walk holding onto an adult's hands

Around the age of 2 months, babies lie flat when placed face down on the floor with their legs extended behind. They can lift their heads off the floor for a few seconds at a time but, a month later, they can hold the weight of their upper bodies on their forearms and lift their heads for much longer periods. At the same time, if babies are held upright, they cannot support themselves at all whereas, at 6 months, they can bear their full weight when held.

At 10 months, most babies will be able to crawl using their hands and knees and be able to stand without being held, but by holding on to furniture. Just before their first birthday, many can walk holding an adult's two hands, gradually needing only one. A big occasion is when a baby takes his or her first steps alone. This is usually around 13–15 months of age. Some babies 'bear-walk' in-between crawling and walking – this is

moving on all fours using both hands and feet. Others never crawl, but move around on their bottoms in a sitting position, so-called 'shuffling', using their arms to push them around.

Fine motor skills from birth to 1 year.

Fine motor skills mean learning to use small muscles to control an action. This is more difficult for babies to do than gross motor actions.

Almost from birth, babies will look at bright lights and shiny objects. By the second month, they will gaze intently at the carer's face and begin to reach out to get hold of a finger. By 3 months, babies turn their heads to follow an adult, can hold a rattle for a few moments and play with their own hands.

By 9 months, objects can be transferred from hand to hand and the pincer grip between thumb and forefinger is developing to pick up small objects. Babies now look for fallen objects and explore everything they can by putting things in their mouths – the most sensitive area for touch.

At the end of the first year, babies throw things deliberately, can eat with their fingers and can manage a spoon, if allowed. The pincer movement is well developed, enabling even small things to be picked up, and babies love to point to and to copy the actions of other people.

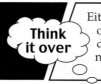 **Think it over** — Either by yourself or in pairs, think of babies you know well and discuss the developments you have noticed in the last few months.

At the end of the first year, how have the standard height and weight measurements changed? (If you need to refresh your memory about these charts, look back to Unit 2.)

Babies now weigh three times their birth weight and have grown half as much again as their birth length. Their limbs have increased in size so that their heads are smaller in proportion to the rest of their bodies, but their heads have not shrunk (Figure 3.3)!

Both gross and fine motor skills develop rapidly between 1 year and 18 months.

With increasing confidence in walking, and a growing ability to carry things around and climb steps, infants are likely to fall down a lot and can

Age in months	Stage of motor development
Birth	Primitive reflexes only
1	Lifts up chin
2	Lifts chest up
3	Reaches for but does not grasp objects
4	Sits supported
5	Grasps objects
6	Sits on chair, reaches for and grasps objects
7	Stands with support
9	Stands alone but holding on
10	Crawls quickly
11	Walks holding one hand
12	Pulls up on furniture to stand
13	Crawls up stairs
14	Stands alone unsupported
15	Walks alone
24	Runs, picks things up without falling over
30	Stands on toes, jumps
36	Stands on one leg
48	Walks down stairs with one foot on each step

Figure 3.2 Average rates of motor development

now come down stairs backwards on their tummies. In playing, they can arrange toys on the floor, hold a pencil in the palm of their hands to scribble and can place up to three blocks in a tower. Infants love action songs like *pat-a-cake* and can turn several pages of a book together. They are also much more expert at eating with a spoon.

Intellectual development

Babies appear to prefer the sound of human voices as opposed to other sounds and soon learn to recognise their mother's voice. Within a few weeks, babies show an interest in human faces. Babies seem to be ready to feed and make relationships with carers soon after they are born.

Language

Infants begin to recognise words before they can talk or say words. At 6 or 9 months of age an infant may recognise and respond to words like 'clap-hands' and 'bye-bye'. Around the first year of life infants may produce **babbling** sounds that begin to sound like words. Some writers call these sounds pre-words, because sounds like 'nan' can mean 'I don't like that', or 'da' might mean 'I like that'.

Infants begin to say recognisable words at different ages. Many infants may say whole words as young as 1 year old, although others will take longer to develop their first word. By the age of 2 years most infants will combine two words together and begin to communicate their needs using the language they hear around them.

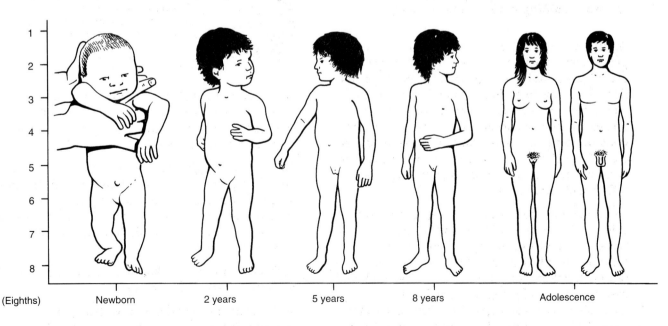

(Eighths)   Newborn   2 years   5 years   8 years   Adolescence

Figure 3.3 Growth profiles from birth to adolescence

Although it can be 2 years or more before infants begin to combine words, infants do communicate with others using their face, their eyes and the sounds they make.

Thinking and memory

The development of thinking and memory is an important part of **intellectual development** (this is also sometimes known as **cognitive development**). This has been studied by many psychologists, perhaps the best known being Piaget.

To begin with, a baby will rely on in-built patterns for sucking, crawling and watching. A baby will adapt this behaviour to explore a wider range of objects. Babies explore by sucking toys, fingers, clothes and so on. In this way they are slowly able to develop an understanding of objects.

According to Piaget, thinking is at first limited to memories of actions. For example, babies will remember grasping a particular toy. If handed the toy again, they may repeat the action.

Piaget believed that infants could not understand that objects existed on their own. For instance, if an infant's mother left the room, the infant would be afraid she had gone for ever. Piaget thought that an infant was not able to understand that his or her mother still existed if the infant could not see, hear, smell or touch his or her mother. This stage is called the 'sensorimotor' stage and lasts until the infant is between $1^1/_2$ and 2 years of age.

At the end of the sensorimotor period, Piaget thought that infants could at last understand that objects and people continue to exist, even if you cannot see them.

However, modern research suggests that many 8-month-old infants can understand that people and objects still exist, even when you cannot see or hear them. Infants are more able than many people once thought!

Piaget's theory
(See Figure 3.4 below.)

Emotional development

Emotional development considers how people develop a sense of themselves as well as how they develop feelings towards others.

During their first year of life, infants can recognise the emotional expressions for happiness, distress and anger. It seems that, by 12 months of age, infants not only react to the facial expression of their carers, but they are also guided by the emotions they see on the faces on their carers. Studies show that infants behave differently with new toys depending on whether their mothers smile or look worried – infants will usually move towards a toy if mothers smile, but back away from it if their mothers look worried. It seems that infants come into the world with an in-built ability to recognise and to react to basic feelings in other people. Infants use this ability to attract attention and to build an emotional attachment with their carers.

Bonding

During the first 18 months of life, infants develop an emotional bond of love with their carers. This **bonding** process ties the infant emotionally to familiar carers. Some theorists think it is very important that children are not separated at any time from their mothers during infancy, so that this

Figure 3.4 Piaget's theory of child development

Stage of development	Age	Key issue
Sensorimotor	0–18 months/2 years	Children do not understand how objects exist
Pre-operational (pre-logical)	2–6/7 years	Children do not think in a logical way
Concrete operational	7–11 years	Children can understand logic if they can see or handle objects. Children do not fully understand logical arguments in words
Formal operational	11 years onwards	People can understand logical arguments and think in an abstract way

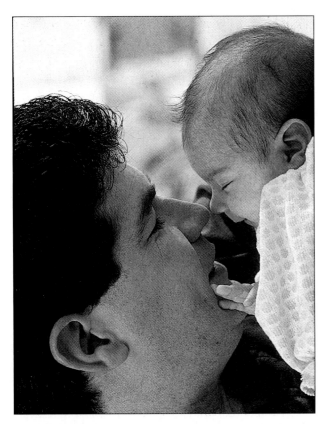

Infants need to experience a loving attachment with a carer

emotional bond can develop. Other theorists argue that an infant's main emotional attachment is not always with the mother; fathers and other carers are also important. Some theorists say it is the quality of love and care that matters most, and not whether carers ever leave their child (for example, to go to work). There is agreement that infants need to experience a loving attachment with a carer and, if this does not happen, then a child's social and emotional development will be damaged.

Sense of self

Young infants probably do not have a sense of being an 'individual' person. As infants grow they gradually learn they can influence their carers with the actions they make. At around 2 years of age, however, infants may develop the idea they are an individual person with a fixed gender. This idea of being a person is called **self-awareness**.

Social development

Social development explores humans' social behaviour and the social skills we need to communicate and make relationships with others.

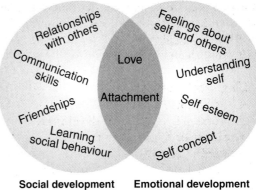

Figure 3.5   Social and emotional development overlap

Emotional development explores how we express our feelings and develop **self-esteem** and **self-concept**. It can be difficult to tell the two areas apart because these areas overlap (see Figure 3.5).

Our social relationships influence our emotional development and our self-esteem can influence our relationships with others. Hence such issues as love and attachment can be looked at from the point of view of both social development *and* emotional development. Infants soon learn to recognise their mother's voice and smell, and can probably recognise her face by 2 months of age. As we have already seen, infants try to attract attention by smiling and making noises.

At about 12 months of age infants often develop a fear of strangers and will protest if they are separated from their parents. After the first year of life infants feel safe with familiar family members if they have formed the necessary social bonds.

Talk it over

Do you think infants should always be looked after by their own mothers or fathers? Or can they be left with carers while their mothers or fathers go to work?

Early childhood

The term 'early childhood' does not have a fixed meaning in terms of age. Here, it is used to cover 2-12 years of age, although exactly where early childhood ends and adolescence begins is difficult to establish.

Physical development

18 months to 4 years

Toilet training usually starts between 18 months and 2 years. Children will show that they are ready, perhaps by telling the carer when they are wet or have a dirty nappy. At first, children will be dry during the day but will often wear a nappy at bedtime or be carried out during the night to sit on the potty.

Children are now very mobile and are able to run, to climb and to descend stairs. Kicking a ball is also now possible, but the skill of catching does not come until around 4 years old. A sense of balance is developing and children are able to ride a tricycle, move on tiptoe and climb on frames. At the end of this period, children can thread small beads to make necklaces, use scissors, copy shapes and draw recognisable people. The tower of bricks can now be built tall and straight, and painting becomes a favourite pastime. Tying shoelaces and fastening buttons are still a challenge for 4-year-old children.

4 years to 7 years

Children start school in this period, become increasingly co-ordinated in their physical activities and have generally lost their 'puppy fat'. By 5 years of age, head size and therefore brain size has just about reached adult size. The sense of balance is such that children can skip, jump off apparatus and learn to ride a two-wheeled bicycle. Growth in height and weight increase

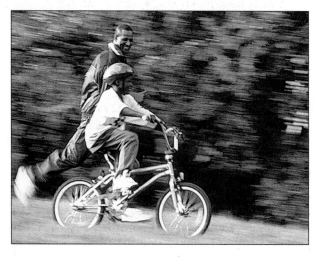

Young children acquire a well-developed sense of balance by the ages of 6 or 7 years

steadily, but not as rapidly as before.

Both girls and boys are usually continent of urine or completely dry during the day and night by the time they are 5 years old.

8 years to 12 years

As milk teeth are replaced by permanent teeth and the jaws grow rapidly, facial features take on their permanent characteristics. Physical growth continues, muscles build and co-ordination is now such that musical instruments, swimming, football and gymnastics can be taken up with proficiency. Many girls begin **puberty** in this period, with the appearance of secondary sexual characteristics such as development of the breasts and sexual organs.

Intellectual development

Language

At around 2 years of age most children have started to speak, using two-word phrases such as 'Zoe sleep' (meaning Zoe wants to go to sleep). As children grow they start to use their own type of language pattern to communicate, such as 'I want drink' and 'the cat goed' (the cat has gone out). Young children of 2 or 3 years of age do not use adult language and it is probably best not to correct what they say. Children may go through stages of language development, such as the ones listed below:

1	Two-word statements	'Cat goed.'
2	Short phrases	'I want drink.'
3	Being able to ask questions	'What that?' 'Where is cat?'
4	Using sentences	'Jill come in and the doggy come in.'
5	Adult sentences	'I would like a drink and a piece of cake.'

By the age of 5 or 6 years, children can use adult speech and have a reasonable knowledge of words. However, children continue to develop their knowledge of words and their ability to understand and use speech throughout childhood.

Thinking and problem-solving

Between the ages of 2 and 7 years, most children learn to count and to explain how much things weigh. Young children do not always fully understand the logic involved in counting and weighing things.

Piaget called the period 2–7 years of age the '**pre-operational**' period. Pre-operational means 'pre-logical'. Young children may make decisions based on what things look like rather than the logic of counting.

Older children do not make the mistakes younger children do. However, 7–12-year-olds can often only understand logical problems if they can see what is involved. For example, you could ask a 9-year-old: 'Tanya is taller than Stephen, but Tanya is smaller than Tolu. Who is the smallest out of these three people?' Obviously Stephen is the smallest. A 9-year-old might not be able to work this out without looking at pictures of the people (see Figure 3.6).

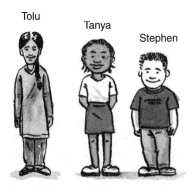

Figure 3.6   Pre-operational thinking

Piaget called the period 7–12 years the '**concrete operational**' period, because older children can only work out logical problems if they can see 'concrete' examples to help them.

Emotional development

Children who have made good emotional bonds with a carer will start to feel safe getting to know other children or adults. All children take time to adjust to changes in their setting, and starting in a play group or school can still be stressful, even for 5-year-olds.

Self-esteem

Young children find it very difficult to explain feelings and emotions, but this may be because their language and thinking abilities are not fully developed. Research during the past 20 years suggests that young children do have the ability to understand and to respond to the feelings of others. Three-year-old children will sometimes try to comfort younger brothers or sisters who are upset. Children also need to feel they are valuable to their friends and family. Feelings of **self-worth** or self-esteem are very important if people are to grow up feeling emotionally secure.

As children grow, it seems they use their imagination to copy the behaviour of others. Children might copy the behaviour of parents or of people they see on TV. Children as young as $2\frac{1}{2}$ years can imagine dolls as talking and having wishes and feelings. By 4 years, children can imagine dolls as being characters who play with other characters. Because children can imagine the things they see others doing, they can also begin to imagine who they are and to start to create an idea of 'self'. More details of the development of self-concept are given in the section on self-concept later in this unit.

Social development

Children's attachment to parents and carers is just as strong as in infancy, but they no longer need to cling to carers. As children grow older they start to make relationships with other children and learn to become more independent. However, young children still depend very much on their carers to look after them, and they need safe, secure, emotional ties with their family. Emotional ties provide the foundation for exploring relationships with others.

Play

Play activities at any age can help us to:

◇ develop our practical skills and abilities

◇ develop social skills and relationships with others

◇ make us feel better – play can provide a feeling of control or of relaxation.

Types of play
The word 'play' can cover many different types of activity. Children's play mainly involves exploring, practising, social learning and pretending (see Figure 3.7).

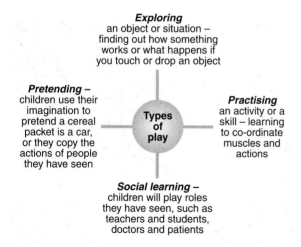

Figure 3.7   Types of play

The development of play
Before 2 years of age, children tend to play alone. At around 2 years of age, children may play side by side with other children, although they may still concentrate on their own activity. Children may start to share activities with other children at about 3 years of age. By 4 or 5 years of age,

children may play in small groups and follow activities or games with simple rules.

By 7 years of age, most children develop same-sex friendship groups. Children may often prefer being with their friends rather than doing other activities. By 10 years of age, friendship groups often share similar attitudes and values. Friendship groups start to have an influence on children's beliefs and behaviour during childhood.

Puberty and adolescence

By 'adolescence' we mean the age range 12-18 years (18 is the age when people are first allowed to vote and, by implication, take on adult responsibilities).

Physical development

Any time from 8 years old onwards, a girl's breasts start to enlarge. This happens well before menstruation and is usually the first sign puberty is starting. In both sexes hair starts to grow in the pubic area and under the armpits (and on the chest in boys), and there is a rapid growth spurt in an individual's overall growth.

Girls tend to reach puberty two years before boys (generally between the ages of 11 and 13 years). In both sexes there is rapid growth in the primary sexual organs (ovaries in girls and testes in boys) and also of the secondary sexual organs, such as the uterus (or womb), vagina and breasts and the penis and scrotum. Girls start to menstruate (the onset of menstruation is called the *menarche*), often irregularly at first with slight bleeding, and the first eggs are produced up to a year later.

Hormonal control

The changes outlined above are caused by hormones secreted by the pituitary gland. These hormones stimulate the production of **oestrogen** from the ovaries in girls and **testosterone** from the testes in boys. The oestrogen and testosterone cause the growth of the genital organs, skeleton, muscles and body hair. When ovulation is well established, a second female hormone is produced – progesterone. This is influential in causing glandular development in the breasts and the development of the uterine lining, whereas the action of oestrogen mainly affects the growth of these structures.

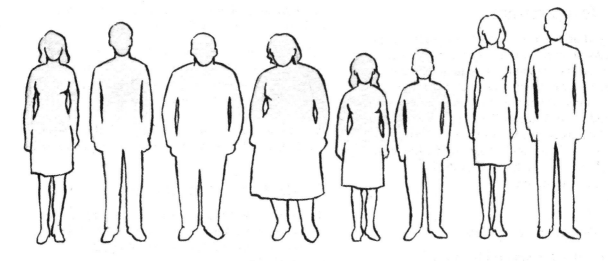

Figure 3.8   The body shapes of mature males and females

These hormones cause changes in body shape: a girl's pelvis widens, making her walk differently with swinging of the hips. She develops a curvy outline and fat is deposited under the skin and around the breast, giving her an hour-glass type of silhouette. Boys, on the other hand, retain their slim hips but they develop wide shoulders and a well defined muscle structure. Testosterone in boys is also responsible for the rapid growth of the voice box (larynx), causing the voice to 'break' and become deeper in pitch.

It is during puberty that boys catch up and overtake the girl's two years' head start in growth. Hence boys end up heavier and taller than girls, although there is a wide variation in mature adult heights and weights in both sexes. The tonsils and adenoids which protect against infection have steadily grown through childhood, but now surprisingly start to shrink quite rapidly. This is why surgeons are now reluctant to remove tonsils as readily as they used to in the 1950s and 1960s, because tonsils rarely give problems after puberty unless they are heavily infected.

The chart opposite shows a summary of how different parts of the body grow at different rates.

Intellectual development

Adolescents are able to imagine and think about things they have never seen or done before: they can imagine their futures and how they might achieve things in the future. Children are not able to plan and think ahead in this way.

Adolescents can solve problems in the same manner as adults.

Returning to the ideas of Piaget once more, Piaget called this stage of development the **formal operational** (or formal logical) period. Formal

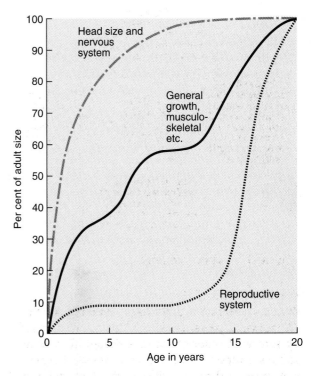

Figure 3.9   Some body systems have different growth rates

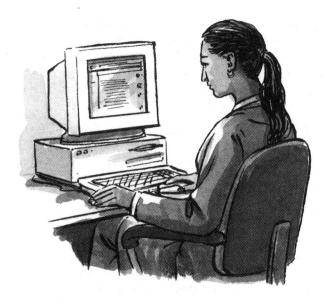

Figure 3.10   Solving problems in software writing involves the use of formal operational (logical) thinking

logic helps people solve problems at work and in daily life. Whereas children often make guesses when they have to solve problems, adolescents can often work things out logically (see Figure 3.10).

Although adolescents can reason in an adult way, they may often not know enough to make the right decisions. Decision-making skills are something we acquire throughout the course of our entire lives.

Emotional development

Adolescence is a period of rapid social and physical change. Some adolescents feel a loss of self-esteem as they transfer from school to work, and becoming independent of your parents can involve conflict and stress. Similarly, the search for love and affection from a sexual partner is not free of stress.

The psychologist Eric Erikson (1902–94) believed that a successful adult life depends on people developing a secure sense of their selves (their self-concept). During adolescence, people have to acquire a concept of themselves that will guide them through leaving home, obtaining work and perhaps learning to live permanently with a

partner of their own choice (see the section on self-concept later in this unit for further details).

Social development

Adolescents become increasingly independent of their families; hence friendship groups become more important than family for the development of social skills. This phase of development is called secondary **socialisation** (see Figure 3.11).

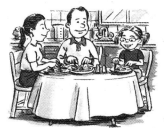
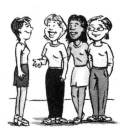

Figure 3.11   During adolescence friendship groups become more important than the family in the development of social skills

Between 12 and 18 years of age, most adolescents begin to explore their sexuality which includes testing out relationships and sexual behaviour with others. In late adolescence people begin to think about, or to take on, job responsibilities.

As young people take on adult roles they may experience trouble and conflict with their parents. This is the stage at which adolescents are trying to assert their adult **independence**.

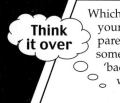

Think it over

Which is more important to you, your family or your friends? If your parents wanted you to stop seeing someone because he or she was a 'bad influence' on you, what would you do?

Adulthood

In the UK people have the right to vote at the age of 18 years, so the age of 18 might be considered the age at which people achieve adulthood.

Physical development

People in their 20s and 30s are at the height of their physical powers and at their reproductive peak. In our 40s we tend to put on weight and become less physically active. Men may start to lose their hair and, in both sexes, grey hairs start to appear. The fine focussing power of our eyes declines so that most people become long-sighted and need reading glasses for close work.

Women continue to menstruate (i.e. are able to conceive children) until about the age of 45 years.

After this age they slowly reach the **menopause**, when menstruation stops. Consequently their bodies produce less of the hormones oestrogen and progesterone (which were formerly needed for menstruation), and hence the organs of the reproductive system shrink and the vagina becomes less elastic.

Both sexes lose skin elasticity, and this leads to wrinkles, particularly around the face.

Men can still father children into their 70s and even into their 80s, although sperm production and sexual performance will have declined.

Intellectual development

Intellectual skills and abilities may increase during adulthood if these skills and abilities are exercised. Older adults may be slightly slower when it comes to working out logical problems, but increased knowledge may compensate for slower reactions. Wisdom is perhaps our ability to use knowledge more effectively as we become older. Wisdom comes from many years of experience of life and so age may help people to make better decisions.

Emotional development

People's concepts of themselves and their feelings about their own self-esteem continue to develop throughout adulthood. During early adulthood many people struggle to develop the confidence they need to share their lives with a partner. Some may finally decide to live alone, feeling that partnership relationships are too demanding. People's experience of their family life as a child may strongly influence the expectations they have of a partner.

Research has suggested that adults often feel more confident and satisfied with their lives in their 30s and 40s than they did in their 20s. This may be because many young adults experience stress while they are trying to establish a satisfying lifestyle for themselves.

Some theorists have suggested that older adults may struggle to stay interested in and involved with other people after their own families have grown up. They may get into 'a rut' and withdraw from active social involvement. The menopause itself is not without its problems: women may become depressed and irritable, perhaps because there is now an imbalance in their hormones. Hormone replacement therapy is often advised to counteract these and other problems associated with the menopause.

Successful ageing, therefore, might be regarded as remaining involved with other people in an emotionally satisfying way.

Social development

Early adulthood is often a time when people continue to develop their networks of personal friends. Most young adults will have sexual relationships and may develop more or less permanent partnerships: marriage and parenthood might be important life events. Some may decide to have children later in their lives, prioritising their personal development and careers instead.

Many people experience stress when trying to cope with the demands of being a parent, partner and worker. Many individuals work long hours or even have more then one job in order to achieve a high standard of living. Going to work while maintaining a family home can create social and emotional problems. Adult life often involves trying to balance the need for money with the needs of partners and other family members (see Figure 3.12).

Older adults may find that, as well as pressures of work, they also have to provide support not only for their own children but also for their parents. Some older adults feel thay are sandwiched between different pressures. When their children leave home they may feel some of the pressures have been removed but may also feel they have lost part of their social purpose now their children have gone.

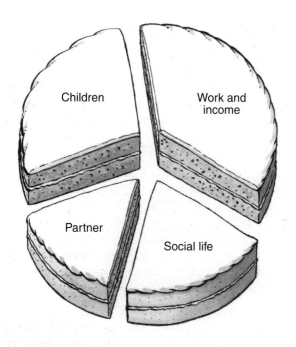

Figure 3.12   Adults have to work out how to divide up their time in order to meet different needs

In one study, 59% of people in the UK stated they 'never seem to have enough time to get things done', and 21% stated they were very concerned about the amount of free time they had!

Although the official retirement age for men is 65 and for women 60, many people now retire in their 50s. Depending on how retirement happens to you – i.e. forced or taken out of choice – retirement can be regarded as a positive release from the pressures of work or as an end to your usefulness to others.

Old age

As we have already mentioned, most people retire by the age of 65, and therefore the period of life after the age of 65 is generally understood as old age. Most 65-year-olds do not see themselves as 'old', however. Some writers make a distinction between the 'young-old' (65-80 years) and the 'old-old' (80 years and over). Many 80-year-olds, however, still claim they are not old!

Currently about 8% of the population is aged between 65 and 74 years. Seven per cent are aged 75 and over. By 2021, 11% of the population are expected to be between 65 and 74 years of age, with 9% over 75 years of age.

Physical development

The ageing process is subtle, and the changes it brings are so slow and so tiny we tend not to notice them. However, once we reach our mid 60s we begin to notice some changes:

- Our skin becomes thinner, less elastic, wrinkled and acquires blemishes.

- Our bones are more brittle and more likely to fracture, particularly in females.

- Our joints become stiffer and may become painful as the cartilage on the bone ends becomes worn away; the ligaments which reinforce our joints become more loose.

- Our height is reduced because the pads of cartilage that separate the vertebrae become compressed, causing the vertebrae to be closer together; the spine may also become more rounded.

- Our muscles are weaker and power is lost.

- Our sense of balance becomes impaired, particularly when turning round.

- Our taste and smell receptors deteriorate.

- Our vision can be further impaired because the lens of the eye starts to block light. This can be the forerunner of cataracts. Night vision is not as good as it used to be.

- We fail to hear high pitched notes, and we may become a little deaf.

- There is a general reduction in the skin's sensitivity, so that we are susceptible to burns and hypothermia. Hypothermia is when the body temperature falls too low. Some older people do not realise they are cold and this can be life threatening.

- The muscles that help food to pass down our digestive tract are weaker. Constipation is a common problem.

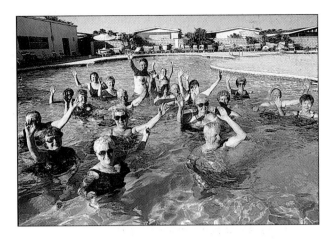

Older people's quality of life can be good

- The heart is less efficient at pumping blood around our body, so our bodily tissues do not function as well as they did.

- Our blood pressure is higher because the walls of the arteries have become hard and less elastic. This means we have a greater risk of strokes and brain haemorrhages.

- Nutrients from food are not absorbed as well as before. This can cause anaemia and vitamin deficiency diseases.

- Our breathing is less efficient because our respiratory muscles are weaker.

- Gas exchange in the lungs is impaired as the elastic walls of the alveoli become damaged.

- The glands that provide hormones (endocrine glands) do not function as well as they used to. The rate of metabolism (the chemical reactions in the body cells) is reduced due to a reduction in thyroxine (a hormone needed to regulate metabolism). Lack of effective insulin from the pancreas frequently leads to diabetes, particularly in elderly people who are overweight.

For all this apparently depressing list of ailments, older people can live healthy and fulfilling lives. People now live much longer than they used to and, with the right support and help, their quality of life can be good.

Intellectual development

In later life, some people may become less able at solving problems and coping with difficult, intellectual challenges. To some extent our mental abilities are influenced by our physical health: for example, poor blood circulation can interfere with the brain, causing difficulties with mental activities, such as problem-solving.

On the other hand, people who enjoy good health and who exercise their minds often retain their mental abilities and continue to develop their store of knowledge. Some older people seem to have an increased ability to make wise decisions and judgements. Even if thinking slows down, the opportunity to develop wisdom may increase with older age.

The risk of developing **dementia** or Alzheimer's disease seems to increase with age, but dementia is not part of normal ageing – most old people never develop dementia or Alzheimer's disease. There are different types of dementia but, in general, dementia can cause a range of disabilities:

- a loss of ability to control emotion

- difficulty in understanding other people

- difficulties in communicating and expressing thoughts

- loss of memory

- difficulties in recognising people, places and things

- problems with making sense of where you are and what is happening

- problems with daily living activities, such as getting dressed.

The reasons why some people develop dementia are not fully understood, but bad health habits such as persistent heavy drinking and smoking may increase the risk of dementia for some people. Other people may inherit a 'risk factor' for dementia because of their genetic pattern.

Emotional development

People's concepts of themselves continue to develop as life progresses. Some theorists have suggested that the main challenge of old age is to retain a strong sense of one's own self-esteem, despite the problems that can arise with age.

Older people may not only develop health problems but they can be stereotyped by other people, who assume they are less able than they are. Some older people may be at risk of losing their self-confidence and self-esteem because of the way others treat them.

Social development

Older people can lead very varied, different lives. Many retired people have a greater opportunity for meeting and making new friends than when they were working and bringing up a family. A network of family and friends can provide vital, practical and emotional support. Alternatively, health problems and impairments can sometimes create difficulties that result in social isolation.

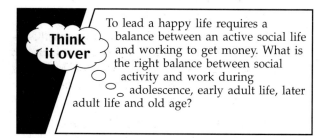

Think it over

To lead a happy life requires a balance between an active social life and working to get money. What is the right balance between social activity and work during adolescence, early adult life, later adult life and old age?

Moral development

Finally, perhaps moral development deserves a section on its own, as our moral development changes throughout all the stages of our lives.

Children's beliefs about what is right and wrong are strongly influenced by the beliefs of the people they live with and mix with. The way children talk about what is right and wrong is influenced by their level of intellectual development. In 1976 a theorist called Kolberg published his ideas about how children and adults go through six different stages of moral thinking. These stages are outlined below:

1   *Punishment and obedience* Things are wrong if you get told off or punished for doing them. You should do what you are told because adults have power.

2   *Individualism and fairness* You should do things that make you feel good or get praised, and avoid things that get punished. It is important to be fair to everyone. For

example, 'If I help you, you have to help me!', 'If I get pushed in a queue, then I have the right to push other people!'

There is a simple belief that everyone should be treated in exactly the same way. For example, if everyone gets the same food, this must be fair. Children at this stage will find it hard to work out that 'the same food' is not fair because it will discriminate against some people and not others. If everyone is given meat, this will be good for some people, but not for vegetarians!

3   *Relationships* As children grow older, relationships with others become important and children begin to think about the way they are seen by others. At this stage, children start to think about 'good' behaviour as behaviour that pleases others. Being good is about meeting other people's expectations of you. Ideas of loyalty, trust and respect come into children's thoughts and feelings. For example, a child might think 'I can trust my friend to keep a secret because they are a "good person".'

4   *Law and order* Adolescents and adults start to think in terms of a 'whole society'. Rules and laws are seen as important as they enable people to get on with each other. Being good is not only about relationships with friends and family, but also about relationships with people in general.

5/6   *Rights and principles* When adults reach these stages they decide what is right or wrong in terms of values and principles. Adults at these stages may argue that laws need to be changed. Adults take personal responsibility for working out what is right or wrong.

Social and economic factors

People do not all have an equal chance to develop their skills and abilities: some are born into a life that holds fewer opportunities than the lives of others.

In 1999 the DSS published a report called *Opportunity for All*. In this report the government states: 'Our aim is to end the injustice which holds people back and prevents them from making the most of themselves.' The government says its goal is 'that everyone should have the opportunity to achieve their potential. But too many people are denied that opportunity. It is wrong and economically inefficient to waste the talents of even one single person'.

The *Opportunity for All* paper also states that:

⬧ The number of people living in households with low incomes has more than doubled since the late 1970s.

⬧ One in three children live in households that receive below half the national average income.

⬧ Nearly one in five working-age households has no one in work.

⬧ The poorest communities have much more unemployment, poor housing, vandalism and crime than richer areas.

The report goes on to say that the problems which prevent people from making the most of their lives are as follows:

⬧ *Lack of opportunities to work.* Work is the most important route out of low income. However, the consequences of being unemployed are far more reaching than simple lack of money. Unemployment can contribute to ill health and can deny future employment opportunities.

⬧ *Lack of opportunities to acquire education and skills.* Adults who are without basic skills are substantially more likely to spend long periods out of work.

⬧ *Childhood deprivation.* This is linked with problems of low income, poor health, poor housing and unsafe environments.

⬧ *Disrupted families.* The evidence shows that children in one-parent families are particularly likely to suffer the effects of persistently low household incomes. Stresses within families can lead to exclusion and, in extreme cases, to homelessness.

⬧ *Barriers to older people living active, fulfilling and healthy lives.* Too many older people have low incomes, a lack of independence and poor health. Lack of access to good-quality services is a key barrier to social inclusion.

⬧ *Inequalities in health.* Health can be affected by low income and a range of socioeconomic factors, such as access to good-quality health services and shops selling good-quality food at affordable prices.

⬧ *Poor housing.* This directly diminishes people's quality of life and leads to a range of physical and mental problems. It can also cause difficulties for children trying to do their homework.

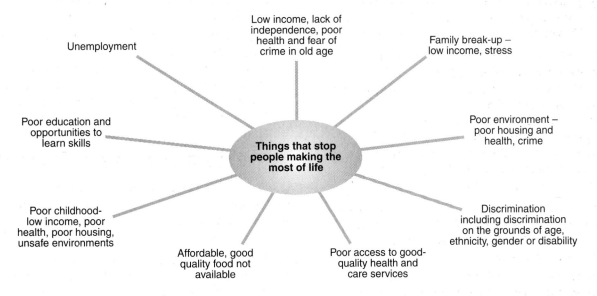

Figure 3.13   Factors that affect whether people are able to make the most of their lives

⋄ *Poor neighbourhoods*. The most deprived areas suffer from a combination of poor housing, high rates of crime, unemployment, poor health and family disruption.

⋄ *Fear of crime*. Crime and fear of crime can effectively exclude people within their own communities, especially older people.

⋄ *Disadvantaged groups*. Some people experience disadvantage or discrimination, for example, on the grounds of age, ethnicity, gender or disability. This makes them particularly vulnerable to social exclusion.

Figure 3.13 summarises some of the factors that stop people making the most of their lives.

Culture

The way we behave, the language we speak, the diet we eat, the way we dress and our lifestyles are all part of our **culture**. The concept of culture also includes those things that make one group of people different and distinctive from others.

Our culture gives us a set of rules or expectations that should help us to understand each other, and to know how to react in certain situations. Very often we do not even know we are working or living within a culture: we just 'do what is normal' and fit in. Because society is made up of various sorts of people, brought up in different circumstances or places, and following different beliefs and religions, different people's culture can vary enormously. We all tend to follow the way we were brought up and are perpetually influenced by the people around us. We follow a 'culture' (see Figure 3.14).

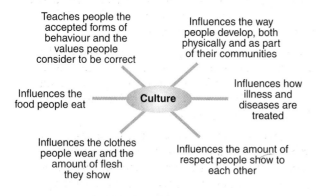

Figure 3.14   How our culture can influence us

Within any culture there are a number of **subcultures**, which have slight variations from the main culture but which still adopt many of those things considered usual or 'correct' in the main culture.

Not everyone shares the same culture, and there are many different cultures in the UK. For example, travellers have made a different **lifestyle choice** from most other people. Most people live in a house and pay the charges and taxes associated with that. Travellers do not conform to this pattern. As a result of travellers frequently moving (either through choice, to follow work or because land owners and local authorities move them on), their children are moved from schools and benefits are difficult to claim (a fixed or permanent address is required to claim child benefit). Their health is put at risk because it is difficult to register with medical services when you are continually moving. The travellers' health, welfare and education consequently suffers. Travelling is a culture, an established way of life, and yet is not always recognised as such.

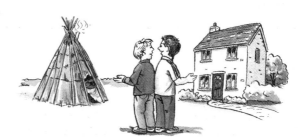

'This is the right way to live'

Gender

It was only in 1928 that women were granted the equal right with men to vote in elections. Before that, women were considered to have a lower social status than men. The assumption was that women should look after the children, do the housework, cook and tidy, and do light jobs. Men did the more valuable administrative, management and heavy labouring jobs such as building and loading ships.

Great changes have come about in the workplace and in the nature of family life since 1928. Women are now generally given equal opportunities in education and employment – and the Sex Discrimination Act 1975 makes it illegal to discriminate against women in education or employment.

However, current studies show that women's pay is as much as 17% lower than men's. Women still hold fewer top jobs and seem not to be promoted. Women far outnumber men in such jobs as nursing and primary school teaching – but, often, these jobs are not highly paid. Men often get the more highly paid jobs, even in areas of work dominated by women. When it comes to domestic work, men still generally do less of the child care, washing and cooking – although they may do more gardening and maintenance jobs.

Think it over

Women often feel there is a 'glass ceiling' which stops them achieving further promotion at work. They cannot really see what it is that is stopping them, but there is something there that prevents them getting on. In what ways might discrimination and stereotyping create an invisible ceiling that holds women back? For further information on these issues see pages 120–22.

Access to services

There is a great deal of evidence which shows that people on low incomes tend to have worse health than people who are on higher incomes. People who live in households where no one has a job often have worse health than people who are employed. Statistics show that people who stay poor or unemployed for most of their lives often have a shorter life expectancy than wealthier people.

The differences in health and length of life are probably caused by the problems people on low incomes face. Problems such as:

- poor housing, crowded living conditions, noise

- poor diet – unhealthy eating

- stress from crime, poor living conditions, debt

- negative thoughts about themselves (see the section on self-concept later in this unit).

Another problem is that people on low incomes and people who are unemployed may not be able to access services as easily as wealthier people.

Access to health services

There is some evidence that, in the past, doctors spent more time with wealthy and well educated people and less time with poorer people. However, most doctors probably do not intend to give a different quality of service to different people: it may be that more confident and well educated people can persuade doctors to take a greater interest in their needs.

There is some evidence to suggest that there are more health care professionals in wealthy areas than in poorer areas. This might have arisen because poorer areas are more difficult or more stressful to work in, or perhaps because it is easier to build new clinics and facilities in wealthy areas. Wealthier, employed people also seem to take more notice of health education advice and to live healthier lifestyles. Wealthy people can afford private health care and health checks.

What we can conclude from this is that being poor or being unemployed for a long period of time may mean not getting your health needs met as effectively as other people.

Access to education

Everyone has to go to school, and colleges are open to everyone. Even so, there is evidence to suggest that schools in wealthier districts often achieve higher standards and sometimes offer more opportunity to their students. Some parents even move house in order to send their children to what they think is 'a good school'.

Wealthy parents often pay for their children to attend private schools, because they think this will give their children better qualifications and skills, and also friends who will be able to help them with their careers.

The government claims it is trying to raise educational standards, to improve services for young children and to create special projects to improve facilities in deprived areas. This may help to even out some of these differences.

The family

The kind of family we are born into can have a great influence on our development.

What is a family?

A family is a social group made up of people who are 'related' to each other. This means that other people (society) recognise that this group is related. In British society, 'family' is the word used to describe groups where adults act as parents or guardians to children. **Belonging** to a family can have many advantages – family relationships can provide a safe, caring setting for children. Family groups can guide and teach children, and they can provide a source of social and emotional support for adults and older family members (see Figure 3.15).

Sociologists have identified four different types of family.

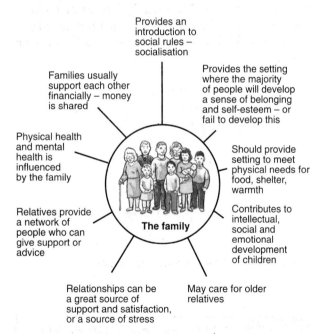

Figure 3.15   How the family can help people

Extended families

An **extended family** is where the parents, children and grandparents all live together or near each other so that they are in constant contact with each other. In England, between 1800 and 1900, many families lived in this way because everyone could help with the agricultural work that was necessary to make a living. The extended family can have many advantages. The parents might be able to work all day without worrying about who is looking after their children – the grandparents can help with this. If the grandparents need care, then the parents or even the older children can help. The extended family provides a network of people who can support each other. (See Figure 3.16.)

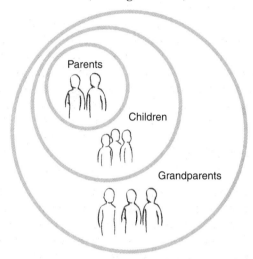

Figure 3.16   The extended family

Nuclear families

Many people now no longer live with their grandparents, and the term **nuclear family** is used to describe this smaller family arrangement, which usually consists of a husband, wife and their children. A nucleus is something's core: hence this family structure consists only of the core members of the family. Historically, the husband would go out to work, while the wife looked after the children while they were young.

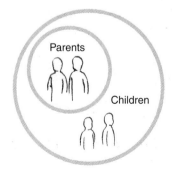

Figure 3.17   The nuclear family

Today, many couples no longer fit this description: often both parents have full-time work and the children are cared for by childminders, nannies or nursery services. Male and female roles have also been changing – men and women are now usually seen as equally responsible for household tasks. However, studies suggest that women still undertake the majority of child care and household tasks. See Figure 3.17.

Reconstituted families

Approximately one marriage in every three now ends in divorce, some people think this figure will rise. Many young people live together before marriage and have children, but there is evidence that a large number of these couples will also split up. Over a third of marriages each year are likely to be re-marriages, and about one million children live with a step-parent. Roughly a quarter of children below the age of 16 years might experience their parents divorcing.

The **reconstituted family** is where the couple are not *both* the parents of each child in the family. One partner might have been divorced from an earlier marriage and has now re-married to create a new family. Children from the previous relationships may be included in this new reconstituted family. Or one partner may have been single but is now married to a partner who has children from a previous relationship. (See Figure 3.18.)

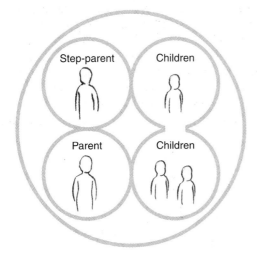

Figure 3.18   The reconstituted family

Lone-parent families

Nearly a quarter of all families with dependent children are now lone-parent families. Of families with dependent children, 21% are **lone-parent families** led by a lone mother, with just 2% led by a lone father.

While some lone-parent families may be well off, many are disadvantaged. Studies suggest 70% of lone parents have incomes equivalent to the poorest 10% of couples with dependent children. Many lone parents rely on benefits or receive low wages.

The type of family a child lives in can change: an extended family can turn into a nuclear family if the grandparents die or move away. Families can become 'reconstituted' if one partner leaves and is replaced by a different person. Few people can guarantee a family style for life. When people leave their partners, divorce or die, a lone-parent family can be created. If the remaining parent finds a new partner, the lone-parent family becomes a reconstituted family. The same child might live in different family structures during his or her childhood and adolescence. (See Figure 3.19.)

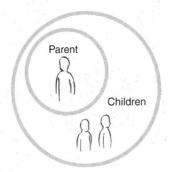

Figure 3.19   The lone-parent family

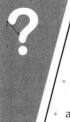
A 1999 report predicts that, by 2010:

- fewer people will form families
- there will be a 33% increase in lone-parent households
- there will be a 55% increase in people living alone
- about 22% of women aged 45 years will not have had children.

How family circumstances can influence lifestyle

CASE STUDY – Anil and Rick

Anil is 8 years old and was born into a family where his parents had good jobs and enough money for lots of toys, books and computers. Anil learned to play on his father's computer when he was only 3 years old. This has helped him to learn. Anil always has someone to talk to at home because he lives with his sister and grandparents in a large house. The family is happy and Anil can go out on his cycle and play with friends in the local park. Anil's family are not afraid of crime in their neighbourhood. Anil is doing very well at school. He has many friends and enjoys school. Anil does not miss school very often.

Rick is 8 years old and was born into a family where both his parents had difficulty in finding work. Because Rick's parents cannot get jobs, there is not much money for toys, books or computers. Rick lives in a crowded block of flats on a housing estate. Rick's mother does not let him out to play because she is afraid of the crime and drug-taking that takes place on the estate.

Rick's mother has periods of depression when she does not talk to Rick. Rick is often unhappy because he has few friends and he gets bored indoors. Rick often gets colds and misses a lot of school. Rick is like one third of children who grow up in low-income households. He does not have the same chance of a happy and wealthy life as Anil.

Questions

Look again at Figure 3.13: 'Factors that affect people making the most of their lives'.

1 Can you see how Rick's story fits with the problems there?

2 Can you see how Anil has been 'born lucky' in that he does not have these problems?

3 What sort of future lives will Rick and Anil have?

Anil's story continues later in this unit, but Rick may not have such a happy life.

Friends

Friends are very important; they can help us to do practical things, such as housework, find a job, repair a car and so on. Friends can also help us emotionally. Friends can listen to us and protect us if we feel stressed. Friends can help us sort out our worries and help us have an interesting and enjoyable life.

Think it over

List all the things you do over a week, such as going to school or college, going out in the evening and so on.

How many of these things could you do without friends?

Friends help us with:

- practical tasks
- emotional needs
- social life.

People without friends will probably have a more difficult and less enjoyable life than people with many friends.

Friends influence the things we believe and the values we hold. As we have already seen, early in life our family influences us (and this influence is called *primary* or *first* socialisation). Socialisation is the process through which we learn social values.

As we get older, such things as school, television and friends come more and more to influence our beliefs and values (this is known as *secondary* socialisation). Our friends can influence the way we behave, and the friends we have during adolescence can have a long-lasting influence on us. If we mix with friends who think it is important to try hard at school, we will probably try hard too. If we mix with friends who take drugs, we may copy what they do.

Low-income housing

People on low incomes often have to live in poor-quality or high-density housing. This kind of housing can mean that people have some of the stresses shown in Figure 3.20. People on low incomes may have trouble paying for maintenance or looking after their homes. Some of the risks connected with poorly maintained housing are shown in Figure 3.21. See Unit 2 for further details on environment and housing.

Ethnicity

For many people, their race is of vital importance as it enables them to understand who they are. Race is not easy to define, however. In the past, people believed that different races were somehow biologically different, but it is now known that it is almost impossible to define racial groups in terms of genetic differences or features

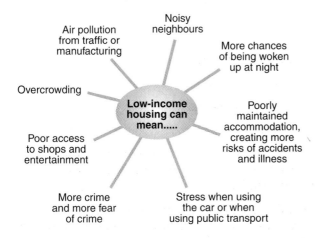

Figure 3.20 The stresses that can arise from low-income housing

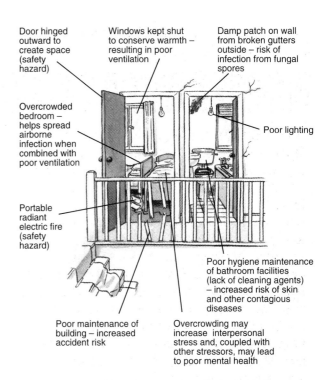

Figure 3.21 Poor housing may contribute to a wide range of hazards to health and social well-being

to do with skin colour or physical appearance. Nevertheless, people do classify themselves and are classified by others in terms of the social and cultural groups to which they belong. A person's culture, religion, style of dress, way of speaking and so on may lead to classification in terms of ethnic group.

A key way people distinguish themselves is in terms of being Black or White: some talk in terms of Black, White or Asian groups of people. However, there is no single Black culture, and no single White culture.

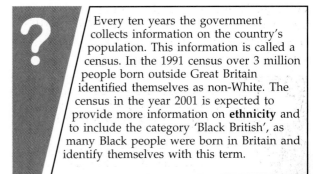

Every ten years the government collects information on the country's population. This information is called a census. In the 1991 census over 3 million people born outside Great Britain identified themselves as non-White. The census in the year 2001 is expected to provide more information on **ethnicity** and to include the category 'Black British', as many Black people were born in Britain and identify themselves with this term.

Since 1965, laws have been in force in the UK to prevent **discrimination** on the basis of race. The Race Relations Act (passed in 1976) set up the Commission for Racial Equality, which seeks to investigate cases of discrimination based on racial or ethnic group. Despite the law and the powers of the Commission, however, there is evidence of inequality between White and Black groups in the UK. Black and Asian people are more likely to be victims of crime than are White people. In general, people from ethnic minority groups are less likely to achieve top professional and management positions than White people.

Unemployment rates vary between Black and White groups but, generally, rates of unemployment are higher for Black people than for White people. In 1991, 12 per cent of White men were unemployed compared with 22.6% of non-White men. Among White women, 7.4% were unemployed, compared to 18.4% on non-White women.

Many Black and Asian people feel that services and employers discriminate against them. A report in September 1998 by the University of Warwick found that four out of five young Black people felt that race relations were getting worse. Employment opportunities and police behaviour are seen by many Black people as the key areas where they are discriminated against.

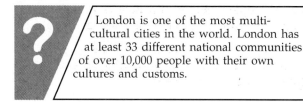

London is one of the most multi-cultural cities in the world. London has at least 33 different national communities of over 10,000 people with their own cultures and customs.

Isolation

Isolation means not having contact with other people.

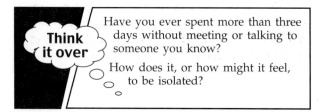

Think it over

Have you ever spent more than three days without meeting or talking to someone you know?

How does it, or how might it feel, to be isolated?

Social isolation

Social isolation is when you are out of contact with friends, colleagues or family, even though there may be many strange people nearby. People who move home or who go into hospital may feel social isolation for a short time until they get to know new people. Social isolation can cause people to feel lonely, depressed, worried or worthless. Extreme isolation may make people want to give up on life and to die. Many older people experience social isolation.

In 1997, more than 55% of women and 30% of men over the age of 75 years lived alone. Living alone does not create social isolation, but some people who live on their own do lose touch with friends and family. Some older people have no children or grandchildren to visit them because:

⋄ some older people may never have had children

⋄ some children and grandchildren live too far away, or are too busy to visit their grandparents

⋄ some children die before their parents, or become ill and unable to visit.

Older people may also lose contact with friends because:

⋄ hearing, visual or mobility problems can make it difficult to go out to meet people

⋄ friends may develop disabilities which make it difficult for them to communicate, visit or phone

⋄ illness and stress can make them withdraw from company and become isolated

⋄ as time goes on, their friends may become ill and die.

Some older people ask for home care or other social services because they are lonely and isolated.

Discrimination

Discrimination means telling things apart – knowing the difference between things that appear similar. It is quite all right to discriminate between, say, a sandwich filling you do not like and one you do. Telling things apart is a vital part of life – if we did not do it we would not be able to live independently.

However, discriminating against people has a different meaning; it does not mean 'telling them apart'. While it is important to realise that all people are different – with different life experiences – discriminating against people means giving people an unequal service or treatment because of their differences.

If an employer did not want to appoint a woman to a job because she might leave to have children, for example, the employer would be illegally discriminating against her. This would be discrimination because she was treated differently from a man who might want to start a family. A man in this situation might be appointed; but the woman is treated unequally.

Common forms of discrimination are based on people's race and culture, gender, age, disability and sexuality. Discrimination is serious because it can:

* damage people's sense of self-esteem and value
* block people from making the most of their lives
* lead to verbal and physical abuse
* cause people not to receive quality care and services.

Stereotyping

Life is very complicated for everyone but sometimes people try to make life easier by considering certain groups of people to be 'all the same'.

For example, a younger person meets an 80-year-old who has a problem with his or her memory. The younger person has seen someone like that before on TV – it hence becomes all too easy to think that 'all old people are forgetful'. This would be **stereotyping** – a fixed way of thinking about a group of people (see Figure 3.22).

People may make assumptions based on stereotyped thinking. For example, a carer working with older people might say 'I'll just go in and wash and dress this next one – I won't ask

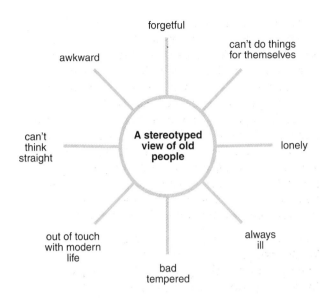

Figure 3.22   Stereotypical thinking

what she would like me to do because she's old and old people don't remember – so it does not matter what I do'. Stereotyped thinking like this may cause us to discriminate against people.

When people say 'all women are' or 'all Black people are' or 'all gay people are' they will probably go on to describe a stereotype of these people. Skilled caring is when we are interested in people's individual differences; stereotyping lumps people together as if they were all the same and stops us from being good carers.

Stereotyping people and discriminating against people can arise from all sorts of apparent differences between people:

* Able people may discriminate against disabled people.
* White people may discriminate against Black people.
* Men may discriminate against women.

Some common bases for discrimination are shown in Figure 3.23. It is always wrong to discriminate against and to stereotype people. Discrimination causes different amounts of damage depending on how it happens.

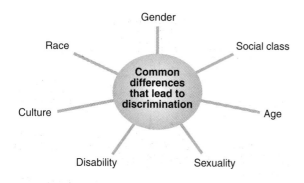

Figure 3.23 Some of the common causes of discrimination

Think it over

Imagine you go into a shop with friends. You have money to spend and you are fit and able. But the shop assistant appears not to like you and does not really want to serve you – how will this affect you?

Now imagine you are alone and in pain lying on a hospital trolley. The nurses appear not to like you and not really to want to help you – how will this affect you?

Consider how you would feel in the situations described in the 'Think it over' above. In the first instance you would feel angry and you would probably choose never to use that shop again! In the second instance you would feel vulnerable. The care staff have power, perhaps your life is in their hands – yet they do not want to give their best. You would probably feel frightened, worried and devalued.

The power people have can make a difference as to how much harm an act of discrimination can cause.

Income

Economic factors that influence people's development include the **wealth** and **income** families have. Wealth includes:

* savings, in banks or building societies
* the value of your home if you own it
* shares, life assurance and pension rights
* any other property that belongs to you.

Income is the money you get each week to live on. Income mainly comes from:

* wages you are paid for working
* profits from your business if you are self-employed
* benefits paid by the government to help people
* money from invested wealth, such as interest on bank accounts
* money raised through the sale of property you own.

Wealth is not shared out evenly in the UK. The poorest half of the population only own 8% of the country's wealth and property. The top 1% of the richest people own 19% of the UK's wealth. The richest 10% of the population own 50% of the wealth. If wealth was a cake, Figure 3.24 shows how it would be shared out.

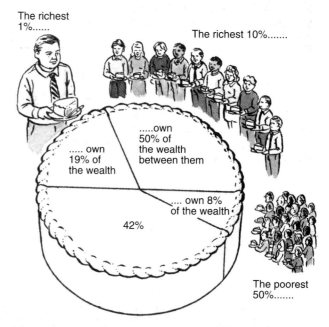

Figure 3.24 The UK wealth cake (based on 1995 figures reported in *Social Trends 1999*)

Income is what really matters to the vast majority of people: your weekly income enables you to pay for your house or flat, and feed and clothe yourself. Wealth, on the other hand, might matter to others. For example, some older people have a low income but own their own house; if necessary, they could raise money on their home through special remortgage schemes or even sell up and move into leased or rented accommodation. Whichever is most important, both wealth and income increase the chances of a person making the most of his or her life.

Availability of money for essential items

Over the last 20 years most people have enjoyed an increasing standard of living. People have better cars, better entertainment and better computers. Many people have more money to spend than ever before. However, studies show that the poorest people have missed out on this prosperity: a 1999 report states that one third of British children live in **poverty** in households that do not have enough income to give children a good start in life.

> **?** In 1995, four out of ten households in the UK felt they could not afford to go on holiday, even for one week.

How much money you have affects where you live and how you live. It affects whether you eat the right diet, whether you can go on holiday, or have savings to fall back on if you lose your job. Low income can cause the kinds of problems shown in Figure 3.25.

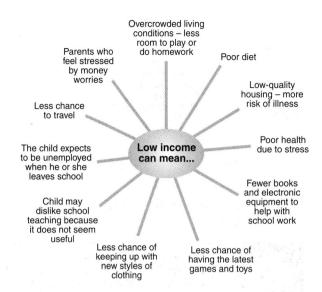

Figure 3.25   Some of the problems a child belonging to a low-income family may face

Availability of money for non-essential items

Budgeting is a difficult skill to learn. Some people never get the hang of it and constantly find they run out of money before they have bought the essentials or paid the bills. Budgeting is really a matter of setting priorities for the income you have (such as paying the rent or the mortgage, feeding and clothing the people in the household), and then seeing what is left to spend on other things.

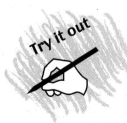

Think about how much money it costs for your family to live for one week. Talk to others in your family and complete the box below, listing everything you and your household spend. Make a guess as to how much each area costs.

1 Essentials	Cost	2 Important things	Cost	3 Luxuries	Cost

Some things are not essential, but they are not luxuries either – they are just things you have become used to having and would rather not do without. Where would you put a magazine or a bar of chocolate – what about a CD player? You could live without them!

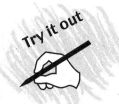

Try it out

See if you can budget for your household for the whole week. Do not forget things which must be paid for, but you do not notice, for example:

◦ light and heat

◦ water rates and council tax

◦ mortgage repayments or rent

◦ house insurance.

Think about food, clothing and other consumer goods.

Could you cope if you lost the main source of income for the household? Where could you start to cut back if someone lost his or her job?

Spending money on non-essentials is a way of 'treating' yourself or other people. You might buy yourself clothes to feel special in, or save up for a holiday. Even a bar of chocolate or a magazine after a hard day can make you feel that life is not just a daily grind to pay the bills. When you are short of money, with no spare cash to spend on non-essentials, this can be depressing and can affect your self-esteem.

Effects of social and economic factors on health

Poverty, a lack of wealth and low income can influence how long you live. For the past 30 years, studies have shown that, in general, poor people have more sudden illnesses and more long-term illnesses than more successful, wealthier people. More babies are born dead to poor mothers than to wealthier mothers. More infants and children born to poor parents die before 14 years of age than children born to wealthier parents. On average, poor people die sooner than wealthier people.

Studies have also shown that people who own their own home have fewer illnesses and live longer, on average, than people who rent their homes. People who have steady employment enjoy better health than people who are unemployed; and mothers from poor housing areas are likely to have low-birth-weight babies. Exactly why a lack of money is linked with

CASE STUDY – Mrs Grahame

Mrs Grahame is a widow aged 83 years. She lives in a second-floor flat in a large house. She has travelled widely in her life – she and her husband lived all over the world. She was the only daughter of a teacher and qualified as a teacher herself, but she has never worked. When living in India and in South America she had servants to run the house and she is accustomed to giving orders.

Since her return to England following the death of her husband 12 years ago, life has not been easy. She does not qualify for a state pension and her savings are gradually being used up.

Friends from the church she attends are getting worried about Mrs Grahame – none of them have even been told her first name. She always feels the cold and seems to be getting more frail. She refuses to see the doctor and last week she shut the door in the district nurse's face, saying 'Mind your own business'.

Questions

1 Why do you think Mrs Grahame is refusing help?

2 How will Mrs Grahame's social and economic problems influence the way she feels about herself?

Figure 3.26 How social and economic factors can affect people's lives

Development	A child born into a low-income family – negative factors	A child born into a high-income family – positive factors
Physical	Poor diet – too much fat and sugar	Balanced diet with the right protein, fibre, vitamins and minerals
	Restricted exercise	Healthy activity
	Overcrowded and dangerous home – risk of accidents and illness	Safe, healthy environment
	Stressful home and community environment (too dangerous)	Safe, relaxed home and community both during childhood and adulthood
Intellectual	Few toys, few books, poor electronic equipment	Toys that help with learning – good learning packages
	Parents stressed, spend little time with children	Parents or childminders spend time with children
	Low expectations of school	High expectations of doing well at school
	Parents have bad experiences of school and do not help	Parents help children with school work
	Low educational achievement and low-paid work as an adult	High educational achievement and better paid work
	Poor skills and worries about coping	Good social skills and education to cope with life's problems
Emotional	Stressed parents may not spend enough time making relationships with their children	Less stressed parents may concentrate on relationships with their children
	Children may feel not as good at things as other children	Children learn to feel successful and competent
	Low self-esteem	High self-esteem
	Trouble finding a good job	Feelings of success at work
	Feeling out of control of own life and feeling controlled by others – unable to choose own lifestyle and place to live	Able to choose own lifestyle and place to live and feeling in charge of own life
Social	Restricted opportunities to play with others	Access to playgroups and social groups
	Friends that hate school encourage others not to try	Friends that value educational achievement and career success
	Friends may be stressed or unable to help	Access to an adult network of friends who can help with work and other needs

shorter life and worse health is not fully understood.

Isolation, loneliness and poverty all have effects on the way a person might think, feel and behave. Poverty can have long-term effects on health. Not having enough money to keep warm or to eat properly will damage your health, especially if you are more vulnerable. Even thinking you might not have enough money may cause stress. Older people, young children, pregnant women and people who are already ill are often at greater risk of long-term damage to health than other people.

Social and economic effects on employment prospects and education

There are many reasons why people decide to discontinue education. To stay in education after the age of 16 years requires interest, ability, opportunity and income. Without these, further or higher education can be very difficult. Even though students aged 16 years and over do not have to pay for further education, a family might rely on a 16-year-old to go out to work to bring some money into the home. Some students help their parents financially, or pay rent to their parents to make ends meet.

The level of education an individual achieves can affect the type of employment they may get. Often, jobs with low-entry qualifications are not highly paid. This can affect the standards of living an individual might be able to reach, the type of housing and diet he or she can afford and so on.

Poor housing and poor neighbourhoods are often found in areas where there are few job opportunities – because many people have no work the area becomes poor. Good job opportunities tend to attract people who will buy property and improve it. Being born in an area of poor housing may sometimes mean that a child will have fewer opportunities for work than a child born in a more wealthy area.

> **?** For each week's work, the average solicitor earns four times the wages of a waiter or waitress (1998 figures).

In many ways, work, housing and education opportunities are often linked. Poor job opportunities may lead to poor neighbourhoods and cause people to believe that education is a waste of time and effort.

Self-esteem

Social and economic forces have far greater effects on your life than just where you live and what you can afford to buy. They affect the way you think about yourself and your life in terms of your feelings about whether you are a success or a failure. If you are struggling to look after yourself because your income is low, you might choose to try to learn new skills, or attempt to find somewhere cheaper to live. If you cannot provide for your family, you might feel you have failed them, as well as yourself. Self-esteem (how you regard yourself) is vital to enable individuals to cope with the everyday pressures of life (self-esteem is covered in more detail in the following section of self-concept).

The way social and economic factors affect people's lives is summarised in Figure 3.26.

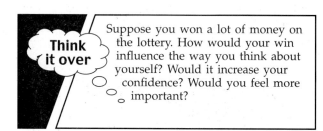

> **Think it over** Suppose you won a lot of money on the lottery. How would your win influence the way you think about yourself? Would it increase your confidence? Would you feel more important?

Self-concept

Self-concept means the way we think about ourselves (see Figure 3.27). How we acquire our self-concept is a very complicated process. However, a simple way of understanding self-concept is to see ourselves as having four 'selves': physical, intellectual, emotional and social. Using this idea of self-concept, you could fill in the questionnaire which follows.

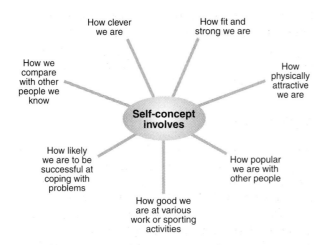

Figure 3.27   Self-concept

The self-concept questionnaire

Thinking about yourself in relation to other people you know, how would you rate yourself on the questions below ? Give yourself a mark out of five for each question; one if you are not very good, five if you are very good! Use the chart in Figure 3.28 to record your scores. For example, if you think you score 3 for question 2 under 'Your physical self', shade in the score 3 under the number 2 in the diagram. Be careful to shade in the correct part of the circle – physical self in the top left-hand quarter!

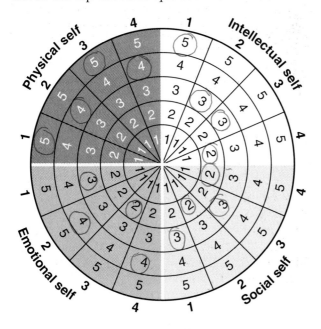

Figure 3.28   Scoring the self-concept questionnaire

Your physical self

1 How attractive are you?

2 How healthy are you?

3 How fit are you?

4 How good are you generally at sport and physical activity?

Your intellectual self

1 How good are you at maths and number work?

2 How good are you at communication and English?

3 How good are you at scientific thinking?

4 How good are you at art, music and general academic work?

Your emotional self

1 How good are you at guessing what other people are feeling?

2 How good are you at understanding your own feelings?

3 How good are you at getting on with other people, including people who are sad or angry?

4 How good are you at making yourself concentrate on work you know you have to do?

Your social self

1 How good are your relationships with members of your own family?

2 How easy do you find it to mix and make friends with new people?

3 How good and satisfying are your close friendships?

4 How good are your relationships with other students or colleagues?

When you have shaded in all your scores on the chart to the left, your 'self-concept pattern' will emerge. Compare your pattern with others. Can you work out why there might be differences or similarities between you?

Some people may have a high score in each area, which might mean they have a very positive self-concept. Other people may have a low score in each area, which might mean they have a poor or negative view of themselves. Many people will rate themselves high on some areas but low on others. This is quite normal: our self-concepts are usually mixed – we think we are good in some ways but not in others. Each person develops his or her own special view of him or herself. This is because of the experiences people have had as they have grown and developed.

Why is self-concept important?

Some psychologists consider our concept of ourselves as being the most important thing in life. Developing and keeping a clear sense of self has been described as 'the goal of living at any age'.

Our view of ourselves is important because it can:

◦   motivate us to do things or stop doing things, for example, doing well at school or at sport

◦   create a feeling of social confidence or cause us to feel anxious with other people

◦   mean that we experience happiness or unhappiness from life experiences

◦   help us lead a successful and enjoyable life, or can lead us into trouble and difficulties in coping with life.

If we think we are good at school or work we will probably enjoy going to school or work. Our concept of ourselves will make us want to be there. If we think we are not good at school or work, we may not want to go there. The way we think about ourselves influences what we do and how we feel (see Figure 3.29).

> **Think it over**
> Do you avoid activities or situations you are not good at or that you feel you cannot cope with? Can you work out why it is you avoid these activities or situations? (It may help if you look back at the scores you gave yourself on the self-concept questionnaire).

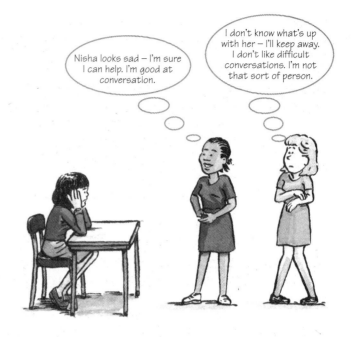

Figure 3.29   Our skills at dealing with the problems of others vary

Self-concept development
Can you change your self-concept?

Yes – because our knowledge of ourselves changes as we go through life. But we cannot change our **self-confidence** or motivation by just wishing things to be different. Our self-concept develops and changes because of the experiences we have. Therefore we should perhaps seek out new life experiences that might help us to change our self-concept.

How does self-concept develop?

When we are born we do not understand anything about the world we are born into – we do not know we are an individual person. The beginnings of self-awareness may start when an infant can recognise his or her own face in a mirror. This happens somewhere about $1\frac{1}{2}$–2 years of age, when an infant begins to demonstrate that he or she is different from other people.

From this point on, children begin to form ideas about themselves. Children are influenced by the

Figure 3.30 The development of self-concept

Age	Stage of development
1½–2 years	Self-awareness develops – children may start to recognise themselves in a mirror
2½ years	Children can say whether they are a boy or a girl
3–5 years	When asked to say what they are like, children can describe themselves in terms of categories, such as big or small, tall or short, light or heavy
5–8 years	If you ask children who they are, they can often describe themselves in detail. Children will tell you their hair colour, eye colour, about their families and to which schools they belong
8–10 years	Children start to show a general sense of 'self-worth', such as describing how happy they are in general, how good life is for them, what is good about their family life, school and friends
10–12 years	Children start to analyse how they compare with others. When asked about their life, children may explain without prompting how they compare with others. For example: 'I'm not as good as Zoe at running, but I'm better than Ali.'
12–16 years	Adolescents may develop a sense of self in terms of beliefs and belonging to groups – being a vegetarian, believing in God, believing certain things are right or wrong
16–25 years	People may develop an adult self-concept that helps them to feel confident in a work role and in social and sexual relationships
25 onwards	People's sense of self will be influenced by the things that happen in their lives. Some people may change their self-concept a great deal as they grow older
65 onwards	In later life it is important to be able to keep a clear sense of self. People may become withdrawn and depressed, without a clear self-concept

environment and culture they grow up in; they are also influenced by the relationships they have with their family and friends. As children's ability to use language develops this will also affect how they can talk and how they can explain things about themselves.

People develop an increasingly detailed understanding of their selves as they grow older. A general outline of the development of self-concept is given in Figure 3.30.

The self-concept we have when we are very young is influenced by our family or carers. Hence primary-school age children are influenced by the adults around them but as we grow older our friends gradually take their place. As adolescents we often compare ourselves with others and choose a particular set of friends accordingly.

Our self-concept doesn't usually settle down until we are ready to go out to work full time or until we plan to leave home and live with a sexual partner. Until this time of life it may be that we experiment with ideas of what we may be like and what we may be good at. Adult commitments perhaps force us into making decisions about ourselves. It could be for this reason that some people may not be able to explain their self-concept clearly until they are in their early 20s.

A clear sense of what you think you are like and what you think you are good at may be necessary if you are to be happy, confident and successful at work and in love (see Figure 3.31).

Influences on self-concept

Age

Age makes a big difference to the way children describe themselves and to the way adults think about their lives. Our self-concept grows and changes as we grow older. Some general differences in self-concept between various age groups are shown in Figure 3.32.

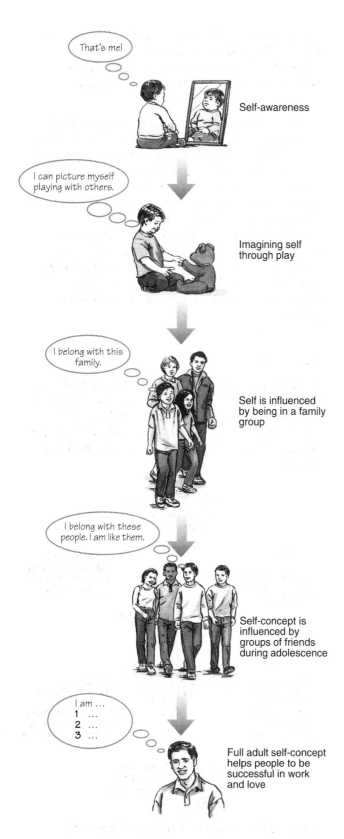

Figure 3.31   The development of our self-concept

Figure 3.32   The differences in self-concept between various age groups

Age	Expression of self-concept
Young children	Self-concept limited to a few descriptions, for example, boy or girl, size, some skills
Older children	Self-concept can be described in a range of 'factual categories', such as hair colour, name, details or address, etc.
Adolescents	Self-concept starts to be explained in terms of chosen beliefs, likes, dislikes, relationships with others
Adults	Many adults may be able to explain the quality of their lives and their personality in greater depth and detail than when they were adolescents
Older adults	Some older adults may have more self-knowledge than during early adult life. Some people may show 'wisdom' in the way they explain their self-concept

Appearance

Somewhere between 10 and 12 years of age, children start to analyse the ways in which they are like or not like others. Children start to work out how they fit in with others – do they look good or not, are they popular with others or not?

The physical shape of our body, our height, weight, hair, eyes and skin colour all influence how we see ourselves and how we think about ourselves. Many people believe there is an 'ideal look' which they should resemble. If we think we look good then we have a positive **self-image**. If we think we do not look attractive we may have a negative self-image. A negative self-image may make us feel bad or have feelings of low self-esteem.

What looks good depends on the culture and the beliefs of the people around us. Take body shape as an example. One hundred years ago, being a bit fat was considered attractive in European culture. A woman who was very thin was seen as poor and unhealthy; a fat man was considered to be someone who was successful. This began to change in the 1950s and 1960s, when looking

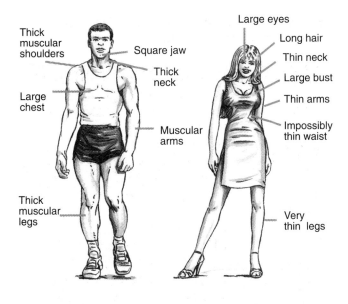

Figure 3.33   Former 'ideal' body shapes

young and thin became the goal to aim for. By the 1980s, children's toys promoted the 'Barbie-doll' look. While very few people ever looked like these ideal shapes, people judged themselves as attractive or unattractive in relation to these shapes (Figure 3.33). Nowadays, TV, videos and magazines tend to promote 'fitness' as beauty. Both men and women should have some muscle but little fat.

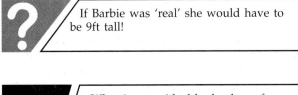

> **?** If Barbie was 'real' she would have to be 9ft tall!

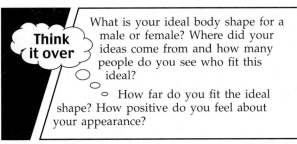

Think it over
What is your ideal body shape for a male or female? Where did your ideas come from and how many people do you see who fit this ideal?

How far do you fit the ideal shape? How positive do you feel about your appearance?

The way you look may indicate you belong to a particular group of people: your hairstyle, dress and behaviour can give other people clues about your gender, age group, wealth, lifestyle, beliefs and culture.

Adolescents usually copy their friends' style of clothing: they often have a need to dress differently from their parents and the 'older generation'. This helps to give them a sense of independence from their families.

Clothes, hairstyle, make-up and body shape are seen differently by different people. No one looks attractive to everyone. What you see as attractive may be attractive because of your own age, culture and lifestyle. The important issue is to feel positive about the way you look. We can easily develop a negative self-image if we do not understand the way other cultures or personal beliefs influence other people's opinion of our appearance (see Figure 3.35). A poor self-image may cause us to lack confidence or to feel depressed about our relationships with other people.

Culture

Different people have different customs and ways of thinking. Your family or the community where you grew up may have different beliefs and expectations from other families and communities. All these things influence the way we think (see Figure 3.34).

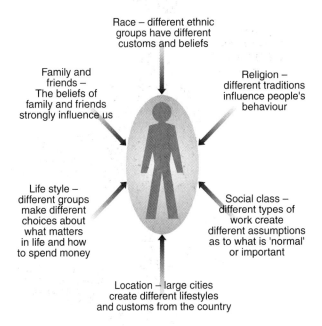

Figure 3.34   **Some of the things that may influence our customs and ways of thinking**

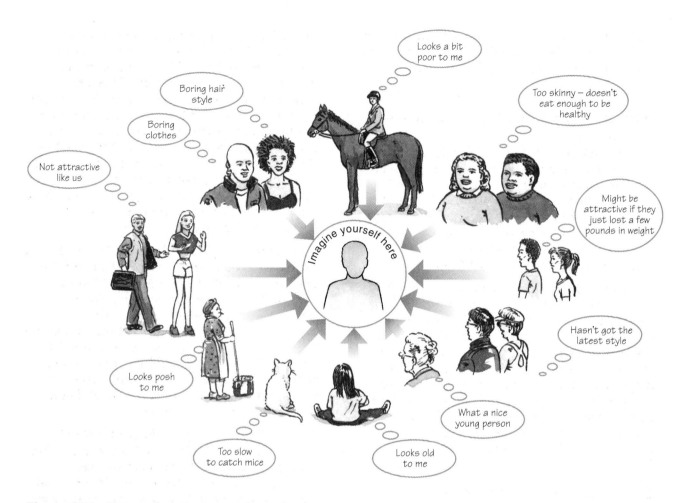

Figure 3.35   No one has the same views about our appearance

People develop different beliefs, values, habits and assumptions because of the social experiences they have had. We call this range of influences 'cultural influences'. Our culture can influence how we understand ourselves because different cultures create different ideas about what is normal or what is right. Sociologists call these ideas **norms**. Some of the norms that influence what we think of as right or wrong are described below.

Different norms about food

Different religions forbid different foods. For example, Muslim and Jewish people do not eat pork, and most Hindus and Buddhists do not eat any meat.

Different ethnic traditions surround the way food is eaten. White Europeans will eat cold food, such as bread, with their fingers but there are limits on eating hot foods with fingers. Asian customs allow certain 'hot foods to be eaten with the

fingers'. Most white British people will not eat snails, frog legs, snake, insects, dog or cat. Snails and frog's legs are eaten by other Europeans. Some other cultures do not restrict what can be eaten.

Different norms about education

Children born into middle-class families are likely to be taught they must do well at school and get a good career. Children in other families may not be brought up (or socialised) in the same way. Asian and South East Asian cultures often stress the importance of educational achievement.

Different norms about behaviour

Some families and communities may emphasise norms about keeping appointments, never being late and being organised for work. Other families may emphasise the importance of relationships and being honest with your friends. Different communities have different views on such issues as drug taking. Some families see using drugs as a very serious crime; others do not think this way.

Different norms about sex, marriage and gender roles

Different religions, families and communities have different beliefs about marriage. Many religions teach that sexual behaviour is only acceptable within marriage. Some communities believe that women who become pregnant outside marriage bring shame on their family. Other families and communities believe that sexual behaviour is entirely a matter for individual free choice.

What you think of as being important, or right or wrong, will be influenced by the norms of the people around you. What you eat, how much you care about education, your attitude to drugs and sex, will be influenced by your culture. Culture will also influence how you think about and judge yourself. For example, whether you think you are good or not will be influenced by your culture. Your self-esteem (how you feel about yourself) will be influenced by cultural beliefs about what is right and wrong.

Developmental maturity

Infants may begin to understand they are a person – that is, different from other people – before 2 years of age. Infants, however, do not have a self-concept. Concepts are ideas we acquire when we start to use language effectively.

Children develop language skills very quickly between the ages of 2 and 6 years, and the way children describe themselves changes as their language skills develop. At $2^1/_2$ years a child may be able to tell you whether he or she is a boy or girl, but may not be able to use other concepts such as how tall or how old he or she is.

By 5 years of age children have developed enough language skills to be able to describe themselves in terms of how tall they are, their age and some of their physical skills, such as: 'I can climb. I can ride my bike.'

The development of language and thinking skills alters the way we can understand who we are. By the age of 8 or 9 years, children may be quite good at describing themselves. They may say

something like: 'My name is Paola. I live at number 58 Birchill Drive. My mum's name is Gina. I have dark hair. I have lots of friends. I like swimming. I love my mum. ' Children between 8 and 10 years can describe lots of things about themselves, but their concept of self may still be limited to simple factual things, such as where they live and the colour of hair they have. Ten-year-olds do not usually have the intellectual skills to answer a question such as 'describe your self-concept'. By 16 years of age, adolescents have usually developed an ability to understand themselves in much greater depth.

A 17-year-old might say: 'Who am I? Well, I'm an individual. I know who I am but it's difficult to put into words. What can I tell you? I'm not going to tell you everything – well, I'm a vegetarian – well most of the time. I am an Aquarian but I don't believe what they say in the 'Stars'. I like mixing with people – even weird people. I love clubbing and I go out a lot. I'm slow to make my mind up – I can't make my mind up about my boyfriend and don't know what I think about relationships.'

What a 17-year-old says is different, not only because he or she is older but because his or her intellectual ability to think about self has developed since he or she was 10. Children may only be able to think in very simple factual ways. Adolescents can often think in more abstract and complicated ways. Adolescents start to think about what they believe: is it right to eat meat or not? What kind of relationships should people have? Adolescents choose causes and groups to belong to – they choose the issues that make up their self-concept.

Adolescents also start to think about what they are thinking! For instance, a child might look at themselves in a mirror and think: 'That's my face.' An adolescent will have more thinking skills – an adolescent might look at him or herself and think: 'I'd like my hair to be different – I want to change how I look – I'll get my hair done at the weekend, just like my friends.' Adolescents not only recognise themselves but they can also use their thinking skills to plan, to change and to develop into whom they want to be.

Physically, people are fully developed by 19 years of age. Some modern psychologists claim that our thinking abilities continue to develop and mature across the adult life-span. People in their 30s and 40s are often able to feel confident and make better judgements about important issues. Some people may become wiser and more able to understand themselves with age. Life experiences and **developmental maturity** may help people to develop more knowledge about themselves as adult life progresses.

Environment

Self-concept is influenced by the people we mix with as we grow up. It is also influenced by the media (TV, computer games, the Internet, newspapers, magazines, etc.). Sometimes the word 'environment' is used to mean all the influences on us which come from other people and from society. When environment is used in this sense it can mean relationships with others, culture, education, gender roles and the media.

Environment can also be taken to mean simply the area where we live. Where we live may influence self-concept in two main ways. First, we may live in a local culture that will influence us and, secondly, the housing we live in may make us feel safe and supported or it may make us feel stressed.

Local culture

The people who live in our neighbourhood may have special customs, habits and ways of speaking. They may include us in social activities. There may be temples, mosques, churches, clubs, centres, village halls or other places where we go to meet friends. We may feel at home in the local culture of our neighbourhood. Many people feel they belong to their own special community. Many develop a concept of themselves as a person who belongs in one special location.

Some people's self-concept would include the geographical area where they grew up. Some people say things like 'I'm a Londoner' or 'I'm a Northerner'.

Housing

People in the top social classes tend to live in more expensive housing and in areas that have good facilities for leisure and education. People with lower incomes may live in more densely occupied housing areas. They may feel they have little choice about where they live. People with money

can choose what kind of house to buy and where to live. The ability to choose where you live may help to provide a sense of control and of self-worth. If you feel 'trapped' where you live, this feeling may lower the value you place on yourself.

Poor-quality or high-density housing can create an environment that has;

- stress-creating noise
- pollution from traffic or local industry
- overcrowding within properties, thus reducing privacy and increasing stress
- poor access to shops and other facilities
- petty crime, again leading to stress
- health hazards as a result of poorly maintained property, such as damp, cold and safety risks.

If you live in an environment that is stressful, it may mean you do not feel valuable or important – you may have low self-esteem. People who live in pleasant areas generally feel more confident and positive about themselves – and their housing may contribute to higher self-esteem.

Education

Our idea of who we are is strongly influenced by our experiences at school. Between 5 and 16 years of age, most people will spend more than half the time they are awake at school, doing homework or meeting with friends from school. Our experiences at school influence our concepts of how attractive, how popular, how skilled and how clever we are. Later experiences at college or university can also confirm or change what we think about ourselves.

Education influences us because:

- we mix with other people and may compare ourselves with them
- the tasks we have to do influence our beliefs about what we are good or bad at
- we may learn theories and ideas that help us to understand our lives.

Mixing with others

Throughout our lives the people we mix with influence what we think is right or proper to do. If we mix with people who think it is important to get good marks in exams, then we will be

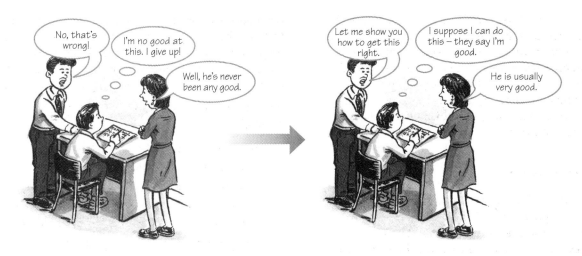

Figure 3.36   The expectations people have of us can affect how much we achieve

influenced to think that exams matter. If we mix with people who think that exams do not matter, then we may not bother to try. If people often want to involve us in their social activities, we may begin to feel confident and positive about ourselves. If people often ignore us, we may begin to feel we are not very valuable.

CASE STUDY – Jai's story

Jai is 15 years old. He is trying very hard to learn a new subject at school and wants to pass his exams. Jai wants to do well because he knows this would please his family. Jai's family believe it is important to do well at school and Jai has been brought up (or socialised) to believe that school work matters.

At first, Jai does not know whether he will be good at the new subject. He works with a small group of other students and realises they do not know what to do. Jai is able to help the other students and thinks to himself: 'I could be good at this.' Two weeks later Jai gives a task in for marking. When Jai gets the task back, it is praised as being clever and well written. Jai is pleased. At break time Jai asks his friends how they got on. Several of them say they found it difficult. Jai thinks: 'I am good at this.' Jai now begins to find the new subject enjoyable and he looks forward to lessons.

Jai feels good about the new subject and therefore he can imagine ways of writing his assignments. He enjoys talking about the subject. Being good at the subject becomes part of his way of thinking about himself. If something goes wrong in a future assignment, Jai will not give up. He has learned he is good at this work and that he will do well in the end.

Jai thinks of himself as a success. Other people think he is good at the subject, so he thinks he is good at it.

Questions

1   What might have happened to Jai's self-concept if he had failed at the work?

2   How has other people's praise or criticism influenced your own beliefs about your own abilities?

The way other people act towards us influences our self-concept.

Success and failure

What teachers, parents and friends expect from you can influence how good or bad you are at school subjects. If children are labelled as 'likely to do well', there is evidence they often do go on to achieve. People's expectations can have a big influence on children. If the people around you expect you to fail, then you are more likely to do badly (see Figure 3.36).

> 'Nothing succeeds like success.'

A sense of self that says we are good at something can motivate us to spend time and effort working hard to achieve good results. If we think we are 'no good' we will probably give up easily.

The stages that lead to achievement

Sometimes people like Jai have positive experiences that work in the following way:

Background: family and friends value achievement, and therefore:

1   the child is motivated to try

2   first experiences are positive

3   the child begins to develop confidence

4   the child receives praise for achievement

5   the child decides he or she is good at the subject

6   the child enjoys doing the subject

7   the child's self-concept includes 'being good at the subject'.

Outcome: a positive self-concept keeps the individual motivated.

Not everyone develops a positive view of his or her ability during his or her time at school or college. Very often the steps outlined above do not happen. Hence people can lose their confidence or get to dislike subjects when they do not feel successful. Some people are not motivated right from the outset because they do not believe that study matters.

Good experiences can lead to a positive self-concept. Just wishing or imagining you are good is

Think it over

How have the ideas about self-concept contained in this book influenced your own understanding of your life story so far?

What are the most important influences that have affected your own self-concept?

If there were no books, computers, school, or college, would you still have developed an understanding of self-concept?

not usually enough. People have to experience positive experiences in order to develop a positive self-concept.

The power of ideas

Understanding such ideas as socialisation, labelling and expectations can help us to understand the influences that have affected our own achievement and performance. Education influences what we think and how we think, and education can help us to develop new ways of understanding ourselves because it gives us new ideas.

Gender

Very early in life children seem to be able to classify themselves in terms of gender – children know whether they are a boy or a girl. Along with ethnicity and age group, gender is a major social influence that affects how we understand ourselves. There are different social expectations of men and women. Men are expected to dress, think and behave differently from women. Men are similarly expected to have different interests and habits from women.

Sociologists see being a man or being a woman rather like having a role in a play. People have gender roles or 'parts' they have to perform throughout life. Fifty years ago in Britain, gender roles or 'parts' were quite rigidly different for men and women (see Figure 3.37).

The nature of society has changed dramatically over the last 50 years, and gender roles have also changed. Both young men and women now expect to go to work and most people do not expect to fight in wars. The Equal Pay Act 1970 and Sex Discrimination Act 1975 brought in the principle that women are equal to men. Before

Figure 3.37 Differences in gender roles in the 1950s

Men	Women
Expected to work full time	Expected to support husband by undertaking household duties (washing, cleaning, cooking, etc.)
Expected to provide money to pay for housing and family	Expected to care for children and older relatives, as necessary
Expected to organise household and to do household repairs	Expected to look after and clean home. Might do part-time or light work to improve household income if no child care work was needed
Expected to fight for country if necessary	Might take on men's work if country went to war and there were not enough men to work in the factories

these Acts, men were often thought to be more valuable employees and were paid more money just because they were men! Furthermore, at the beginning of a new millennium people are no longer assumed to all be heterosexual. The pattern of family life has altered, and many individuals may not live as couples with children during their early adulthoods.

Despite all the changes some gender role differences still exist. Jobs that involve working with young children or cleaning are still mainly done by women. Jobs that involve engineering, building or vehicle repair are still mainly done by men. Women's pay is still 17% lower than men's (on average, between the two groups). Men tend to achieve the top-ranking (highest paid) jobs more often than women.

When it comes to self-concept, women are likely to think differently from men. Career success,

work and making money are standards men may judge themselves against more than do women. More women than men see a successful life in terms of good relationships. Hence the gender roles of 50 years ago still influence how people think of themselves today.

Relationships

In some ways 'we are all other people'. Our idea of self develops because of the way other people talk to and act with us. Self-concept is strongly influenced by the quality of the emotional relationships we make with others. Throughout life, relationships affect how successful and happy we are, and our self-esteem is likely to be influenced by our relationships with others.

If you were about to bring a new baby into the world you would want to make sure the child enjoyed most of the positive things listed in Figure 3.38.

The way we communicate with and get on with other people directly affects our self-concept. We will copy the cultural views of our friends and family. We will judge our appearance in terms of the people we mix with. We may take on a male or female gender role because of the influences of friends, family and the local community.

Our friends, family, relatives, teachers and community are similarly influenced by:

⋄ the local environment

⋄ their education and developmental maturity

⋄ their cultural background and gender roles

> **Think it over**
>
> In your household, who mainly tends to do the following tasks, or are they shared equally between men and women?
>
> ⋄ shopping
> ⋄ ironing clothes
> ⋄ washing clothes
> ⋄ cooking
> ⋄ cleaning rooms
> ⋄ cleaning bathrooms and toilets
> ⋄ earning money to pay bills.
>
> Do you still see some types of activity as part of a male or female role? How does this influence how you think about yourself?
>
> Does your behaviour fit a 'gender role'?

Figure 3.38 The effects of personal relationships at different stages of a person's life

Good relationships can produce:	Poor relationships can produce:
Infancy Secure attachment between the infant and parents A rich learning environment A safe, loving environment which meets a child's emotional needs	A failure to make a secure or safe emotional attachment between parents and the child Neglect, rejection of the child
Early childhood A secure home from which to develop slowly Parents who can cope with the stressful behaviour of young children Friendships with other children	A stressful home situation Neglect or rejection of the child Inconsistent attempts to control a child Parents who become angry or depressed because of the child Isolation from other children
Later childhood Membership of a family or care group Socialisation into a culture Friendships with others at school Increasing independence from parents A feeling of being confident and liked by other people A feeling of being good at things	Stress and change if parents fight each other or separate No clear feeling of belonging with a group or culture Limited friendships Feelings of not being liked by others Feelings of not being good at anything or not as good as others
Adolescence Independence but still with the support of the family A network of friends, a sense of belonging with a group of friends A culture shared by friends A positive environment that has opportunities for the future	Conflict and fighting with parents and family Few friends, feeling depressed and rejected No feeling of belonging with other people No clear sense of who you are The feeling that life is not worth much
Adulthood A network of friends and family who help and support you A secure, loving, sexual relationship Good relationships with work colleagues The ability to balance time pressures between work, partner and other family relationships A feeling of being secure and safe, with other people to help you	Feelings of isolation, loneliness, rejection and no feeling of belonging with friends No support Changing relationships No social protection from stress Low self-esteem
Old age A network of family, friends and partner to provide emotional support Control of own life A sense of purpose	Few friends, no social support No social protection from stress Isolation No sense of purpose

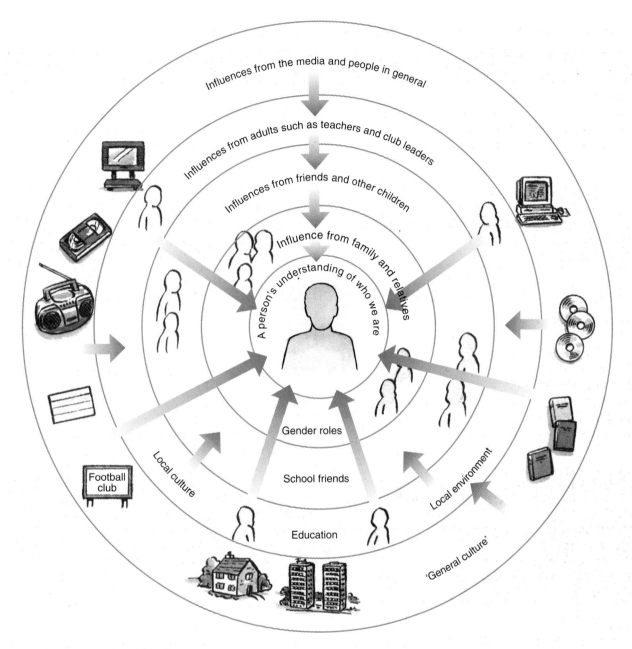

Figures within the circles:
- Influences from the media and people in general
- Influences from adults such as teachers and club leaders
- Influences from friends and other children
- Influence from family and relatives
- A person's understanding of who we are
- Gender roles
- School friends
- Education
- Local culture
- Football club
- Local environment
- 'General culture'

Figure 3.39   Circles of influence

* the wider influences in Western culture, including newspapers, TV, radio, the Internet, computer games and so on.

It is possible to think of these influences working at different levels, like the circles in Figure 3.39.

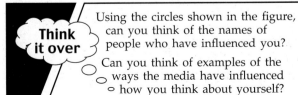

Think it over

Using the circles shown in the figure, can you think of the names of people who have influenced you?

Can you think of examples of the ways the media have influenced how you think about yourself?

Life changes

Living a successful life involves coping with **change**. Many changes during life are predictable. We know they will happen and sometimes we even choose to make the changes. Some examples of predictable change are:

* starting a new school
* growing up and going through puberty
* starting a new job
* leaving home

- marriage
- changing job
- retirement.

Some types of change are unexpected or unpredicted. These include:

- the birth of a new brother or sister
- physical injury or illness
- divorce
- the death of a friend or relative
- redundancy.

Positive and negative effects of change

Change usually involves some level of stress. When people choose to change, for example, when they get married or start a new job, the stress may be experienced as excitement. People may feel 'butterflies in their stomach' on their first day at work, but they may also look forward to meeting new people and learning new things. Some changes, such as the death of a friend, are

experienced as being negative and these will usually cause people to feel very stressed.

Some life events change us for ever. **Life changes** involve some stress because change can cause:

- a sense of *loss* for the way things used to be
- a feeling of *uncertainty* about what the future will be like
- a need to *spend time* and/or *money* and/or *emotional energy* sorting things out
- a need to *learn* new things.

Changes in location
Going to school

Some people are taught at home because of travelling problems or personal needs. Most people, however, go to school and many will remember their first day.

Starting school can involve a sense of loss. This might be the first morning your mother and

CASE STUDY – starting school

David is a black 4-year-old who is starting nursery school. Until now he has always been at home with his mother. He has played with other children many times in his home and also when his mother visited friends. David is an only child. He has a close, loving relationship with his mother.

David's first reaction to school was one of shock – there were so many other children and it was noisy. He had always looked to his mother for guidance, but she was not there and he was on his own. David had been told all about school, but he could not really understand or imagine what it would be like. Another adult who looked very different from his mother was trying to get him to join in a game. David felt frightened and lost. David cried for his mother and told staff he wanted her. A kind teacher who looked a little like his aunt spent time with him and he felt better.

Later in the day, David enjoyed some food and joined in making music with the other children. When his mother came to collect him he was relieved. He did not really feel safe until she appeared. Now he felt tired, but important. He had been to school, he had learned about music and his mother made him feel everything was all right and safe again. This was a real adventure!

Questions

1   Can you remember starting or changing school?

2   Did you feel a sense of uncertainty, tiredness, excitement or fear when you went through this change?

3   Were your experiences positive or negative?

family have left you to cope with lots of other people on your own. You might cry because you miss them. You might also feel uncertain. Where are the toilets? Whom should you speak to? What will happen if you do not like the food?

Starting school can also be stimulating and positive. Some children feel it is exciting to meet new people. They might find school interesting and be proud they are 'grown up' enough to start school activities. Starting school can be a positive experience, involving increasing independence – it all depends on how each child is helped to cope with the change.

David's needs might be summarised as follows:

- *Physical*: David needed food and drink and to be active. The shock and excitement made him feel tired.

- *Intellectual*: David had lots of new things to learn. He needed to feel he was doing well.

- *Emotional*: David was used to feeling safe with his mother. David lost this feeling of safety. David did not know what to expect and was scared.

- *Social*: David needed to feel welcome – to get on with, and be included in the activities of, others.

The teachers and helpers at David's school would understand young children's needs for food, drink and rest. They would use their communication skills to help David understand new activities. Teachers would understand his emotional stress at being parted from his mother. They would do their best to meet his social needs by including him.

CASE STUDY – going out to work

Rahim is 18 years old and has successfully completed an information technology course at college. He wants to design software in the future but decided he would like to get some experience of working first. Rahim wrote over 30 applications to companies in his area asking for work. Most of his applications were unsuccessful and Rahim was very disappointed. Eventually he was successful in getting a temporary job at a local company helping to design spreadsheets and doing data entry.

Rahim felt very anxious on the first day. He wanted to do well and prove he was 'smart'. Rahim did not know what to expect. He did not know what they would ask him to do or how other people would treat him. Rahim was worried about the older workers in the company. Some might see him as a **threat** because he was young; others might be racially prejudiced against him.

On his first day he was warmly welcomed by a senior member of the company who suggested he work closely with a 38-year-old manager. Rahim was nervous at first but soon found his new boss was easy to get on with. During his first day Rahim began to feel the job would be interesting and that the people were OK to work with. At the end of the day Rahim felt exhausted but looked forward to the weeks ahead.

The staff understood how difficult it is to start a new job and therefore they helped him and gave him a guide or 'mentor' to teach him all the new things he needed to know. Anxiety turned into excitement. Rahim felt he could cope. Rahim felt the effort to learn a new way of working would be worthwhile.

Questions

1   What might happen if staff are not sensitive to the needs of new people?

2   How effective would Rahim's work be if he felt that he did not get on with others?

141

CASE STUDY – leaving home

Sarina is 21 years old and works near the centre of the city. Sarina has lived at home up until now but has decided to share a flat with a friend who works with her. Sarina will have her own room and will share the costs of renting and running the flat with her friend.

Before deciding to move out, Sarina had to do a lot of work to find a flat that was suitable and not too expensive. She spent over a month looking around at different flats. Sarina also had to sit down to work out what the running costs would be and how much money she would need to live on her own. She was shocked to find out just how much of her wages would have to be spent on rent, heating and food. Sarina also had to be sure she could trust her friend to look after their flat, pay her share and that they would get on together.

Sarina is sad to be leaving her parents, but she wants to be independent, to invite friends round and to do what she wants without having to involve her parents all the time. The new flat is also much easier for travel to work.

Sarina is anxious about the money and about getting on with her friend. Sarina is not used to looking after her own home – she will have to learn to do housework and plan her own meals and weekly budget.

Questions

1   How might Sarina's move to independence influence her self-concept?

2   Can moving home have an influence on a person's sense of who he or she is?

Rahim's needs might be summarised as follows:

- *Physical*: Rahim's first day was stressful so Rahim became tired.

- *Intellectual*: Rahim had a lot to learn. He was interested and excited by his new job.

- *Emotional*: Rahim was worried about racial discrimination. He was afraid of failure and rejection. Rahim's self-esteem and self-concept were threatened.

- *Social*: Rahim had a need to be included, to become a part of the staff team.

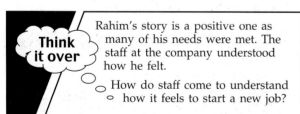

Rahim's story is a positive one as many of his needs were met. The staff at the company understood how he felt.

How do staff come to understand how it feels to start a new job?

Sarina's needs might be summarised as follows:

- *Physical*: searching for a place to live and worrying about money will make her feel tired.

- *Intellectual*: there are a lot of things to learn in order to run your own home.

- *Emotional*: Sarina is sad to be leaving her parents, but excited at being independent.

- *Social*: Sarina will have a new social life when she lives in the new area and can invite her friends round to her flat.

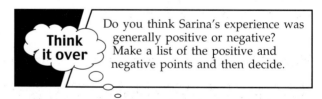

Do you think Sarina's experience was generally positive or negative? Make a list of the positive and negative points and then decide.

Relationship changes

Throughout life, emotional relationships are of central importance to human health and happiness. Research suggests that people who have strong loving relationships are happier and healthier than those without. People who are widowed or divorced are more likely to take time off work and to see the doctor more often than married or single people. Death rates for newly divorced or widowed people are higher than for people of the same age who still have partners.

Relationships with family and friends are also important. Talking with friends, family and colleagues may help protect us from the stresses we might otherwise face in life. Parents protect us in early life, while adult relationships with partners and friends help us to cope with change in adult life. Relationships with family, friends, work colleagues, neighbours and the wider community are important because of the benefits they provide. These benefits are summarised in Figure 3.40.

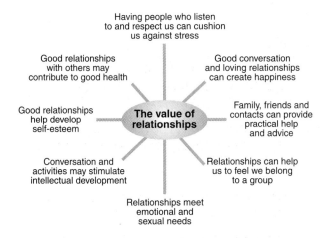

Figure 3.40   The value of relationships

Some changes in relationships, such as marriage, are seen as positive because they may increase many of the benefits relationships bring. Other changes may be viewed less positively because they take these benefits away.

The birth of a new brother or sister

Gaining a new brother or sister changes our relationships with our parents and other family members. Children's reactions to a new member of the family can be very varied, and reactions differ depending on how old a child is and how large the family is. Very often children have mixed emotions. Children may feel pleased they have a new brother or sister, but they may also feel jealous that their new sibling (brother or sister) gets more attention from the others. Some of the positive and negative feelings associated with gaining a new brother or sister are listed in Figure 3.41.

Marriage

In Britain, marriage is the legal union of one man to one woman. Gay and lesbian couples cannot currently be registered as married. Some other cultures permit a husband to have more than one wife or a wife to have more than one husband, but the legal definition of marriage in Britain restricts marriage to one man and one woman.

Many heterosexual couples live together without marrying – some may go on to marry after living together for some years, but about half of all couples who live together do not go on to marry each other. Current trends suggest that perhaps one in five people will never be married during their lives.

Figure 3.41 The positive and negative feelings associated with gaining a new brother or sister

Positive	Negative
Feeling important because you can care for the new infant	Feeling rejected because your parents seem to spend more time with the infant
Feeling pleased because there are more people in your family group	Feeling you have been replaced in the family and are not important
Feeling valued because you are the older child	Feeling your attachment to the family and parents is threatened
Making a relationship or attachment with your new brother or sister	Feeling you are in competition with your brother or sister

Marriage involves a commitment to live with a partner permanently. It ties the financial resources and the networks of family relationships together. Marriage is a big change in life and it can involve moving house and leaving your family. This may cause a sense of loss. Many people feel some anxiety about getting married: are they marrying the right person, will they get on well together, what will living together for ever be like?

Learning to cope with married life takes a lot of time, money and energy. Living with a partner involves learning about his or her needs and ways. For some people marriage is the most positive change that can happen in life. Other people regard it as involving a loss of freedom, or even as entering a relationship where one person dominates or exploits the other.

Talk it over

Discuss with your friends how positively or negatively you view marriage. What rating would you each give it on a five-point scale from one (very negative) to five (very positive)?

Divorce

At present, one in three marriages is likely to end in divorce. In the 1950s many people stayed married despite being unhappy with their partners. In the past, it was often difficult to get a divorce and there were likely to be serious problems over money and finding somewhere to live following divorce, particularly for women.

Divorce is much more common nowadays, but many people who divorce go on to re-marry. Each year, over a third of marriages are likely to be re-marriages. Nearly a quarter of children in Britain may expect their parents to divorce before they are 16 years old.

Although many people experience divorce negatively, it may often be better than living in a stressful situation. Sometimes people develop a deeper sense of self following divorce. Agencies such as Relate provide counselling services to help people to understand the emotions involved in partnerships. Counselling may help some people to decide whether it is best to divorce or not.

Parenthood

Becoming a parent involves a major change in life. Many parents experience their relationships with their child as an intense, emotional experience. There may be strong feelings of love and a powerful desire to protect the child. However, becoming a parent also involves losses – parents can lose sleep because the baby wakes them up, and they may find they cannot go out very easily – they lose touch with friends and their social life. Parents can lose money because they either have to pay for child care or give up full-time work to care for their child. Parents can lose career opportunities if they stay out of full-time work to bring up a family. These losses can sometimes place a relationship or marriage under stress – sometimes a parent can even become jealous of the love and attention a child receives from the other parent.

Becoming a parent can involve some anxiety about the role of being a parent: 'Will the baby be healthy?', 'Is the baby safe?', 'Am I being a good mother/father?' New parents usually seek advice from family, friends, doctors and health visitors. Parenthood involves a great deal of pressure on time, money and energy. A new infant will need nappies, clothes, toys, food, cot, high chair, car seat and so on. An infant needs a lot of attention. Carers will need time and emotional energy to care for the child. Parents often need advice on caring skills – there is new learning involved in being a good parent and always much to learn about the child as the new relationship develops.

Retirement

The nature of work is changing rapidly. Many people will be self-employed or temporary workers in the future, and retirement may become very flexible with some people effectively retiring in their 40s and others continuing to take on work in their late 60s and 70s. Retirement can represent a

Think it over

Retirement provides a mixture of positive and negative possibilities. If you were to talk to people who have been through retirement, what would they say were the main problems and the main advantages?

How positively or negatively would they rate retirement?

major change for people who have worked in a demanding full-time job and then stop working completely.

A sudden break from full-time work might cause a feeling of loss. Work roles influence self-concept, so a person's self-concept and self-esteem can change following retirement. People may lose their routine and perhaps their work friends when they retire, and some people may not be prepared for the leisure time they have and be unsure what to do with their time each day. Some people say that retirement makes them feel redundant – they are no longer of use to anyone. People who have to live on the state pension alone may experience a loss of income. Some older people live below the poverty line.

On the positive side, people with private pensions and savings often have the time and money to travel, study or take up hobbies and so they thoroughly enjoy themselves. Some people see retirement as a time of self-fulfilment, when they harvest the rewards of a lifetime's work. Retirement can lead to greater freedom and the opportunity to spend more time with family, relatives and friends.

The death of a friend or relative

People can lose their partners at any stage of life but, as couples grow older, the chances one person will die increase. **Bereavement** means

CASE STUDY – bereavement

Nathan had been married for 22 years when his partner unexpectedly died of a heart attack. They had been very close. When Nathan was first told about the death he showed little reaction. Friends had to persuade Nathan not to go into work the next day. Nathan had said it would give him something to do – take his mind off things. Later, at the funeral, Nathan said he felt frozen inside and that he did not want to eat. It was some weeks later that Nathan said he felt better because he could talk to his partner, sitting in a chair late at night. Nathan admitted that he never saw his partner, he just felt a presence.

As time went on, Nathan said he felt he could have done more to prevent the heart attack; if only he had noticed some signs, if only they had not smoked. Nathan felt angry with their local doctor. His partner had seen the doctor only two months before. Surely, if the doctor was any good, they should have noticed something! On occasions, Nathan just became very angry and bitter about how badly everything had gone. Perhaps he was to blame?

Months later, Nathan explained he had sorted his life out a bit. Whereas his partner had used to organise things, he had now learned to cope alone. He explained that he spent time with a close friend – ' shoulder to cry on', as he put it.

After a year and a half Nathan still misses his partner but he now says the experience has made him stronger: 'It's as if I understand more about life now. I feel – if I could cope with this loss – well, there isn't much I can't cope with.' Nathan has now become involved with the local voluntary support group for people who are bereaved. He says helping others has helped him: 'It has given me new meaning and purpose in life. I think everything in life has a purpose – things are meant to happen to you. I had a good life before and now I've got a new life to lead.' Nathan says that 'life feels OK now'.

Question

1 How can you help someone who is going through a bereavement? (See pages 148 and 155–57 for further ideas.)

losing someone you have loved and it causes a major change in people's lives. There is a very strong sense of loss – you might lose the main person you talked to, the main person who helped you, your sexual partner, a person with whom you shared your life and a person who made you feel good. Living without a partner can involve great uncertainty. Your partner may have helped with household bills or with shopping or housework – now you have to do it all yourself. Bereavement can mean you have to learn to live a new life as a single person again. Learning to cope on your own can take a lot of time and energy.

People who try to cope with a major loss often experience feelings of:

- disbelief the person is dead

- sadness and depression

- anger or guilt

- stress because they have to learn to cope with a different lifestyle.

Few people describe bereavement as a positive life event, but the final outcome need not only be sadness and grief. Over time, people can take a positive outlook on life again. Read the case study on page 145. Nathan has come through the experience in a positive way even though he will always wish his partner had never died. Bereavement can lead people to start what might feel like 'a new life'. Bereavement need not be understood as totally negative.

Physical changes

As we grow older our bodies change and this change may alter the way we think about ourselves, our self-image and self-concept. Some changes like puberty are expected. Some research suggests that boys who start puberty early tend to gain increased self-esteem, while boys who go through the changes late tend to have lower self-esteem. Girls who start puberty either well before or well after other girls in their class seem to have lower self-esteem throughout their adolescence.

Other changes, such as injury and illness, can be unexpected and very negative in their effects. A sudden disability, such as the loss of sight or the loss of a limb, can cause a person to react in a

similar way to the loss of a friend or relative. As well as a major sense of loss and uncertainty about the future, injury can cause problems with self-esteem and self-image. Older people who lose limbs will often say such things as: 'I'm not going to the doctor – other people will look at me. I don't want to go out, I'm worried that other people will talk about me.' Learning to cope with major physical change can be very difficult for some people.

Types of support

Coping with change is easier if you have other people to help you. Most people have family and friends to help them cope with change. Family and friends can provide help and support to meet different types of needs.

Physical needs

Friends and family can often provide practical help to help meet people's physical needs. For example, moving house or grief can make a person feel very tired. Friends and family might do practical things, such as helping with housework or shopping. Practical help can take the pressure off a person who feels tired. Examples of practical help include:

- helping move furniture when a person moves house

- giving money when a person gets married

- baby-sitting when a person is going through a divorce

- providing transport for a person who is physically disabled.

Intellectual needs

Family and friends can help people to understand change. Sometimes they may be able to offer useful advice or information to help with change if they have coped with similar problems before. Examples of advice and information include:

- advice about managing money when a person moves house

- information about support and adaptations available for a person with a disability

- sharing own experiences of loss or grief.

Emotional needs

Family and friends often give us an emotional 'safe place' to get away from stress and pressure. Friends and family help us to feel valued – to feel we are important. Our sense of self-esteem usually develops out of our relationship with family or carers. Friends can support us through periods of stressful change by helping us to feel we matter.

Examples of emotional support include:

- listening to one another

- using conversation to show that we understand how other people feel

- making other people feel important or valued.

Social needs

Friends and family create groups of people we belong to. Mixing with other people who like us is very important when we have to cope with changes in our life. Friends and family influence our self-concept. Change is easier if we can talk to and be with other people. Examples of social support include:

- visiting relatives in hospital

- being able to talk to parents about marriage or divorce

- talking to friends about new jobs or moving house.

Professional carers

Paid and voluntary care workers can provide many of the types of support friends and family give. Some people do not have friends and family and need professional support. Professional carers may also provide more specialised services. Professional care includes the following:

- Doctors (GPs) who can offer advice and drugs to help with stress.

- Counsellors who can offer skilled listening and emotional support.

- Voluntary services, such as *Relate* which provides counselling about relationships and marriage, *Victim Support* which provides advice and emotional support for victims of crime and *Cruise* which provides support for people who are bereaved.

- Citizens' Advice Bureau which can offer advice on a whole range of issues, including equipment to help people with disabilities.

- Social care services, such as residential care, day care and home care which provides social, emotional and practical care.

- Early years services, such as playgroups and nurseries, which provide for intellectual development as well as other needs.

As well as providing specialised support, professional carers also help people to cope with change by:

- using their understanding of people and change

- using good listening and communication skills (see Unit 1 for details)

- working with values that respect the diversity, rights and confidentiality of clients (see Unit 1 for details).

Support for individuals experiencing life changes

Expected change

Starting a new school

A child's family can help by understanding what is involved. Most children feel a little afraid at leaving their parents and being with different people. Going to school involves learning to be more independent. A family might help their child by the following means:

- Providing playgroup experiences before the child starts school, so that the child is used to meeting others and change is less sudden.

- Praising their child for his or her independent behaviour.

- Talking to the child before going to school and afterwards.

- Showing love and affection – being away from parents does not mean you have lost them.

Professional carers, teachers and classroom assistants might help by understanding the change children face. Carers can help by:

147

- being careful to include all children in social activities
- providing a warm, friendly, emotionally safe atmosphere for children
- learning about individual children's needs – listening to children
- praising children's achievement.

Starting a new job

Friends and family can help by listening and talking. Talking helps people to understand their own emotions and thoughts. There is a saying: 'I know what I think, when I hear what I say.' Starting a new job involves worries about doing well and being accepted. Talking and listening will help to meet a person's emotional needs. Sometimes friends and family may also be able to give helpful advice or practical help with getting to work and so on.

Change is often stressful and stress is tiring. Friends and family may help by understanding this. Colleagues at work can help by listening to and understanding the needs of a new worker. They can help with advice. They can also help by creating a welcoming social atmosphere that will help the new worker to feel included in a new group of people.

Marriage

Marriage can imply a new lifestyle, moving home, developing a deep attachment to a partner and preparing to look after children.

Friends can family can help by:

- listening and talking to help people cope with the emotional need to change
- offering advice
- giving practical help with organising the marriage ceremony and so on
- creating a warm, friendly, social environment where new relatives and relationships are accepted.

Professionals can help by offering counselling and spiritual advice. Most religions will offer some emotional and spiritual support.

Unexpected change

Death of a friend or relative

Friends and relatives can help in the following ways:

- *Listening and talking*: there is an old saying 'A problem shared is a problem halved'. The loss of a person you loved can leave you with the problem of making sense of your life. Being able to talk about it can help.
- *Doing practical work*: grief can make you tired – if other people do shopping or housework this can help you to cope.
- *Providing company*: many people who are grieving need to have other people around them.

Professionals can help in the following ways:

- Listening, talking and showing they respect and value the person.
- Doing practical work: home-care services might help with housework.
- Providing social support and company: self-help groups and day and residential services can meet social needs.
- Specialist help (counselling): some people need expert help in making sense of and adjusting to their loss. Professional counselling can help people to cope with change.
- Specialist help (advice): sometimes the loss of a relative might leave people with practical worries about expenses, loss of benefits, legal issues and so on. Organisations such as the Citizens' Advice Bureau or a social worker may be able to offer help with these worries.

Divorce

The emotions people go through when relationships break up are often not very different from the feelings people have when they lose someone through death. In many ways the help people need will be similar to the help needed in bereavement. People will still need to talk and be listened to. People will still benefit from practical help. People will still want company and may benefit from advice. Sometimes divorce creates special problems to do with looking after children or financial problems. Specialist legal help may be needed in this situation. Some people may have strong feelings of anger, guilt or depression. Counselling may be an important service for these people.

Redundancy

Some people may welcome the chance to change their job, but others may experience emotions similar to those who lose someone they loved. People who have been made redundant from a job they liked may need to talk through their feelings. Practical help and advice may be useful. Some people may need professional counselling or help from employment agencies to help them to cope with the changes they face.

Physical injury or loss of health

Damage to sight or hearing, or a sudden loss of health or mobility, can cause a major change to the way a person sees him or herself. People who experience physical loss will often feel the need for:

- company

- conversation and listening

- practical help

- advice and help with learning to cope with a changed life.

In some ways a loss of health or ability can be similar to the loss of a loved relative in terms of the help needed.

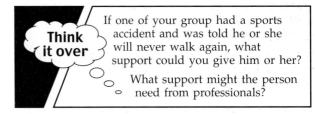

Think it over

If one of your group had a sports accident and was told he or she will never walk again, what support could you give him or her?

What support might the person need from professionals?

Unit 3 Assessment

Unlike Units 1 and 2, this unit is tested externally. To help you with this, this section provides further analysis of the issues involved in personal development. Its focus is on those things you must be able to do to assist you in gaining a merit or distinction grade.

Revision for test

You will be expected to read short case studies and answer questions on:

- the physical characteristics of different life stages
- the social and economic factors that affect development
- the social and economic factors that influence self-concept
- the support individuals may expect when they experience life changes.

Analysing the positive and negative effects of personal relationships on an individual's development and self-concept

Most real people do not have such a happy and positive story to tell about the development of self-concept. Things might go wrong for many people.

CASE STUDY – Anil

Anil is male and was born in 1982. When Anil was young he lived in a large household with his mother and father, older sister and grandmother. Anil received constant attention from these family members and was never left on his own. All the family loved him and had time to play with him. Anil soon learned to recognise his family and he made a close emotional bond with them. Anil's first two years of life provided him with a feeling of being safe and of belonging to the family.

In early childhood Anil was encouraged to play with other children in neighbouring houses. Anil learned to mix and play with others and began to imagine the things they did. Anil felt he mattered and that he was liked by his parents and friends. Anil's parents brought him up to be polite and to behave appropriately. They encouraged Anil to learn to read and write, and play computer games. The family could afford to buy books, a

computer and a TV for Anil. At school, Anil made friends with many other children and usually received praise from his teachers. By the age of 9 years, Anil felt he was good at school and asked if he could do homework like his older sister.

At around 10 years of age Anil began to take an interest in his appearance: he began to be concerned that he had stylish clothes – not old clothes like some of the younger children. Anil also took an interest in his hairstyle.

Anil began to compare himself with other children. Anil decided that he was not the fastest or the cleverest boy in his class, but he was good at football and he was good at maths and most other school work.

By the age of 11 years, Anil had a general sense of self-confidence and a deep feeling of belonging to his family and friendship groups. Anil also felt that he 'looked OK'. Anil had a range of positive feelings about himself. These feelings were due to his earlier life experience.

Anil started secondary school and made new friends there. His school work was often praised and his parents said they were proud of him. Anil sometimes won sports competitions and other boys often asked his advice or wanted to be with him. Anil continued to develop a positive sense of self-esteem and self-worth during secondary school.

Around the age of 15 years, Anil became very concerned about being seen as attractive by the girls he mixed with. By 16 years, Anil decided he was popular and attractive. Anil worked hard for his exams; he did this mainly because his parents

brought him up – or socialised him – to value hard work and educational success.

Anil made friends with a couple of other boys who were very interested in the media and computers. Anil decided to study media and computing, with the idea of making a career in this area.

Now that Anil is older he has set up his own business with one of his old friends and with financial help from his family. Anil has a close, loving relationship with his girlfriend and they plan to marry next year. Anil is a very confident adult; he feels he is good at what he does for a living. He has a very positive self-concept, he feels he is important to his local community, valued by his family, loved by his girlfriend and highly respected by the people he works with.

For a Merit grade you need to be able to analyse the positive and negative effects of relationships on an individual's development and self-concept. Looking at Anil's story above, can you analyse how relationships have had a positive effect on him? You need to think about the following:

◦ Early relationships and attachments in infancy.

◦ Early childhood relationships with parents and family, and the degree of safety and security he felt at home.

◦ Friendships with other children – what values and ways of behaving did he learn?

◦ Relationships with teachers and other adults – how did this influence his self-concept?

◦ Relationships with friends and partners during adolescence and early adulthood.

◦ Friendship networks across life.

You might look for the positive steps in the development of a person's self-concept, as shown in Figure 3.42.

You could use these steps to help you analyse other case studies. The question to ask is: 'Did relationships help the person to achieve a positive self-concept, or did relationships have a negative effect by blocking the development of a positive self-concept?'

Analysing the positive and negative effects of personal relationships on Anil's self-concept

The diagram in Figure 3.43 analyses the many positive influences on Anil's developing self-concept. Even in Anil's story, some issues could be seen as negative (two are noted in the figure). At Distinction level you have to consider which factor has had the most significant influence on the development and self-concept of one person in a case study. To do this you have to make up an argument that one issue is particularly

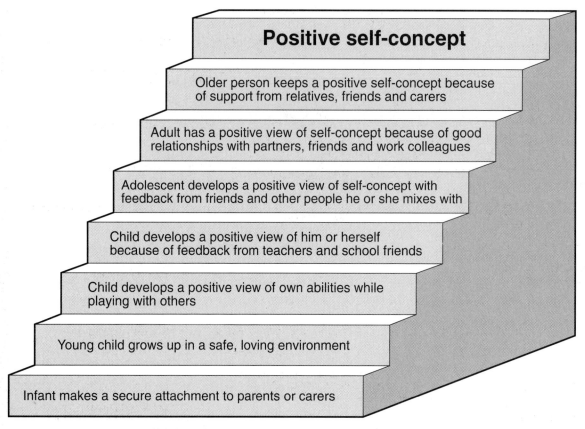

Positive self-concept

Older person keeps a positive self-concept because of support from relatives, friends and carers

Adult has a positive view of self-concept because of good relationships with partners, friends and work colleagues

Adolescent develops a positive view of self-concept with feedback from friends and other people he or she mixes with

Child develops a positive view of him or herself because of feedback from teachers and school friends

Child develops a positive view of own abilities while playing with others

Young child grows up in a safe, loving environment

Infant makes a secure attachment to parents or carers

Figure 3.42   The positive steps in the development of self-concept

important in influencing development and self-concept. This is hard to do because, in real life, all the different influences combine together to influence our development. At Distinction level you have to choose an influence and make an argument that this particular influence can be seen as more important than the others.

When trying to analyse a case study it is important to ask the right questions. You might like to use the diagram in Figure 3.44 to help you think about case studies you work with. Looking back at Anil's case study, we can see the following:

Relationships had an influence: Anil made an attachment to his parents, he was influenced by the norms and values of his family.

Economic factors had an influence: his parents brought him books, a computer and

TV to help him with his learning.

Appearance had an influence: Anil had a positive self-image because he thought many other people found him attractive.

Local environment might have had an influence: Anil mixed with people who valued education and learning.

Culture had an influence: the story does not give details, but Anil was influenced by his family's values and these may have been influenced by class values, and by values associated with religious and ethnic traditions.

Gender role is involved in the story: Anil and his male friends were especially interested in computers. Boys may see computers as a very appropriate thing for men to work with – male gender-role expectations might be involved with this.

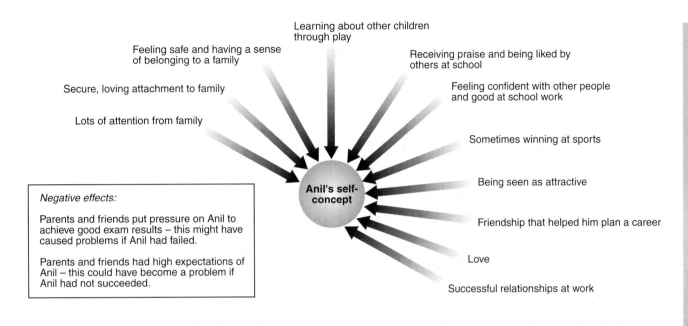

Figure 3.43   The positive and negative effects of personal relationships on Anil's self-concept

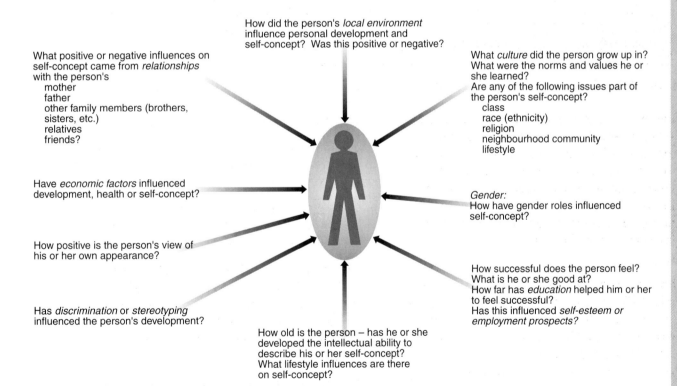

Figure 3.44   Questions to ask about development when analysing a case study

Anil also felt proud of being good at football – perhaps because he was fulfilling expectations of male sporting roles.

Education had an influence: Anil did well at school and started to expect he would do well in his career. His success at school influenced his self-esteem and his future employment prospects.

Which influence was most significant?

Go through the list and decide how strong a case you could make for each factor. Discuss the possibilities with friends. There may not be much you can write about some influences – you could choose to leave these. A particular influence might seem interesting – and this might be the best area to choose. For instance, appearance only started to matter at the age of 15 years – perhaps it was only a small part of what made Anil confident and successful. Anil's parents bought him a computer – but perhaps this was only a small help in developing his self-confidence. The story does not tell us much about local environment or culture, so perhaps it is best not to pick these areas. Gender role is interesting, but it is difficult to explain how Anil's whole concept of self and self-worth is influenced by gender. Perhaps relationships or educational influences might be the best influences to write about.

What could be written about relationships?

Anil had positive relationships throughout his life. He made a secure attachment to his parents which laid the foundation for a happy and positive life. Early relationships may be particularly important, because they are the first relationships we make and they may influence all our later relationships. Looking back to the steps to developing a positive sense of self (Figure 3.42), we could write about the way relationships helped Anil to develop feelings of self-worth, confidence and a very positive self-concept. Looking back at the diagram of the effects of relationships on Anil (Figure 3.43), you can see a wide range of influences.

Using all these ideas you can make an argument that relationships had the most significant influence on Anil's development and self-concept. You could argue that, if he had not had all these positive relationships, he would be a very different person – probably less confident, unsuccessful, with low self-esteem and much less happiness and success in life.

What could be written about education?

Anil grew up in a family that valued learning and that expected Anil to work hard and to do well. Anil's parents bought books and computers to help him. Anil mixed with friends and lived in a culture that encouraged him to learn and to do well at school. Looking back to the section on education earlier in this unit, Figure 3.43 shows how positive expectations can lead to success – this diagram could be used to explain how Anil developed a very positive view of his own abilities. It could be argued that Anil's success at school and at work were caused by family and social expectations of him, and the development of a self-concept which included being confident and successful. Anil's success at school could be argued to be the most significant influence on his development and self-concept. You could argue that, if Anil had not had these expectations and experiences, then he may have developed a sense of being a failure and have grown up to be much less confident, with lower self-esteem and much less happiness and success in life.

When writing about real people you can only guess which factor has had the most significant influence on their development. A Distinction grade is not given for being right, but for the quality of thinking that goes into your answer.

Relevant support

You need to understand case studies that describe people who need support. You need to be able to pick out the major changes that have happened in someone's life and describe what kind of help and support might help a person to cope with expected changes, such as starting school, starting a new job, leaving home, marriage and retirement.

Using a case study, such as Rahim's or Anil's story (pages 141 and 150), pick out key changes and then use the headings Physical, Intellectual, Emotional and Social to describe the help friends, family and professionals might give people to help them cope with change.

For a *Merit* grade you need to cover unexpected change as well as the expected events covered for a *Pass*. This means you should explain some of the emotions that might come with such losses as bereavement, divorce, redundancy, loss of health or ability. You need to explain how talking and listening can help people to cope with change. You should give examples of practical help and advice, and explain how these forms of help are useful.

At *Distinction* level you need to explore different ways people react to change and how these different reactions could affect the type of help and support needed. You might use the following section on reaction to change to help you compare and contrast different case studies that describe people who are coping with change.

Different reactions to change
Most people spend time thinking about their future and wishing for good things to happen. Children often want to start school; adolescents and adults might want to start work. Some people want to get married. Some people even welcome redundancy because they want to stop work. If change is seen as positive, then people do not have the same emotional problems as when change is seen as negative.

If people feel they have lost something, or if people feel they are not the same person any more, then they are likely to see change as negative. When people see change as

negative they try to avoid making a change. Emotionally, people want to 'run away' or 'fight' the need to change.

Coping with negative change and loss (*Distinction* level theory)

A famous author called John Bowlby researched child development during the 1940s. He believed that most people would form close emotional attachments during their lives. When an attachment is broken, the first reaction is the pain of separation and a desperate desire to find the lost person again. When a partner (or close family member) dies, the first phase of grief may focus on the desire, somehow, to find the dead person again. During this first phase, the individual is unable to change. He or she has to let go of his or her past expectations that are focused on the lost person before change is possible. Because the person is denying the fact of death, this phase is called **denial**.

In the second phase of grief, the bereaved person may experience strong feelings, such as guilt, anger or despair. This phase involves developing a degree of detachment from the dead person.

In the third and final phase, the grieving person reorganises his or her sense of self, expectations and habits. This is the stage when an individual starts to rebuild his or her life. This rebuilding or reconstruction is, perhaps, like reconstructing a tower of cards after it has fallen down (see Figure 3.45).

In summary, grief may often involve three phases:

- denial and searching for the lost person
- feelings of despair, anger and guilt
- rebuilding a new life.

Going through a bereavement involves coping with a massive amount of unwelcome change. An expert on grief, Colin Murray Parkes, explained that going through a change involves a need for

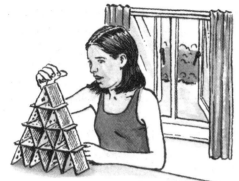

The development of a sense of self takes time and effort

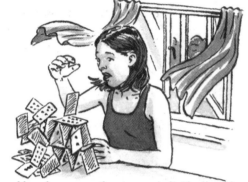

A sudden change can threaten an individual's self-concept

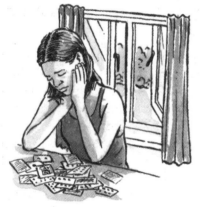

Reconstruction takes time

Figure 3.45   The construction of identity may be like building a tower of cards

psychological work and this takes time and effort. Much of the pain and sorrow associated with loss may be connected with people's reaction to resist change. Parkes wrote: 'Resistance to change, the reluctance to give up possessions, people, status, expectations – this I believe, is the basis of grief.' *Bereavement,* C. Murray Parkes (Penguin, 1995).

Parkes described the process of grieving. Each person experiences the struggle of grief differently, but there may be some general components of coping with change that might be identified. Some reactions are listed below.

Denial

If a person is told a relative is dead, or that he or she will be made redundant, or has a serious illness, that person may react with denial. Denial means the person may refuse to believe the information, saying such things as:

- 'No, it's not him that's dead – you must have the wrong name.'
- 'No, this is a bad joke, I've always worked here.'
- 'I can't have diabetes, no one else in my family has it.'

Sometimes people will deny the importance of what they have been told:

- 'Oh, it's terrible that he died, but I'm all right, I can cope. It doesn't make any difference to my life.'
- 'Oh, they're getting rid of me soon, but I'm all right, it doesn't matter.'
- 'Oh, lot's of people have my illness – it won't really affect me.'

People often deny the seriousness of a problem when they are stressed and in a state of shock. At this stage it may be very important not to challenge people or argue with them about their feelings. Very often the most helpful support is to offer to:

- provide practical help with day-to-day tasks
- provide company
- listen if the person wants to talk.

Professional counselling may help some people to cope without needing to deny a loss or the seriousness of that loss.

Anger or guilt

Coming to terms with loss is a difficult process and some people will try to cope by wanting to blame others or blame themselves. Blaming and being angry with others can sometimes help a grieving person to make sense of what has happened. Blaming others may also help some people to avoid experiencing the full pain of their loss. Guilt can be a similar emotion. By blaming yourself it helps to make sense of things. It may also help some people to change their view of themselves and slowly recover from a loss. Although anger and guilt can help people to adjust, they can also be very unpleasant emotions.

Ways of helping people who feel angry or guilty include the following:

⬥ Listening may help them understand their feelings. It is possible to listen and be good company without agreeing with everything a person says, or arguing with a person.

⬥ Practical help can be very important if they feel stressed and tired because of their emotions.

⬥ It is usually important not to agree with statements about blame, or argue with people who feel anger or guilt.

Professional counselling may help some people who find it hard to cope with their emotions. People who are seriously stressed may be helped by their doctor, who may be able to prescribe drugs or refer the person for counselling or other specialist help.

Withdrawal

Sometimes people 'give up' when very serious things go wrong. Some grieving people refuse company, become depressed and sometimes stop looking after themselves. People who seriously neglect themselves might benefit from an assessment of their mental health or care needs. Care staff may try to build an relationship and to provide practical help to people who are depressed or withdrawn. It may sometimes be appropriate to encourage a person who is withdrawn to see his or her doctor.

Sometimes people experience a feeling of **depersonalisation**. Depersonalisation is the feeling you are not really there, that you are watching yourself from outside. Things that happen seem unreal.

As with other reactions, listening and showing respect and value are key care skills. Practical support and providing company – to meet social needs – are also important.

Trying out or testing ways of coping

As people begin to come to terms with loss, they may experiment with new behaviours, ideas or lifestyles. Very often a person may want to talk about new activities or places they could go to. Some people may ask your advice about clubs or interests they could take up, or just want to talk through their memories of their past life as they come to accept their life has changed. Talking and listening may help people to imagine a new or different life. Care of some older people involves **reminiscence work** where people are encouraged to remember and talk about their past. Reminiscence activities may help some people to test ideas for coping.

Unit 3 Test

Scenario one

Anil is 2 years old and lives with his mother and father, his older sister and grandmother in a large semi-detached house. Anil's mother goes to work, but while she is at work his grandmother looks after him. Anil is well looked after and has developed as expected for a 2-year-old.

1   Think of one way in which children develop in each of the following areas during the first two years of life:

- physically
- intellectually
- emotionally
- socially.

2   Put the following stages of physical development into the order in which they generally occur:

- toilet training
- sitting
- crawling
- walking alone
- bear-walking.

3   Explain ways in which Anil's family might help him to develop his intellectual abilities.

4   Anil always has a member of his family with him. Explain one way in which this might be positive for Anil's emotional development.

5   Anil's sister is 5 years old. Think of one way in which she will be more developed than Anil intellectually.

6   Anil's mother and father both work in order to have enough money to run the home; they often look tired and complain they do not have enough time to do the things they want. If Anil's parents become very stressed because of this, how might this stress affect Anil?

7   Anil's grandmother is 70 years old. Think of three physical changes that are common in old age.

8   Anil's grandmother chooses to live with the rest of the family. How might living with the rest of the family influence her self-concept?

9   Anil's grandmother spends a lot of time praising him and his sister. She is very interested in helping them to develop. How will praise and interest be likely to affect the development of the children's self-concept?

10   Anil's grandmother grew up at a time when it was assumed that women would usually look after the home and children while men went to work. What is the difference between men and women's social role usually called?

11   Name three things which will be important to help Anil develop a positive self-concept by the time he is 18 years of age.

12   Which issues listed below will be cultural influences on Anil's self-concept?

- going with his family to worship at the local temple
- mixing with other children at school
- eating a balanced diet
- taking regular exercise.

Scenario two

Tola is 16 years old and she lives with her mother in a flat on a low-income housing estate. Tola has many friends at school but she is looking forward to leaving and getting a job. Tola's ambition is to move into a flat with her boyfriend once they have enough money.

13   Tola's household does not have much money. Name four different types of stress that may be more common in low-income households than in better-off households.

14 Tola's mother is going through the menopause. Which of the following is responsible for the menopause?

- her children are grown up and have left home
- there are no eggs left in the woman's ovaries
- she has stopped having sexual intercourse
- she has reached the age of 45 years.

15 Tola passed through the life stage of puberty a few years ago. Name two physical changes she will have experienced at this time.

16 If Tola succeeds in getting a well paid job, how will this affect her self-concept?

17 If Tola moves out of the flat she shares with her mother, name two examples of change Tola may be likely to experience in relation to her self-concept.

18 Tola's mother cares for Tola's grandmother, who lives two miles away. Tola's grandmother recently slipped and fell over at home. Why might older people be more at risk of accidents than younger adults?

19 Think of one example of each type of need Tola will have if she starts a new job:

- physical
- intellectual
- emotional
- social.

20 Tola's mother may miss her after she has moved out. She may feel a sense of loss, or even grief. Name three emotional reactions people often experience when they have to adjust to change.

Introducing human body systems

This unit covers the knowledge you will need in order to meet the assessment requirements for Unit 4. It is written in three sections.

Section one outlines the main human body systems, their functions and how each system relates to the other systems. It also contains details of the heart, lungs, skin and joints. Section two discusses those things we must take into account when we are monitoring the well-being of clients in our care. Finally, section three suggests ways we can apply our knowledge of the systems of the body to the people in our care.

Advice and ideas for meeting the assessment requirements for the unit and for achieving Merit and Distinction grades are at the end of the unit.

Also at the end of the unit is a quick test to check your understanding.

Body systems

The cardio-vascular system

The heart and blood vessels create a system which permits the continuous flow of blood around the body to provide the body tissues with oxygen and nutrients (food materials).

The heart pumps blood around the body and to the lungs. It is located in the thorax, behind the sternum (breastbone) and ribs, and between the lungs. It lies slightly to the left, with its apex about 12 cm from the midline of the chest. Blood vessels must supply all tissues with blood (see Figure 4.2).

Blood vessels come in many sizes. The largest are those nearest the heart. There are also three types of blood vessels. Vessels which leave the heart are known as *arteries* and usually carry oxygenated blood (red blood, full of oxygen) from the lungs around the body. *Veins* bring blood back to the heart, and usually carry deoxygenated blood (most of the oxygen has been removed) ready to be pumped by the heart to the lungs again. The exception to the arteries/oxygenated blood, veins/deoxygenated blood rule are the vessels supplying the lungs themselves. These are the

pulmonary artery and vein and they carry blood of the opposite type. *Capillaries* are microscopic vessels with single-celled linings which lie very close to all body cells. They lie between the arteries and the veins, and have walls through which the fluid part of blood can pass. Oxygen and nutrients are delivered to the cells by passing through the capillary walls.

In addition to the functions already described, the circulatory system forms the main transport system for:

- the distribution of heat around the body

- hormones produced by the **endocrine** glands

- antibodies from white blood cells which help to neutralise invading foreign **micro-organisms**

- digested food materials for storage or **metabolism** (chemical reactions occurring in the body)

- raw materials for use by various cells in the body.

The respiratory system

When we breathe, we should breathe through the nose because the nose contains a series of folds covered with special linings that warm, moisten

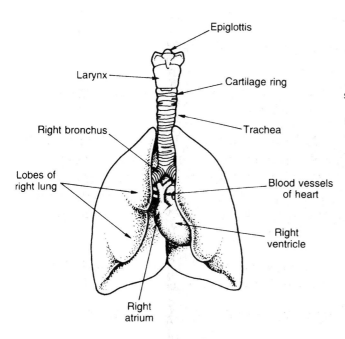

Figure 4.1 Diagram of lungs showing position of heart

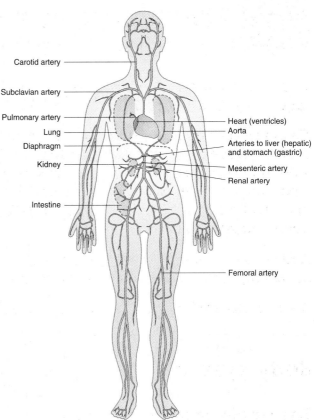

Figure 4.2 The arterial system

and filter the incoming air. This ensures the inner fragile linings of the air sacs in the lungs (alveoli) do not get infected, dirty or dried. After passing down the back of the throat, the air travels through the windpipe (trachea) into the bronchi. The bronchi divide into many smaller branches, the bronchioles. Rings or plates of cartilage support the trachea, bronchi and bronchioles so that they remain open when the head is turned or when food passes down the oesophagus (gullet), which is positioned behind the trachea. Each bronchiole enters an air sac that contains a number of alveoli. The total number of alveoli is enormous so that the actual surface area in contact with the air is about the size of a football field. This is packed into your chest cavity!

Air is a mixture of gases (NB: these percentages have been rounded up):

- nitrogen (80%)

- oxygen (20%)

- carbon dioxide (trace)

- water vapour – (the amount depends on the weather conditions).

The nitrogen we breathe in is of no use to our bodies in gaseous form, and the water vapour we breathe in is of no real benefit to us because the nose adds a great deal more water to the air as we breathe it in. It is the oxygen and carbon dioxide we need to remember, and both these gases dissolve readily in water.

The alveoli are only one cell thick. They are lined with a film of moisture on the inside and, on the outside, by densely packed blood capillaries. Blood entering the lung (pulmonary) capillaries is low in dissolved oxygen. It has unloaded its oxygen to the body cells. It is, however, high in carbon dioxide because this is a waste product of cell **respiration** (the process whereby cells break down nutrients to produce energy). It is one of the jobs of blood to collect carbon dioxide and to take it back to the lungs. In the lungs, oxygen dissolves in the alveolar moisture and passes by a process called **diffusion** through the two thin walls of the alveolus and the capillary to enter the red blood cells. Here it combines with a special pigment called **haemoglobin** to make oxyhaemoglobin (haemoglobin combined with oxygen). At the same time, carbon dioxide passes in the reverse direction – from the fluid part of the blood, through the two thin walls of the alveoli and into the lungs. This is also achieved through the process of diffusion.

Diffusion is the passage of chemical molecules from a region of high concentration of that chemical to a region of low concentration of that chemical. The process of diffusion is at its most efficient in the human body when:

◇ it takes place at body temperature

◇ the linings in between the two regions are only one cell thick

◇ there is a large surface area

◇ the difference in concentration between the two regions is great.

This exchange of carbon dioxide and oxygen between the alveoli and the blood is referred to as a 'gaseous exchange'. If for some reason the concentration of carbon dioxide or oxygen became the same on both sides of the diffusion process (i.e. in the air in our lungs and in the blood in the capillaries of the alveoli), gaseous exchange

would stop. There would no longer be a difference in concentrations and diffusion would not take place. However, the blood in our bodies circulates and moves on, air is continuously refreshed and so a state of equilibrium (balanced concentrations on both sides of the diffusion process) is never reached.

This is how blood circulates within our lungs and how one gas is exchanged for another, but how is the air we breathe refreshed? In other words, how *do* we breathe?

Breathing is accomplished by the muscles and rib bones that surround the airtight chest cavity. Impulses from the brain stem pass down the nerves and cause the dome-shaped diaphragm muscle to contract and to move downwards. At the same time, the muscles attached to the ribs contract, moving the ribs upwards and outwards. These two movements increase the volume of the chest cavity. As the volume of the chest cavity increases, the pressure of the air inside it becomes less than that of the air outside the chest cavity. To equalize the pressure on the inside and on the outside, air passes into the chest through the nose (and mouth). This process is called **inhalation** (Figure 4.3a).

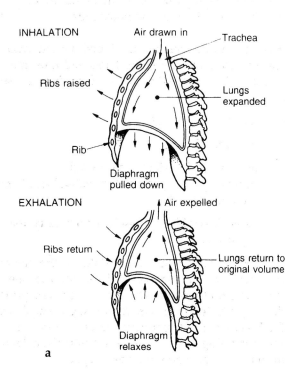

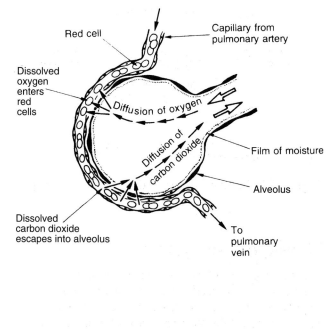

Figure 4.3 The respiratory system: *a* **Inhalation and exhalation;** *b* **Gaseous exchange in the alveolus**

Alveoli (Figure 4.3b) have elastic fibres around them and we all know that, when elastic is released, it recoils. When the nerve impulses stop arriving from the brain, the alveoli and the diaphragm and rib muscles relax. They return to their former positions, which causes the chest cavity to decrease in size. The pressure inside the chest cavity rises once more and air rushes out. This process is called **exhalation** (or breathing out).

Once oxygen-rich blood leaves the lungs it circulates to all parts of the body. Because the oxygen concentration in the body cells is lower than that in the blood, diffusion once more takes place. Oxygen leaves the blood to enter the cells, and carbon dioxide leaves the cells and enters the blood stream.

Inside the cells, respiration is a continuous process, releasing energy so that the cells can perform their jobs. When the cells combine sugar (glucose) with oxygen in the process of respiration, the result is the release of carbon dioxide, water and energy.

All body cells require energy to support the chemical reactions that are taking place inside them (see Figure 4.4).

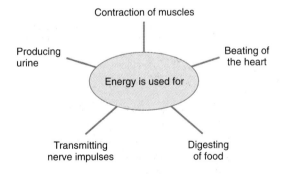

Figure 4.4 Bodily processes that require energy

The digestive system

The sugar (glucose) needed for the process of respiration is acquired by our bodies through **digestion**. Digestion occurs in the alimentary canal – a long tube that runs from the mouth to the anus. Along its way, the alimentary canal changes in size and structure (see Figure 4.5).

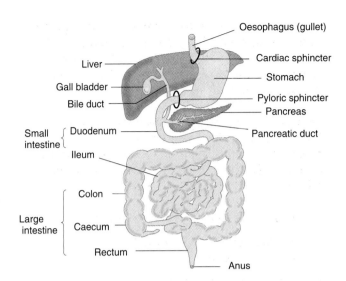

Figure 4.5 The alimentary canal

As we have already seen in Unit 2, food which contains energy is composed of carbohydrates, proteins and fats. These chemicals can all be broken down in various parts of the alimentary canal to produce glucose and other simple nutrients. This breakdown is achieved through chemicals secreted by the linings of the different parts of the alimentary canal (**enzymes**). When broken down, the resulting sugar and other chemicals are absorbed into the blood stream which carries them to the body cells.

Absorption of sugar into the blood stream takes place in the small intestine. The small intestine (Figure 4.6) is specially adapted for this purpose by:

⋄   its very long length

⋄   its folded lining

⋄   its increased surface area (by villi – microscopic projections that extend out from the lining cells)

⋄   its capillary blood vessels, which carry the sugar away.

Diffusion is once more responsible for the passage of sugar from the interior of the small intestine into the blood vessels. The blood then transports the sugar to the liver, where any sugar surplus to the body's current requirements can be stored. The remaining sugar then passes into the cells by diffusion, in the same way as oxygen.

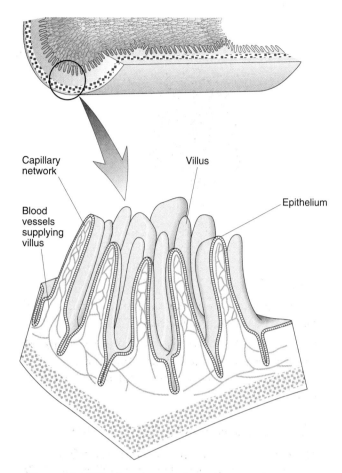

Figure 4.6 The structure of the lining of the small intestine

Digestion can be summarised as the breaking down of complex food substances into simple, soluble materials the body can use for energy and for the other processes necessary to keep our bodies in good condition.

The reproductive system
(See Figures 4.7 and 4.8.)

Male

The testes are contained in a skin bag (the scrotum). This bag is outside the abdominal cavity because cool temperatures are required for the formation of spermatozoa (the male sex cells). When a man ejaculates as a result of sexual stimulation, the spermatozoa leave the testes in a fluid called semen.

The penis has two functions: to transport urine out of the body, and to introduce spermatozoa

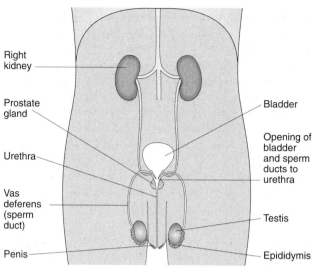

Figure 4.7 The male reproductive and urinary system

into the vagina. These two functions, however, never happen at the same time. The tubes that take semen out of the testes are called the vas deferens. Vasectomy is an operation whereby the vas deferens are cut to stop the flow of spermatozoa from the testes. This operation effectively **sterilises** a man.

The penis contains a special spongy tissue that fills with blood during sexual excitement. When engorged (filled) with blood, the penis becomes stiff so that it can penetrate the vagina.

Female

The female's egg-producing organs are the

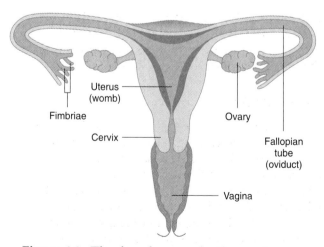

Figure 4.8 The female reproductive system

ovaries. These produce one egg every month during a woman's fertile years (about 13–48 years of age – although this varies widely). The egg slowly travels down the fallopian tubes (oviducts) towards the uterus (womb). If on its journey to the uterus the egg (ovum) comes into contact with a spermatozoon (a single male sex cell deposited in the vagina during sexual intercourse), it may become fertilised. Fertilisation is the union of a female and male sex cell, and this process of fertilisation is necessary for the ovum to have the potential to develop into an **embryo**.

If fertilised, the egg embeds itself in the lining of the uterus. The embryo (as the fertilised egg is now called) receives all it needs to grow and develop from the blood supply to the mother's uterus. An unfertilised egg, however, does not become embedded in the uterine wall. It passes out of the woman's body during the next period of menstruation (the uterus sheds and renews its lining about once a month if an egg has not been fertilised).

After about two months of growth, the embryo is known as a **foetus**.

As well as nourishing the foetus during its development, the uterus is the organ that discharges the foetus out of the woman's body after about 40 weeks of its growth. The uterine muscle contracts rhythmically and strongly until the cervix **dilates** (enlarges). It then contracts even more strongly to push the foetus into the vagina (which is capable of great extension).

The man's testes and the woman's ovaries also produce hormones that stimulate the body's growth and development as well as controlling the body's reproductive system.

The nervous system

The nervous system (see Figure 4.9) is the means by which the body co-ordinates all our bodily systems and tells us about changes in our environment. From the central nervous system (the brain and the spinal cord) nerves extend to all parts of the body. These nerves carry brief electro-chemical messages that trigger appropriate responses in the various parts of our bodies. The messages (**impulses**) make the muscles contract

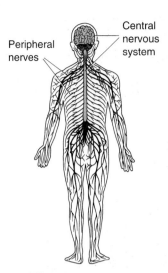

Figure 4.9 The nervous system

(as in breathing), the glands secrete and the blood vessels widen or narrow, etc.

The brain is the organ that enables us to think, to sense things and to remember things. It also controls our rate of breathing, our heart beat and our body temperature.

The musculo-skeletal system

The skeleton is the body's bony framework to which our muscles are attached (see Figure 4.10). It is the structure that holds our bodies together and that enables us to move (without bones, our muscles would not be able to function properly: see the section on levers below). It is important that you know the names of the major bones so that you can report fractures and injuries using accurate terms and describe lever systems accurately.

The place where two bones meet is called a joint. Again, it is important you understand the features of a joint and how these can affect a client's lifestyle (Figure 4.11).

The muscles are attached to the bones by tendons. Tendons are not elastic like ligaments (the tissues that join bones together) but they are equally as strong. When a muscle contracts, it shortens and pulls on the tendon. The tendon, in turn, pulls on the bone, which moves at the appropriate joint. Muscles only pull bones; they never push. Hence they must act in pairs. One muscle pulls the bone into its new position; the other returns it back. It is the impulses from our central nervous system that cause our muscles to contract.

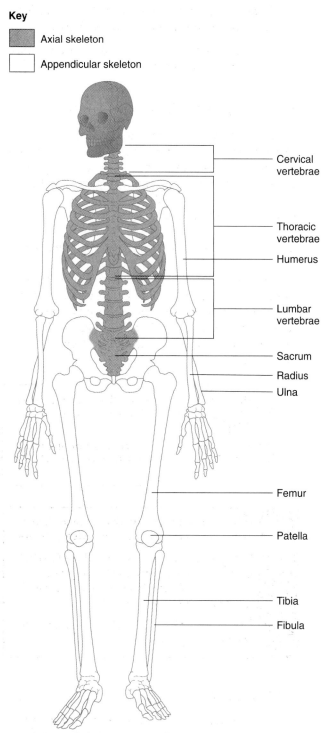

Key

Axial skeleton

Appendicular skeleton

- Cervical vertebrae
- Thoracic vertebrae
- Humerus
- Lumbar vertebrae
- Sacrum
- Radius
- Ulna
- Femur
- Patella
- Tibia
- Fibula

Figure 4.10   The structure of the human skeleton

When the protective cartilage covering the bone wears down through years of use, the joint becomes stiff and painful – this is known as osteo-arthritis and occurs mainly as people get older.

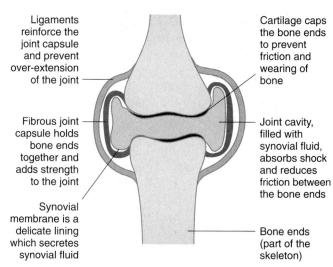

Ligaments reinforce the joint capsule and prevent over-extension of the joint

Fibrous joint capsule holds bone ends together and adds strength to the joint

Synovial membrane is a delicate lining which secretes synovial fluid

Cartilage caps the bone ends to prevent friction and wearing of bone

Joint cavity, filled with synovial fluid, absorbs shock and reduces friction between the bone ends

Bone ends (part of the skeleton)

Figure 4.11   The structure of a joint

Rheumatoid arthritis can affect all ages and the joints become hot, red, swollen, painful and frequently deformed. Current thinking believes that people can produce antibodies against their own joint tissues – called an auto-immune disease.

Lever systems

We come across levers everyday of our lives: when we open a door, turn a key in a lock or change gear in a car.

A lever is any device that can turn about a pivot or a **fulcrum**. In a lever, the force we apply is called the **effort**, and this effort is applied to overcome a resistance, the **load**. Imagine you are trying to lift a stuck slice of pie out of a pie dish. You push the knife under the slice and rest the remainder of the blade on the rim of the pie dish. You then push down on the knife's handle. If you push down too hard, the slice on the end of the blade flicks into the air; if not hard enough, the slice doesn't move. The slice of pie is the **load**, your pushing down is the **effort**, the knife is the **lever**, and the rim of the pie dish where you rest the knife is the **fulcrum**. And we must get the balance between the load and the effort correct if we are to move the slice at all or prevent it from flying into the air!

There are three types of levers, depending on the arrangement of the load, effort and fulcrum:

- *First-order levers* are arranged effort, fulcrum, load (as with the slice of pie).

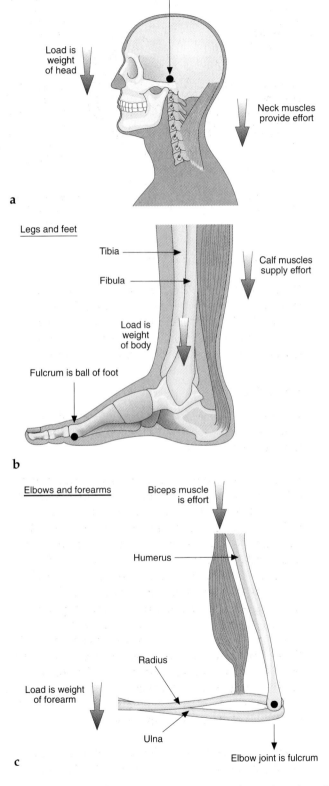

a

b

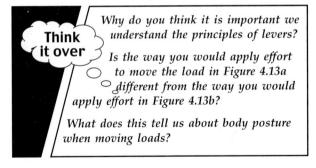

c

Figure 4.12 Levers in the human body: *a* Head and neck (first-order lever); *b* Leg and foot (second-order lever); *c* Elbow and forearm (third-order lever)

* *Second-order levers* are arranged fulcrum, load, effort (as when moving a wheel-barrow).
* *Third-order levers* are arranged fulcrum, effort, load (as in pulling up a draw-bridge).

Levers in the human body

Most of the muscle actions in our bones are third-order levers (see Figure 4.12c), but there are also first and second-order actions (see Figure 4.12a and b). Note carefully in Figure 4.21 the order of load, effort and fulcrum in each example of muscle action.

Lever systems are also used in care equipment.

Having looked at the different systems within the human body, we must now study the ways these systems work together. Hence we need to understand the relationships between the features and functions of the heart, lungs, skin and joints.

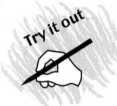

Try it out

Study the three examples of levers given in Figure 4.13.

Which order of levers does each belong to?

Think it over

Why do you think it is important we understand the principles of levers?

Is the way you would apply effort to move the load in Figure 4.13a different from the way you would apply effort in Figure 4.13b?

What does this tell us about body posture when moving loads?

The heart

The heart (Figure 4.14) is conical in shape and is the size of a closed fist. It is protected by the sternum and ribs. It consists of four chambers, two upper and two lower, and it is completely separated into right and left halves. The right side contains deoxygenated blood and the left side oxygenated blood. The upper chambers on both sides are called the atria (singular 'atrium')

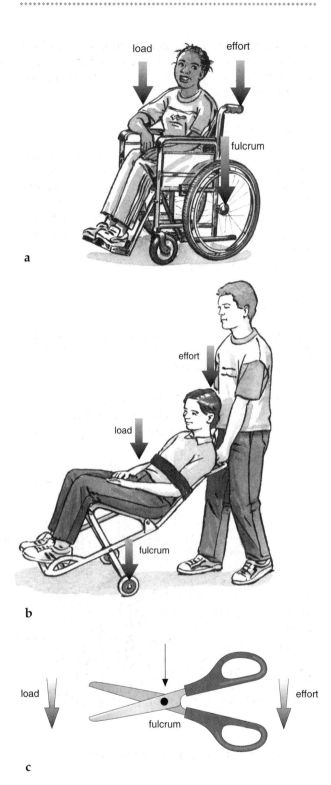

Figure 4.13 Levers in common use in a care setting: *a* **A wheelchair;** *b* **A carrying chair;** *c* **Scissors**

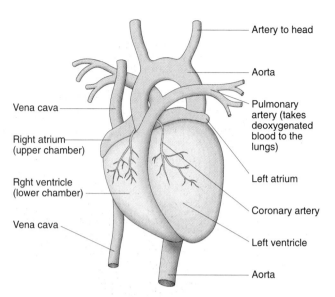

Figure 4.14 The external structure of the heart

and the lower chambers are called ventricles. Blood comes into the upper chambers, passes through valves into the lower chambers, and is then pumped out through the exit arteries. In between the two chambers on each side are sets of valves which, when closed, prevent blood flowing backwards from the ventricles into the atria during the forceful contraction of the ventricles: blood can flow only onwards into the two exit arteries. The atria have thin muscular walls as they contract for a short time only in order to push blood into the ventricles. Ventricles, on the other hand, have thick muscular walls to force blood into the *exit arteries*.

On the right side of the heart, blood is pumped up the pulmonary artery to the lungs for oxygenation. On the left side the newly oxygenated blood (returned via the pulmonary veins to the left atrium) is pumped around the whole of the rest of the body by the large aorta.

Both these large arteries contain sets of semi-lunar (moon-shaped) valves that prevent blood flowing backwards into the ventricles while they rest momentarily between contractions. Not surprisingly, the wall of the left ventricle contains much thicker muscle than the right as it must force blood both up to the head and down as far as the toes!

The heart valves

The valves between the atria and ventricles are larger than the semi-lunar valves and they are

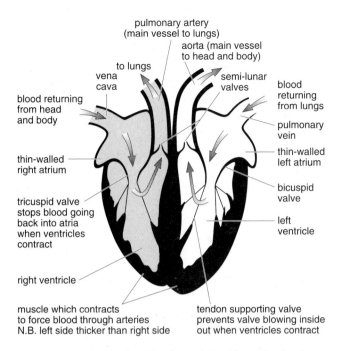

Figure 4.15 Longitudinal section through the heart

double the thickness of the membrane that lines the heart. The valve on the right side is called the tricuspid valve (as it has three flaps). The valve on the left side has only two valves (the bicuspid valve). These valves do not have any muscle in their flaps, and they open and close simply as a result of the differing pressures between the blood in the atria and ventricles. However, both need help to stop them blowing inside out when the ventricles contract – rather like an umbrella blowing inside out on a windy day.

Attached to the edges of the valves are tiny valve tendons which are tethered to tiny papillary muscles on the inside walls of the ventricles. These contract just before the main bulk of the ventricular muscle contracts, helping the valves to stay in position. This is like having strings tied to the points of an umbrella to stop the spokes bending the other way round in the wind, and holding these strings in your hand.

Nothing happens to the composition of the blood when it is in the heart – the heart is just a double pump to give the blood a boost so that it reaches its destinations successfully.

The coronary vessels

The heart itself also requires blood full of oxygen and nutrients because it works very hard indeed. Blood vessels run all over the outside surface of the heart muscles. These are called coronary vessels (because they look like a crown). When these become blocked, the heart muscle becomes damaged. This condition is called a heart attack or **coronary thrombosis**.

The skin

The structure of the skin is shown in Figure 4.16. Figure 4.17 outlines the skin's features and the function of these features.

Finally, Figure 4.18 outlines the major systems of the human body, their functions and their relationships to other bodily processes.

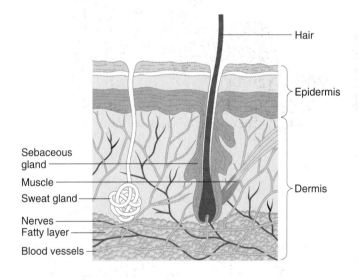

Figure 4.16 The structure of the skin

Figure 4.17 The skin's features and their functions

Feature	Function
Epidermis	
Outer layer of dead cells	Forms a waterproof barrier
	Forms a barrier to invasion by micro-organisms
Inner layer of cells	Constantly dividing to replace cells lost from outer layers
	Contains black pigment cells that protect from harmful, ultra-violet light in the sun's rays
Hair follicle	Little use in humans, but has a cosmetic effect and signals cold, fright, etc. ('goose-pimples')
Sebaceous or oil glands	Pours down the hair on to the skin surface to help waterproof the skin
Dermis	
Sweat gland	Pours sweat on to the skin surface when too hot; evaporation of the water in sweat cools the surface and aids temperature regulation
Nerves and nerve endings	The skin is an important sense organ, detecting temperature changes, pressure, touch and pain; sends impulses to the central nervous system, which promotes responses
Blood capillaries	Bring nutrients and heat, and remove waste products (the diameter of the capillaries alters to adjust to heat loss by radiation, convection, etc.)
Fatty layer	Acts as a shock absorber
	Makes vitamin D when directly exposed to sunlight
	Stores vitamins A, D, E and K
Innermost muscle layer	Contracts rhythmically (shivering) to generate heat when the body temperature is decreasing

Earlier in this unit, you have learned about the inter-relationships between the respiratory system, circulatory system and musculo-skeletal system; Figure 4.18 shows the inter-relationships between other major systems of the human body and bodily processes.

Figure 4.18 The inter-relationships between some of the major systems of the human body and bodily processes

Name of system	Major organs	Position and location	Functions	Inter-relationships
Nervous system	Brain	Within the skull, which lies in the head	1 Receives and interprets all the nerve impulses from sensory organs (such as the eye, ear and tongue) 2 Begins voluntary motor impulses, which make muscles contract	Interprets sensory impulses from receptors to enable the process of homeostasis to occur (the regulation of the body's internal environment, such as temperature)

Name of system	Major organs	Position and location	Functions	Inter-relationships
			3 Site of all the thinking and learning humans do **4** Co-ordinates muscle actions **5** Controls organs (such as the stomach), heart rate, breathing rate	Starts and co-ordinates all muscle actions in the body so that we can move, breathe and food can travel through the alimentary canal Parts of the brain control the secretion of hormones from the endocrine system Controls the amount of water allowed to pass into the urine Controls the thirst and appetite centres
	Spinal cord	Lies inside the large opening of the vertebrae of the spine and runs from the brain to the lower border of the first lumbar (back) vertebra	**1** Allows nervous impulses running to and from the lower part of the body to reach the brain **2** Allows rapid automatic movements to occur to prevent further injury – these are called reflexes **3** It is the source of all spinal nerves	It is the route taken by all nerves passing to and from all organs below the head
	Peripheral nerves	These run from the spinal cord to each organ or muscle they serve	**1** Contain the motor or effector axons which run to the muscles **2** Contain the sensory or receptor dendrons which carry impulses from the sensory receptors	Allow protective reflexes to occur Allow muscle action to occur Allow sensation to be received by the central nervous system (brain and spinal cord) Assists in the control of body temperature
Endocrine system	Pituitary gland	Hangs below the brain in a cavity in the skull, in the centre line	Secretes hormones which control reproduction, other endocrine glands, growth, water balance, birth process and breast-milk production	Relationship with reproductive processes including birth and breast-milk production Relationship with water balance and the kidney and renal system Relationship with body growth and locomotor system Relationship with the nervous system as it is closely linked with a part known as the hypothalamus

Name of system	Major organs	Position and location	Functions	Inter-relationships
	Adrenal glands	Small conical glands sitting on top of the kidneys	**1** The inner part secretes adrenaline which prepares the body for stress **2** The outer part secretes a type of cortisone which is anti-inflammatory **3** Secretes sex hormones	Adrenaline makes the heart beat stronger and faster, blood pressure rises and there is a shift in the distribution of blood Adrenaline raises blood sugar by taking stores from the liver, part of the digestive system Adrenaline causes more blood to flow to the muscles of the locomotor system Cortisone helps in the defence of the body Sex hormones help in reproduction
	Ovaries	Within the pelvis, close to the fallopian tubes which arise from the uterus. One lies each side of the midline	**1** Secrete oestrogen and progesterone which prepare the uterus to receive a fertilised egg **2** These hormones also produce secondary sexual characteristics at puberty, such as breast growth, pubic hair, growth of the sexual organs and menstruation	Related to growth in the locomotor system Related to the nervous system, as they influence emotions Closely related to the reproductive system of the female
	Testes	Lie in skin bags (called the scrotum) behind the penis outside the abdominal cavity	Production of the male sex hormone called testosterone, which is necessary for sperm production and male secondary sexual characteristics such as deepening of the voice, increase in stature, pubic hair and growth of the sexual organs	Related to all systems as it influences the rate of respiration Closely related to respiration and the locomotor system
	Thyroid gland	Lies in the neck over the trachea	Produces the hormone thyroxine which controls the rate of metabolism including cell respiration and growth	Related to all systems as it influences the rate of respiration Closely related to respiration and the locomotor system

Name of system	Major organs	Position and location	Functions	Inter-relationships
Reproductive system – female				
	Ovaries	Within the pelvis, close to the fallopian tubes which arise from the uterus. One lies each side of the midline Oviducts or fallopian tubes	1 Production of ova or eggs 2 Secretes oestrogen and progesterone (for the functions of these, see above under endocrine system)	Related to growth in the locomotor system Related to the nervous system as they influence emotions Closely related to the endocrine system
	Oviducts or fallopian tubes	Lie in the pelvis, one on each side coming from the uterus	1 Transports the ova from the ovary to the uterus 2 Site of fertilisation 3 A fertilised ovum begins development here	Closely related to the male reproductive system
	Uterus	Lies in the midline, deep in the pelvis	1 Receives the fertilised ovum and allows it to bury itself in the uterine lining 2 Shelters the foetus during pregnancy 3 Through strong muscular contractions expels the foetus during birth 4 Renews its lining every month in preparation for pregnancy	Is influenced by hormones from the ovary and pituitary gland, so it is closely related to the endocrine system Closely related to the male reproductive system
	Vagina	Lies below the uterus in the midline, deep in the pelvis and open to the outside	1 Receives the male penis during insemination (intercourse) 2 Semen containing sperms is deposited high in the vagina during insemination 3 Forms part of the birth canal during the birth process	Closely related to the male reproductive system

Name of system	Major organs	Position and location	Functions	Inter-relationships
Reproductive system – male				
	Testes	Lie in skin bags (called the scrotum) behind the penis and outside the abdominal cavity	**1** Production of sperm **2** Secretes hormones (see above under endocrine system)	Related to the locomotor system, producing growth Closely related to female reproduction
	Vas deferens	Tubes (which come from the testes) loop around the ureters and enter the base of the urethra within the prostate gland	Transport the sperms from the testes to the urethra during insemination	Closely related to female reproduction
	Prostate gland	Lies in the midline below the bladder around the urethra in the pelvis	Produces fluid which matures sperms and which forms part of the semen	Closely related to the female reproductive system Is connected to part of the urinary system
	Penis	Lies in the midline, mainly outside the abdominal cavity in front of the testes	**1** Contains the urethra along which urine passes from the bladder to the outside **2** Contains the urethra along which semen passes during insemination **3** Contains spongy tissue which fills with blood during sexual excitement to make it stiff enough to penetrate the vagina during insemination	Closely related to the female reproductive system Forms part of the urinary system

Monitoring clients in care

When carers are looking after clients in any setting, it is important they are always alert to changes in people, and whether change indicates deterioration or improvement in the client's condition. Clients may deteriorate slowly and this may put their lives in danger, or indicate that their quality of life is not as good as it used to be. An alert carer should be able to recognise such changes and ensure these are brought to the attention of appropriate people, such as line managers, doctors or even the emergency services.

Improvements in conditions should also be noted, as these might mean there should be changes in the client's care package, that different aids could improve the quality of life (including increasing independence), or that some services may no longer be required.

In a busy care environment it can prove difficult to monitor large numbers of clients, so routine observations and measurements are carried out and recorded. When a client enters a care environment for the first time, it is important to carry out an assessment of his or her health so that later changes can be monitored.

Routine observations and measurements are undertaken by a variety of health professionals to monitor the growth and development of babies and children from birth until adulthood. Any change from normal may need to be acted upon to prevent further physical or emotional damage. For example, visual and auditory tests are regularly carried out on babies and schoolchildren.

Increasingly, adults are encouraged to have regular health checks (such as measuring blood pressure, breast screening, cervical smears, etc.) to pick up any deviations in health and to arrest any serious illnesses before they become life-threatening. Family, school, work and hospital doctors all carry out routine checks to help diagnose any illnesses among their clients.

Observing clients

Posture

The client's **posture** while walking, standing or sitting can be observed by a carer quite quickly.

A person's posture is affected by pain, muscle and bone disorders, condition of joints and any disorder of the nervous system. People may try to disguise their pain, but altering position often results in a grimace, a sharp intake of breath or holding the body in a different way.

Complexion

Complexion is the colour and texture of a person's skin. It is frequently the complexion of the face we notice first, as this is uncovered.

Beware of signs of disguise by heavy make-up. Pallor (paleness) can be checked elsewhere, such as in the pink part of the fingernails or in the inside of the lower eyelid. Pallor most commonly indicates anaemia and a blood examination will confirm this condition. Anaemia is a lack of oxygen-carrying capacity in the blood and it leads to fatigue and breathlessness. If a client has a heart or lung disease, anaemia can seriously complicate his or her condition.

Conversely, an unusually high colour can indicate various skin conditions, infectious diseases (such as measles) or an **endocrine** (gland) disorder (such as **hyperthyroidism**). You are not expected to diagnose, just to observe, report and be alert if necessary. It is always important to notice bruising or capillary damage anywhere on the body, and to remain vigilant for possible signs of physical abuse or blood disorders.

Skin

The **skin** might be dry due to age or **hypothyroidism**, for example. It may be wet, infected, spotty, scaly or scabby as a result of highly infectious diseases (such as impetigo) or treatable skin disorders (such as dermatitis, psoriasis or eczema).

It is important to notice when parts of the skin look bluish. This is known as cyanosis, and is most commonly seen in the lips, tongue and nails, where blood capillaries run close to the surface. It is due to poor oxygenation of the blood and requires medical investigation. There are several causes, the most common being heart and lung disorders.

If the skin is inflamed (red, hot, swollen and painful), look for wounds or breaks in the surface of the skin and clean these with antiseptic lotion and cover with a sterile dressing. Observe the progress daily and if there is no improvement after 2 or 3 days refer the client for medical assistance. The client may require antibiotics or other treatment.

Hair

Many **hair** disorders are purely cosmetic problems, but they can also indicate a more serious disorder (such as hypothyroidism or malnutrition) when the hair is brittle and dry. Infection with head or pubic lice causes itching, which leads to scratching. Scratching can lead to impetigo and dermatitis.

Eyes

The **eyes** can be red, watering, infected or swollen, and causes of these conditions include foreign bodies, injuries, infectious diseases or eye disorders. All need reporting and treating to prevent permanent damage. Aged eyes appear faded and a white ring is often clearly visible on the outer edge of the iris – this is called the arcus senilis. Cataracts appear as a white opacity where the blackness of the pupil used to be. Cataracts are painless but affect the ability to see. The inner lens of the eye, normally transparent, becomes opaque due to degenerative changes in lens substances. Many eye conditions can signify disturbance of the body systems, so observe them carefully.

Mouth

In the **mouth** (apart from deformities such as cleft lip and palate), the most common problems are infections and ulcers. Thrush (a fungal infection giving rise to cream-coloured patches on the lining of the mouth) is common in the young and the old, in people taking antibiotics and in those who are taking drugs to suppress the immune system after organ transplants.

Fingernails

With the **fingernails** (as well as checking for signs of changes in skin colour as mentioned above), it is important to note any early indications that the fingernails are regularly bitten, which could be a sign of stress or nervousness.

The above list is by no means complete nor is anyone expecting you to diagnose illnesses. But remember to be alert and to observe changes! Apart from these physical signs, you should also observe the level of consciousness in individuals, and any changes in their mood.

Consciousness

Consciousness is an awareness of our self and of our surroundings. If consciousness starts to deteriorate a person may end up in a stupor, where he or she can be aroused only briefly by vigorous external stimulation, or in a coma, where the individual is unconscious and unresponsive. There are many causes, both accidents and illnesses, but it is clearly very important to draw an appropriate person's attention to a client whose consciousness levels are altering.

Changes in mood

Change of mood may be perfectly normal – we all experience times when we feel down or 'blue', and other periods when we feel good or even elated. Some people, particularly those prone to mental illness, may experience rapid mood swings for little or no cause. Carers need to learn to recognise these signs and to anticipate when medical intervention is necessary.

Taking measurements

Measurements are extremely useful in care situations because they are more precise than observations. Observations are usually qualitative – reflecting our ideas and opinions in words – whereas measurements are usually quantitative (they are based on numerical values). Carers are somewhat limited in the range of measurements they can take because they do not wish to cause extra stress to the client and must usually use non-invasive techniques. The most useful measurements that can be easily obtained include the following:

- The client's weight in kilograms.
- The client's height in metres or centimetres.
- Body temperature in degrees Celsius (Centigrade is another name for this scale, and the Fahrenheit scale is obsolete – this is not used any more).
- Pulse measurements in number of beats per minute.
- Breathing or respiratory rate in number of breaths per minute.

- Vital capacity in litres.
- Tidal volume in litres.
- Fluid input and output in litres and millilitres.

Expected range of measurements

Weight and height

The weight and height of children are checked as a routine index of growth, and these measurements are included in routine physical examinations.

Divergence from normal weight for height at any age may have medical implications. Ideally, a person should be weighed before breakfast wearing light clothing or none at all. The weight should then be compared with charts that show an individual's height and sex. You probably did this in your work for Unit 2.

Serious deviations from the norm may be the result of malnutrition, disease, mental illness (such as anorexia or bulimia), endocrine disturbance or accumulation of fluid.

Body temperature

Although 37 °C is often quoted as the normal body temperature, in truth very few individuals, when measured, would register that temperature – it is merely an average. The accepted normal range of temperature is from 36.5 °C to 37.2 °C, depending on where it is measured (the mouth, armpit or rectum), and on the subject's activities (including exercise, sleep, eating and drinking). The time of day also influences body temperature. Temperatures are lowest around 3 am and during sleep; they are highest after exercise and after taking hot food and drink.

A temperature higher than 37 °C in the mouth or 37.7 °C in the rectum is usually defined as fever (or pyrexia) and this is mainly caused by bacterial or viral infection. Temperatures lower than 35 °C result in the condition known as **hypothermia**. This is a serious medical condition which leads to lowered heart and breathing rates, lowered consciousness and even death. Urgent medical treatment or first aid is required.

Pulse rate

Pulse rates are covered more fully in Unit 2. Normal pulse rate is said to be 70 beats per minute, but again this is an average figure. Rates higher than this (say over 80 beats per minute) will be normal during or after exercise, but abnormal at rest, usually indicating a heart disorder. Low rates of below 60 beats per minute can also indicate heart problems. Hypothermia produces lower heart rates. Athletes have lower pulse rates than average people, at around 65 beats per minute. Pulse rates are increased by fever and infections. Babies and children have much higher pulse rates than adults (over 100), and these gradually decrease with age.

Breathing or respiratory rates

Babies also have a higher breathing rate than adults, about 30–40 breaths per minute compared to a normal adult range of 13–17 breaths per minute. During vigorous exercise, this can increase up to 80 breaths per minute. At rest, higher breathing rates occur in fever, shock, anaemia, hyperthyroidism and lung disorders, where effort is being made to carry more oxygen around the body. Lower breathing rates occur in hypothyroidism and hypothermia.

When checking someone's breathing, look for the rise and fall of the chest or listen to the flowing in and out of air. It is also good practice to check for difficulty in breathing (such as in asthma, whether there is a cough present and whether the breath is dry, rattley, hoarse, etc.) and whether sputum has been produced. Blood or pus in sputum indicates serious lung disease and needs medical intervention.

Lung volumes

The quantities of air flowing in and out of the chest can be measured quite easily with special apparatus, or in a laboratory using calibrated bottles, water and rubber tubing.

Vital capacity is the maximum quantity of air that can be breathed out, and the amount varies with the size of the chest. It is usually 5–6 litres. Females have smaller chest capacities than men, and clearly children are smaller still. A shortfall in vital capacity signifies a lung disorder.

Tidal volume is the amount of air that ebbs and flows with each breath during rest – it normally measures 0.5 litres.

Fluid input and output

Normally, the amount of fluid taken in by the body matches the amount put out in urine, expired air and sweat. Some individuals may have an imbalance and need to have their fluid input and output logged on charts.

If fluid input is greater than output, fluid is collecting somewhere in the body. This may put an extra strain on the heart, or produce swollen tissues called **oedema**. People with heart failure readily develop this condition. If output is greater than input, another serious condition may develop – **dehydration**, and the organs will function less well as a result. Dehydration can eventually cause death.

Applying knowledge of the systems of the body to caring for clients

Factors affecting body temperature

Just as fluid needs to be balanced, so does the amount of heat taken in by the body and the amount given out (Figure 4.19). This is so in order that body temperature can be maintained within the narrow limits previously described.

An individual has some control over heat gain because he or she can take cold food and drink or choose shade rather than sun. We can also choose to remain inactive, which further reduces heat gain. Heat loss, on the other hand, can only be controlled by the skin. Some of the technical terms relating to loss are as follows.

Conduction

The body warms up anything it comes into contact with by **conduction**. We all know that a recently vacated seat is warmed by conduction from the person who has just left it, and so are our clothes, bedding, etc.

Convection

The body warms up a thin layer of air close to the skin which becomes less dense and moves upwards to be replaced by colder air from the floor. This is why a room is always warmer near the ceiling than the floor. When a lot of people are in a room together there are many **convection** currents moving towards the ceiling. When the warm air hits the ceiling it moves sideways, becomes colder, and slides down the walls to the floor again.

Conduction and convection can both be modified by wearing thick clothes in winter and light clothes in summer.

Radiation

Heat flows from a warm body to a cold one. If we make our skin hot, more heat will be lost by **radiation** from it. If the skin is cold, less heat will be lost. If more blood flows to the skin it warms the skin, and the skin becomes pink and warm to the touch. So when we need to lose heat through radiation, the capillaries in the skin widen and more blood flows nearer the surface, causing more heat to be lost.

On the other hand, when we need to conserve heat because our body temperature is falling, the skin capillaries narrow and less blood flows to the skin surface. Our skin now feels cold to touch

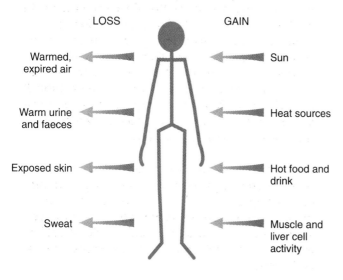

Figure 4.19 The means by which our bodies gain and lose heat

and looks white or even bluish. In these circumstances, less heat is lost by radiation and more heat is retained in the body.

The brain and nervous system control the blood vessels and respond to skin receptors which send messages to the brain about rises and falls in body temperature.

Sweat or evaporation of water

This is the most effective way of increasing heat loss from the body. Sweat glands in the skin are excited by the brain and nervous system and they pour out sweat (a very dilute mixture of salt) on to the surface of the skin. To convert the water in sweat to water vapour (which will move off into the atmosphere), a heat source is needed – and this is the hot skin surface itself.

Heat is used to convert the water into water vapour, and so the skin surface becomes cooled. When the body is cold and heat needs to be conserved, sweating stops.

Variations in radiation and sweating are the chief ways the body controls its temperature range.

Effects of extreme variations in body temperature

New-born babies and elderly people are unable to control their body temperatures as well as other people because their nervous systems are not fully developed or are worn out. This is why these client groups are more susceptible to hypothermia than others. Athletes and walkers produce a lot of heat through muscular activity, but they also lose a lot of heat through sweating. Athletes tend to wear very light clothing and can easily become chilled after a race is over – hence the use of space blankets to reflect the heat back on to their bodies.

Have you ever let yourself dry naturally after swimming on a hot day? Do you remember how cold you felt an hour or two later? This is because the drying process took heat away from your body surface and made you cold. Exposure to cold weather and to the wind clearly removes extra heat from the body and increases the risk of hypothermia (particularly in walkers and climbers). We must remind ourselves that most people can alter their behaviour to suit external conditions

(such as putting on extra clothing, curling up to reduce exposure, sheltering, switching on sources of heat and so on). But one susceptible client group – people with learning difficulties – may be unable to anticipate changes or may travel unsuitably clad. Hence the responsibility for preventing exposure and hypothermia may lie with carers. Also, people with mobility difficulties cannot use exercise to warm themselves up, and may become colder than the rest of us.

Pyrexia (overheating) is often a sign of infection. It is particularly dangerous in babies and young children, and can produce fits.

Effects of pressure on the skin and ways of relieving pressure

Someone who has a disease or who has damage to part of the body, or anyone confined to bed or to a wheelchair, can develop deformity through the stiffening of the muscles and the shortening (contracture) of the muscles and tendons. This is the result of continuous pressure from being in the same position. Regular turning of bedridden clients helps to prevent these problems.

Babies' skulls are often slightly deformed by pressure in the womb and at birth. They rapidly correct themselves within a few weeks after birth, however, and are not a cause of concern.

Pressure sores are ulcers that develop on the skin of clients who are bedridden, unconscious or immobile. They start as red, painful areas which become purple. The skin then breaks down and an open sore develops. Once the skin has broken, the sores enlarge, deepen and prove very difficult to heal. Prevention is very important as sores can become very extensive and infected, particularly if the client is incontinent of urine.

Pressure sores are most common where the skin is over bone, as pressure from the weight of the body compresses the blood supply to that patch of skin and it becomes vulnerable to breakdown. Typical sites for breakdown include the shoulders, elbows, lower back, hips, buttocks, knees, ankles and heels.

A client should be turned every two hours, kept clean and dry, and barrier creams may be used if the client is incontinent of urine. Cushions and pillows placed between the knees and under the shoulders relieve the pressure of the weight of the body. Ripple-bed mattresses are often used – these pump air in and out of cylindrical sections to stimulate blood flow. Water beds are also useful for redistributing body weight. Sheepskin pads under the buttocks and around the heels and ankles are also effective in cushioning against pressure.

Causes and effects of friction on the skin and ways of reducing friction

Friction occurs when one surface moves over another. It can be helpful or a nuisance. If we did not wear shoes with soles that grip, our feet would tend to slip on the ground, so friction is helpful here. If carers drag a person in a bed, friction is created between the heels and other body parts and the sheets. This friction can cause pressure sores.

Any weight on a moving surface (such as body weight) increases friction and causes heat to develop. Special materials can be used for making sheets to reduce friction with the body. These can be natural fibres (such as cotton), artificial ones (such as polyester) or mixtures of both (polycotton). Getting rid of the old practice of starching sheets has also helped to reduce friction, and lubricating surfaces with creams or gels is helpful.

Causes and effects of poor circulation

Poor circulation may result from various disorders, some of which are shown in Figure 4.20.

Causes and effects of poor lung capacity

Lung capacity is the volume of air the lungs can hold, so poor lung capacity results when the lungs are shrunken, filled with something else, diseased or surgically altered. Some causes and effects of poor lung capacity are shown in Figure 4.21.

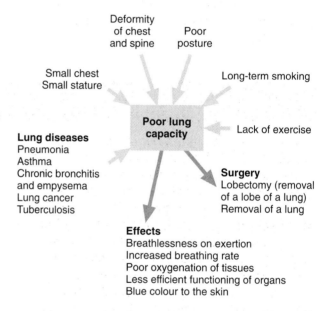

Figure 4.21 Some of the causes and effects of poor lung capacity

Disorders of arteries
• Narrowing (atherosclerosis) ⇒ tissue damage – pressure sores, confusion, cramp, dizziness
• Obstruction ⇒ tissue death – coronary thrombosis, stroke
• High blood pressure ⇒ coronary thrombosis, stroke, embolism
• Raynaud's disease ⇒ grey-blue skin colour, numbness, 'pins and needles'

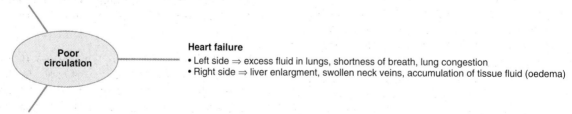

Disorders of veins
• Varicose veins ⇒ aches, swelling, itchiness, haemorrhoids
• Phlebitis (inflammation of veins) ⇒ swelling, tenderness, clot formation

Figure 4.20 Some of the effects of poor circulation

Unit 4 Assessment

Obtaining a Pass grade

You are required to produce an investigation into two major body systems and to describe their inter-relationships. Examples of these might be:

* the cardio-vascular and respiratory systems
* the cardio-vascular and digestive systems
* the nervous and musculo-skeletal systems.

These pairs of systems would enable you to gather relevant information about inter-relationships.

You are also required to describe the observations you could make to monitor a healthy client. You are asked to make observations involving two body systems, but you may carry out some of these observations on a fellow student or member of your family if you cannot gain access to clients or if there is likely to be a breach of confidentiality. State clearly why you made the observations on someone other than the client him or herself. Remember, you are asked to monitor healthy functions, not those of an illness.

The next task involves describing the state of a client's health and linking this to the care the client receives. The case study on Sammy should help you to understand what you have to do.

CASE STUDY – Sammy

Sammy has just been brought into hospital because he has hypothermia. He has not been using fuel to heat his flat as he has very little money. He has been put to bed in flannel pyjamas with a woolly hat on his head. As he is conscious he has been given a bowl of hot soup. Although Sammy was very pale when he came in, his skin is beginning to look a little pinker. Every half-hour, Sammy has his temperature and pulse taken and his breathing rate recorded. He was very quiet at first, but is beginning to talk a little; what he says doesn't always make sense, but he is getting better.

Explain how the care Sammy received is related to his state of health

You might start by connecting his low body temperature with the poor functioning of his organs (such as confusion, lack of interest, pallor of skin, etc.) When the surroundings cool the body cells, the chemical reactions inside the cells slow down. If the cooling continues, these reactions will eventually stop and life will cease. Confusion and lack of interest are signs that the brain is not working as it should be. Pallor of the skin shows that the skin capillaries have shut down in order to preserve heat for the vital organs – the brain, heart and kidneys.

It is important not to warm the skin first as doing so takes vital blood from the major organs (the heart, lungs, brain, liver, etc.). The bed warms the whole of his body without causing skin dilatation. The woolly hat stops further heat loss from his head. The hot soup passes to his stomach and warms him up from the inside.

Sammy's temperature is monitored regularly at short intervals to check there is no further decrease and to make sure it has started to rise. His pulse is monitored to check his heart is now beating more strongly and that the rate is increasing. His skin colour is monitored to check improvement in the circulation in the blood under the skin and to check heat distribution. Sammy's respiration is monitored to check his respiration rate is returning to normal.

After his body temperature has returned to normal range, Sammy will be monitored at longer intervals. The hospital would arrange for a welfare officer to discuss the financial side of heating his flat – or else Sammy will be back in hospital again in the next spell of cold weather.

Obtaining a Merit grade

To obtain a *Merit* grade, you must demonstrate you have a good understanding of the two body systems you have chosen. To do this, you will need constantly to ask yourself how? What? Why? When? Where? You will also have to put much more detail into your work.

Your understanding of the inter-relationships must also be deeper. An example of how you could demonstrate this would be to study the inter-relationship of the cardio-vascular and respiratory systems at rest, during mild exercise (such as stepping on and off a step 20 times) and during severe exercise (such as running round the block). Be careful – make sure it is all right for your 'client' to undertake such exercise!

Finally, you are asked to link the type of care a client receives to two body systems. The case study used above as an example would come into this category. For example, if a client has infected pressure sores, you would need to link this with the lack of blood supply to the skin surface. The capillaries have been unable to function properly due to the pressure – the client's weight has been compressing them for a long period of time. This is probably because the client is bedridden due to illness. The skin surface has broken down as a result of this and infection has occurred. The client may be incontinent and bodily waste has contaminated the area. The care received by the client would involve the circulatory system and the skin because they would need turning regularly to improve the skin circulation, antibiotics to overcome the infection and hygienic cleaning of the skin surface to prohibit further contamination.

Obtaining a Distinction grade

You must demonstrate a fluent use of technical language throughout your work, including explaining to your client the reasons behind making the observation and taking the measurements.

You will also need to make suggestions as to how the care a client receives could be improved to give maximum benefit to one body system and to minimise harmful effects on another. For example, using the case study of Sammy again, you could explain how eating energy-rich foods (such as potatoes, rice, bread and pasta) and taking some mild exercise twice a day would lessen the chances of hypothermia developing again, would improve his heart and circulation and reduce the stiffening in the joints of his musculo-skeletal system.

Unit 4 Test

1   In what state of oxygenation is the blood in the following blood vessels (high or low)?

  ◦   Aorta.
  ◦   Pulmonary artery.
  ◦   Coronary artery.
  ◦   Pulmonary vein.

2   State the function of the following parts of a joint:

  ◦   Cartilage.
  ◦   Synovial fluid.
  ◦   Ligaments.

3   Suggest one inter-relationship between the musculo-skeletal system and the nervous system.

4   At what time during pregnancy does an embryo become a foetus?

5   You have a client who is confined to bed. What options do you have to prevent the formation of pressure sores?

6   You are on holiday in a very hot place. Which main methods of heat loss would you use to cool your body down?

7   What is oedema?

8   Describe the arrangement of the fulcrum, load and effort in a first-order lever.

9   Describe the features in the small intestine that make it a suitable place for the absorption of the end products of digestion.

10   Suggest one cause of a low pulse rate.

Planning and preparing food for clients

This unit covers the knowledge you will need in order to meet the assessment requirements for Unit 5. It is written in seven sections.

Section one describes those things that make up a healthy diet and explains how to plan a balanced diet. Section two discusses the effects an unbalanced diet can have upon our health. Section three explores those things that influence an individual's choice of diet. Section four considers food hygiene and storage and the problems concerning food contamination. Section five outlines the procedures involved in food planning, preparation and handling. Section six suggests ways we can help clients who need assistance with eating. Finally, section seven discusses the safety issues involved in all aspects of handling food.

Advice and ideas for meeting the assessment requirements for the unit and for achieving Merit and Distinction grades are at the end of the unit.

Also at the end of the unit is a quick test to check your understanding.

Diet

The constituents of a healthy diet and the sources of nutrients

Unit 2 discusses those things that constitute a balanced diet. This unit, however, goes further, considering such things as recommended dietary intakes, specific vitamin and mineral requirements, and good sources of nutrients. Figure 5.1 outlines the basic constituents of a healthy diet and why our bodies need these substances.

(*Note:* The tables in this unit are for reference only; you are not expected to learn them!)

'Recommended dietary intake' is that quantity most nutritional experts agree is necessary for people in general to maintain a healthy lifestyle. However, as we have already seen, people are not all the same and, hence, dietary intake will vary from one person to another. For example, female adolescents and adults need more iron than males because they lose iron-containing blood during menstruation (and during childbirth.) Their recommended dietary allowance of iron must, therefore, take this into account.

Although most nutritional experts agree about the broad principles that constitute a balanced diet, there is still controversy over the *amount* of some of the substances we must consume. For example, the recommended daily allowance of energy-giving foods (such as fats) varies depending upon an individual's level of activity. Our energy expenditure will influence how much of these foods we need.

Where we can be more certain, however, is in the amount of vitamins and mineral salts we need. We can also be a little more precise about our need for protein and about the energy requirements of different age groups.

Mineral salts and minerals

In Figure 5.2, you will find the most common mineral salts and the reasons why our bodies need these salts, together with the daily recommended intake for 5-year-olds, 15-year-olds, people aged over 50 years and the *extra* needs women have when they are pregnant. You will notice these amounts are given in milligrams. A milligram is one thousandth of a gram – a very small quantity indeed!

Figure 5.1 The basic constituents of a healthy diet

Nutrient	Comments
Carbohydrates	The two main types of carbohydrates are the sugars and starches. These provide the energy for all bodily processes. At least 60% of the diet should contain carbohydrates, preferably in their natural (unrefined) state, e.g. wholemeal flour rather than white flour
Fats	Fats also provide energy for bodily processes and are necessary for the formation of some hormones and for the formation of parts of the membranes that surround body cells. About 20% of the diet should be in the form of fats but no more than 30%. Polysaturated fats (found in meats and dairy products) tend to increase the amount of cholesterol in the body, whereas monosaturated and unsaturated fats (such as those found in olive oil, sunflower oil and fish) tend to decrease cholesterol levels. We do not need to supply our bodies with extra cholesterol: it makes enough for its own use. Too much cholesterol can lead to heart and circulatory problems
Proteins	Proteins are the main constituents of the body's organs and cells, and so are important for their growth and repair. Each protein is made up of chemicals called amino acids, of which there are 20 known types. The body cannot make eight of these amino acids itself and therefore these must be present in the food we eat (these are known as essential amino acids). About 20% of the diet should consist of protein foods.
Vitamins	Vitamins help to control the body's chemical reactions and some help in the release of energy from fats and carbohydrates. They do not provide energy in themselves and, consequently, they are required in only small amounts. Vitamins A, D, E and K are found dissolved in fats. Vitamins B and C, on the other hand, are water soluble. Vitamin deficiencies are fairly rare. Most people who eat a variety of foods have no need to take vitamin supplements
Mineral salts	Like the vitamins, mineral salts do not supply energy but are necessary to keep the body in good condition. For example, calcium is needed to make strong teeth and bones; iron is needed to make haemoglobin which carries oxygen round the body; zinc and magnesium help in the body's chemical reactions; and sodium and potassium are important constituents of body fluids
Fibre	Fibre, in the main, consists of the cell walls of plants. It passes through human intestines unchanged but is necessary to prevent constipation and bowel disorders
Water	Water is found in nearly all foods and drinks. It is essential to life as it enables substances to dissolve, blood to flow and the body's temperature to be regulated, etc.

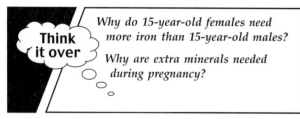

Think it over

Why do 15-year-old females need more iron than 15-year-old males?

Why are extra minerals needed during pregnancy?

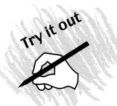

Try it out

Study Figures 5.2 and 5.3 to try to find the answers to the following questions:

1 Why are mineral salt deficiencies rare in people who eat a wide variety of foods?

2 Why is breakfast a very important meal?

3 Why are vegans (people who eat only plant products) at risk of iron deficiency?

Figure 5.3 lists the sources of these mineral salts.

The way vitamins work is explained in Figure 5.4.

Vitamins are found in a wide range of foods. A summary of rich sources of vitamins is given in Figure 5.6.

Figure 5.2 The most common mineral salts our bodies need

Mineral salt	Why we need it	Recommended daily allowances (milligrams)			
		5 years of age	15 years of age	50 years of age	Pregnancy (extra amounts)
Calcium	Strengthens the teeth and bones	800	1,200	800	400
Iodine	Used in the making of the hormone thyroxine, which regulates the rate of cell metabolism	90	150	150	50
Iron	Used in the making of haemoglobin, which carries oxygen round the body	10	18 (f) 10 (m)	10	50
Magnesium	Also contributes to bone and teeth formation, as well as to muscle contraction and enzyme reactions	200	300 (f) 400 (m)	300 (f) 350 (m)	150
Zinc	For growth, reproduction and enzyme activity	10	15	15	10

Note: f = female, m = male.

Figure 5.3 Sources of the most common mineral salts our bodies need.

Mineral salt	Red meat	Dairy products	Green vegetables	Whole-grain cereals	Pulses (peas, beans, etc.)	Fish	Water (hard)
Calcium		✓	✓		✓		✓
Iodine		✓		✓		✓	
Iron	✓			✓		✓	
Magnesium			✓	✓	✓		✓
Zinc	✓	✓		✓	✓	✓	

Note: An important source of iodine is iodised salt (ordinary salt which has had iodine added to it).

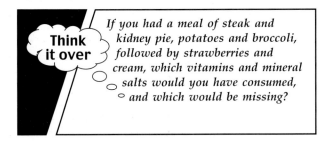

Think it over

If you had a meal of steak and kidney pie, potatoes and broccoli, followed by strawberries and cream, which vitamins and mineral salts would you have consumed, and which would be missing?

Figure 5.4   Vitamins and their effects upon the body

Vitamin	Effect on the body	Recommended daily allowances			
		5 years of age	15 years of age	50 years of age and over	Pregnancy (extra amounts)
Fat-soluble vitamins					
A	Protects against infection, helps with night vision, helps in the formation of bones and teeth	500 mcg	1,000 mcg	1,000 mcg	200 mcg
D*	Aids calcium absorption, promotes healthy bones and teeth, regulates the balance of calcium in body	10 mcg	10 mcg	5 mcg	5 mcg
E	Helps in enzyme activity and in red blood cell formation	6 mg	10 mg	10 mg	2mg
K	Promotes blood clotting	The quantities are not known because natural deficiencies of this vitamin are rare; it is made by bacteria present in the body's own large intestine			
Water-soluble vitamins					
C	Helps wounds to heal and prevents scurvy which causes bleeding in soft tissue, muscle and bone	45 mg	60 mg	60 mg	20 mg
B12	Helps in the production of red blood cells; helps to maintain the nervous system	2.5 mcg	3 mcg	3 mcg	1 mcg
Folic acid	(As for B12) Plus helps in the body's growth and in reproduction	200 mcg	400 mcg	400 mcg	400 mcg
Thiamine	Helps in enzyme activity and in the body's use of carbohydrates	0.9 mg	1.4 mg	1.2 mg	0.4 mg
Riboflavin	(As for thiamine)	1 mg	1.7 mg	1.4 mg	0.3 mg

Note: *1 microgram (mcg) is one thousandth of a milligram. Vitamin D can also be made in the skin when it is exposed to the ultraviolet light present in sunlight.

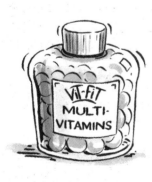

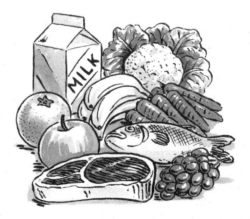

Figure 5.5   Which would *you* rather have?

Figure 5.6 Good sources of vitamins

| Vitamins | Main food categories | | | | | | |
	Meat	Dairy products	Fish	Green vegetables	Cereals/ bread	Fruit/ nuts	Non-green vegetables
Fat-soluble vitamins							
A	Liver	✓	Liver oils			Oranges	Carrots
D	Liver	✓ (especially butter and margarine)	Liver oils, oily fish				
E	✓			✓	✓	Nuts	Vegetable oils
K	Pork, liver			✓			Vegetable oils
Water-soluble vitamins							
C				✓		Citrus fruits, strawberries, blackcurrants	Potatoes
B12	Liver, kidney	✓	✓		✓		
Folic acid	Liver			✓	✓	Nuts	
Thiamine	Liver, kidney, pork		✓		✓	Nuts	
Riboflavin	Liver, kidney	✓			✓		

Protein

The amount of protein a person needs varies widely: some people can live healthily with a low protein intake while others may not. However, if our diet does not have sufficient carbohydrates and fat to meet our energy requirements, our bodies will break down protein to provide us with energy rather than using protein for the body's growth and repair. Protein foods are expensive whereas carbohydrates and fats are cheap. For example, bread and butter cost less than beef or ham.

A 5-year-old child needs about 45 g of protein per day, compared to 60–75 g for 15-year-olds and 55–70 g for the people over the age of 50. Adult males require more protein than females but, in all cases, the more active the individual, the more protein is required.

Carbohydrates and fat

Carbohydrates and fats supply our bodies with energy, and in Unit 2 you learned that about 60% of our diet should be starches and sugars and 20% should be fats. But how do we work out what an individual's energy requirements are?

Figure 5.7 Daily individual energy requirements

Age/activity/status	Daily energy requirements (kJ)
New-born baby	2,300
1-year-old baby	4,200
5-year-old child	7,500
15-year-old adolescent	12,600 (m) 9,600 (f)
Adult undertaking light physical work, e.g. office work	11,550 (m) 9,450 (f)
Adult doing moderate work, e.g. house-work	12,100 (m) 10,500 (f)
Adult undertaking strenuous activity, e.g. footballer, labourer	15,000-20,000 (m) 12,600 (f)
Pregnant mother in the last months of pregnancy	10,000
Mother who is breastfeeding an infant	11,300
An older person aged 75 and over	8,000-9,000

Note: m = male, f = female

Energy requirements are calculated based on an individual's age, gender and degree of activity (and also on such factors as whether she is pregnant or breast-feeding). Figure 5.7 suggests the energy requirements different people might need – these are expressed in kilojoules (kJ). Values used to be expressed in 'calories' (Cal) or kilocalories (Kcal). One calorie (Cal) or kilocalorie (Kcal) equals 4.2 kJ.

Our bodies can convert protein, carbohydrates and fat into energy. Each gram of protein and carbohydrate we consume is converted into 17 kJ of energy, and each gram of fat into 35 kJ.

CASE STUDY – Jennifer

Jennifer is a very active 8-year-old who seems always to be hungry. Her mother wonders if she is getting enough energy-containing food but does not know how to check this.

Based on tables of energy requirements, Jennifer's need is for about 8,800 kJ of energy per day. As noted earlier, 60% of this should come from carbohydrates:

$$8,800 \times \frac{60}{100} = 5,280 \text{ kJ}$$

To work out the number of grams of carbohydrate Jennifer needs, we divide 5,280 by 17 (remember, 1 g of carbohydrate = 17 kJ of energy):

5,280 ÷ 17 = 311 g or carbohydrate

Some 20% of her energy needs should come from fats:

$$8,800 \times \frac{20}{100} = 1,760 \text{ kJ}$$

Remembering that 1 g of fat is converted into 35 kJ of energy, we can work out the quantity of fat Jennifer needs:

1,760 ÷ 35 = 50 g of fat

To work out if Jennifer if getting enough energy from her food, her mother should look carefully at what Jennifer eats in a typical day and, using tables of energy values, plan a diet for Jennifer that will fulfil her requirements. (Some food labels supply information about kilojoule contents; otherwise tables listing the kilojoule content of specific foods can be obtained from food tables in books on nutrition – see page 190).

Figure 5.8 An analysis of Mrs Singh's current diet

| Food | Nutritional content | | | | | |
	Energy (kJ)	Protein (g)	Carbohydrate (g)	Fat (g)	Vitamins	Mineral salts
Tea with milk and sugar – one cup	80 (milk) 168 (sugar)	1.	1 (milk) 10 (sugar)	1 (milk) 0 (sugar)	Thiamine, riboflavin, trace of A and D	Calcium iron, (trace)
Bread	600	4.	23	0.75	Thiamine, riboflavin	Calcium, iron
Honey	200	0.	12	0	Riboflavin	Calcium, iron
Rice	1,530	6.2	86.8	1	Thiamine, riboflavin	Calcium, iron
Chicken	400	18.	4	0	Thiamine, riboflavin	Calcium, iron
Digestive biscuit	300	1.	10	3	Thiamine, riboflavin	Calcium, iron

CASE STUDY – Mrs Singh

Mrs Singh is an elderly widow who lives alone. Over the past three years, she has been steadily losing weight and has become quite frail. Her family doctor believes she may not be eating properly. This could be a result of a combination of factors, such as dental problems, a lack of interest in food generally and difficulty in shopping. The GP has asked Mrs Singh to list those things she eats in a typical day.

This is the list Mrs Singh gave to her doctor:

Breakfast: two cups of tea (with milk and one teaspoon of sugar)

Lunch: one slice of bread and honey, and one cup of tea

Evening meal: one portion (about 1 cupful) of boiled rice, $\frac{1}{2}$ cupful of cooked, chopped chicken and one cup of tea

Supper: one digestive biscuit and a cup of tea

Questions

1   Does Mrs Singh eat the right food each day (and in the correct quantities) to supply her with enough nourishment (energy, fat, protein and carbohydrates)?

2   Based on her current diet, work out Mrs Singh's vitamin and mineral intake.

3   What improvements could the doctor suggest to Mrs Singh's diet?

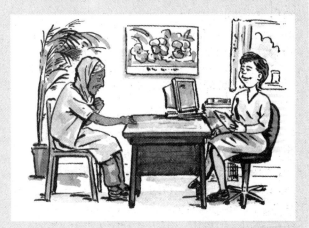

Figure 5.8 summarises the nutritional content of Mrs Singh's current diet. Figure 5.10 lists valuable sources of protein, carbohydrates and fat. Use these tables to help you decide your answers to these questions.

Fibre (roughage or cellulose)

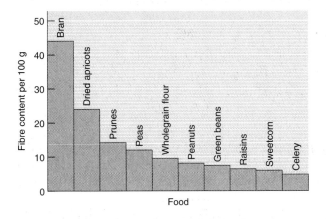

Figure 5.9 Good sources of fibre

As noted in Unit 2, our recommended daily intake of fibre is 25–30 g. Figure 5.9 lists the amount of fibre (in 100 g portions) contained in

Figure 5.10 Valuable sources of protein, carbohydrates and fat

Protein	Carbohydrates	Fat
Meat/liver/kidney	Sugar/sweets	Butter/margarine
Fish	Syrup/jam	Eggs
Eggs	Cereals	Bacon
Milk	Cakes	Oils/lard
Cheese	Bread	Cheese
Soya beans	Biscuits	Oily fish (herring, salmon)
Peas	Rice	Nuts
Beans	Pasta	Meat
Nuts	Potatoes	Whole milk
Bread	Beans	Liver

those foods that are good sources of this dietary requirement.

Water

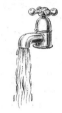

How much water we need depends very much on the temperature. When we are cold, we need to drink between 1.5 and 2 litres of water a day. When hot, this amount should be doubled because we sweat a great deal of water out of our bodies to keep our body temperature under control.

Water is essential to all forms of life

Approximately half the water we need we obtain from food; the remaining half we obtain through the process of respiration – through the air we breathe. This is the case no matter what the climatic conditions we live under.

Planning balanced diets

Planning a balanced diet is a complex process. You will need to consult the tables contained within this unit as well as the guidelines given in such standard sources of dietary requirements as the latest editions of:

Manual of Nutrition: Reference Book 342, Ministry of Agriculture, Fisheries and Food (London: HMSO, 1995. 10th ed. ISBN: 0112429912).

The Composition of Foods, D. A. T. Southwell (editor) (Cambridge: Royal Society of Chemistry, 1991. ISBN: 0851863914).

McCance and Widdowson's The Composition of Foods, Margaret Ashwell (editor) (British Nutrition Foundation, 1993. ISBN: 0907667074).

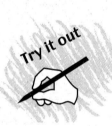

Try it out

One way to help you plan a balanced diet is to devise a diet for yourself (you will already have a good idea about how to do this from the case studies of Jennifer and Mrs Singh given earlier in this unit). You could devise this diet for a work day or for a day over the weekend. Remember to bear in mind the activities you plan to do on that day because this will affect your energy requirements. Figure 5.11 suggests a way you might go about planning your diet for your chosen day.

Once you have gone through all the steps listed in Figure 5.11, ask yourself the following questions:

1   Are the energy-providing foods you have listed in the correct proportions?
2   Have you taken into account your own gender?
3   Does the diet contain some fresh foods, such as fruit and vegetables?
4   Are all the required vitamins present, particularly the water-soluble types as these are difficult to store in the body?
5   Is there an adequate mineral salt and fibre content?
6   Is the amount of fluid you have allowed consistent with recommended daily allowances?
7   Do you need to change anything to improve your diet's nutritional content?

For example, you might need to consider the following:

◦   If you think the protein content is too low, you could add cheese to potatoes or change a drink of tea to milk or hot chocolate.

·   If you think the fibre content is too low, you could change white bread to wholemeal bread, or change a pudding for an apple or add an apple after a particular meal.

Remember, you do not have to be precise about the amounts of food you need to eat but you do need to be precise about the reasons why you have included them.

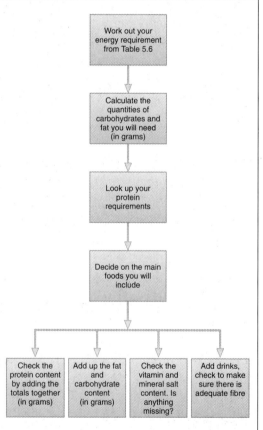

Figure 5.11 The steps involved in planning a balanced diet for yourself for one day

Figure 5.12 An analysis of some common foods (in 100 g portions)

Food	Energy (kJ)	Protein (g)	Carbo-hydrates (g)	Fat (g)	Vitamins	Minerals
Grilled bacon	1,850	25	0	40	B12	Calcium, iron
Pork chop	1,400	30	0	25	B12, thiamine, riboflavin	Calcium, iron
Sausage	1,250	10	12	25	Thiamine, riboflavin	Calcium, iron
Chips	1,115	4	40	11	c, thiamine, riboflavin	Calcium, iron
Beefburger in bun	1,115	14	55	10	B12, thiamine, riboflavin	Calcium, iron
Chicken	621	25	0	6	Thiamine, riboflavin	Calcium, iron
Liver	1,020	25	6	14	A, D, C, B12, thiamine, riboflavin	Calcium, iron
Butter	3,000	25	0	40	A, D	Calcium, iron (trace)
Cheese	1,800	25	0	35	A, D, B12, thiamine, riboflavin	Calcium, iron (trace)
Egg (1)	612	12	0	11	A, D, B12, thiamine, riboflavin	Calcium, iron
Milk	274	3	5	4	A, D, C, thiamine, riboflavin	Calcium, iron (trace)
Cod in batter	850	20	8	10	B12, thiamine, riboflavin	Calcium, iodine, iron (trace)
Rice	1,531	6	86	1	Thiamine, riboflavin	Calcium, iron (trace)
Bread (white)	1,068	8	55	2	Thiamine, riboflavin	Calcium, iron
Bread (wholemeal)	1,025	10	47	3	Thiamine, riboflavin	Calcium, iron
Banana	326	1	20	0	A, D, thiamine, riboflavin	Calcium, iron (trace)
Apple	1,970	0	12	0	A, C, thiamine, riboflavin	Calcium, iron (trace)
Baked beans	270	5	10	0	A, C, thiamine, riboflavin	Calcium, iron
Carrots	100	0	6	0	A, C, thiamine, riboflavin	Calcium, iron (trace)
Apple pie	1,180	3	40	15	A, C, thiamine, riboflavin	Calcium, iron (trace)
Cola (medium)	567	0	0	0	0	0
Fruit yoghurt	410	5	18	1	A, C, D, B12, thiamine, riboflavin	Calcium, iron (trace)

Textbooks on catering and biology (particularly human biology) might also be of help, but these may not be as detailed as the books listed above.

The effects of an unbalanced diet

As we have already noted, a balanced diet is one that supplies us with energy-giving foods in the correct proportions and that provides us with adequate amounts of protein, vitamins and mineral salts. It should also contain plenty of fresh fruit and vegetables and the correct amount of water.

But why should we be concerned about a balanced diet? Because if our diet has too much of one food and not enough of another, we will sooner or later begin to show signs of physical ill-health.

Figure 5.13 lists some of those conditions that must arise as a consequence of an unbalanced diet. It is important to remember that several of these conditions, if left untreated for a long period of time, could be fatal.

Loss of appetite

People might lose their appetites temporarily for several reasons. Some of the most common of these reasons are listed below:

- Depression can cause a lack of interest in most things, including food.

- Strong emotional feelings (such as grief, being in love, excitement or fear) tend to depress our digestive secretions and, consequently, our desire for food.

- Mouth problems (such as pain from gum disease, dental decay, poorly fitting dentures, inflammation or tumours) will cause a loss of appetite.

- Frail physical health is often reflected in a poor appetite (for example, extreme old age or chronic illness).

- Over or under-cooked food is unappetising.

- Some food looks unappetising because it lacks colour. Cauliflower, fish and potatoes can look insipid; sloppy food running over the side of the plate similarly looks tasteless and bland.

---

1 Diets that contain too little or too much energy-giving food will result, in the long term, in a change of body weight.

2 A diet that does not provide sufficient energy will make a person feel tired, cold and less inclined to exercise or work. This will happen very quickly.

3 Diets that contain too much energy-giving food will result in fat being deposited under the skin and round the organs. The person will feel less inclined to be active as a result, which will make the situation worse in the long term.

4 A low protein intake will eventually make a person more vunerable to infections, and bodily functions will become less efficient.

5 A too high protein intake will cause extra work for the liver and kidneys. This is wasteful as protein foods are expensive. Proteins cannot be stored in the body – unused proteins are broken down and excreted.

6 A lack of vitamins will mean the enzyme systems are less efficient, the body is more prone to infections, certain types of anaemia may occur, and bones and teeth may become fragile. Vitamin deficiencies take time to manifest themselves.

7 A lack of vitamin D can produce rickets in children (rickets makes children's bones become deformed). A lack of vitamin C causes scurvy, which means bleeding gums and poor wound healing.

8 Over time, a lack of iron leads to anaemia (tiredness and breathlessness on exertion, pallor, and a tendency to dizziness and fainting).

9 Similarly, the bones can become brittle if the calcium intake is low. A lack of iodine can lead to a swollen thyroid gland (goitre).

10 An imbalance in fluids can lead to dehydration or over-hydration, and extra work for the kidneys in excreting the surplus.

11 Diets that are too low in fibre can lead to bowel problems in later life, and constipation in the short term.

12 Lastly, but by no means least, too much fat in the diet leads to heart and circulatory problems.

Figure 5.13 Some of the health problems associated with an unbalanced diet

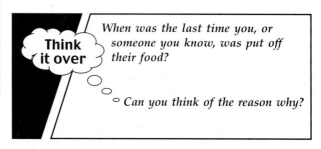

Think it over

When was the last time you, or someone you know, was put off their food?

Can you think of the reason why?

The dietary needs of clients

People do not eat the same food all their lives. Dietary needs change with age.

Changing needs with changing life stages

Newborn babies first take either breast milk or formula milk and, after a few months, start to take more solid food. This is because the reserves of nutrients they received from their mothers during pregnancy are getting low. They hence need to eat food that will supply them with sufficient energy to support their fast rate of growth and increasing activity. Milk alone cannot provide the sufficient quantity of kilojoules for their energy needs.

This process of turning to solid foods is called weaning and can last for several months as new foods and textures are slowly introduced into the baby's diet.

Toddlers are usually capable of joining in with most family meals, providing the food is cut up into small pieces. There are, however, some meals young children will not eat (for example, salads).

Older children readily eat most family meals but will probably have special favourites – usually soft foods such as jelly, custard and spaghetti.

Teenagers are usually very busy. They often like to meet up in fast-food restaurants, where they enjoy eating beefburgers, and chips and drinking milkshakes and cola. They frequently miss out on family meals and make up for this by eating snacks.

Adults prefer slower, more traditional meals (such as roast dinners and casseroles) but they may occasionally indulge in fast foods such as fish and chips. They also tend to be more aware of the need to include fresh fruit and vegetables in their diets.

Older people may take advantage of fast-food outlets to save themselves the time and effort of preparing and cooking meals. They are more likely to eat snack meals, especially if they live alone. The quantity of food eaten is usually much smaller than in earlier adult life as their need for kilojoules is reduced.

Influences on dietary needs
Gender

As we have already seen (Figure 5.7), women need less energy than men do. This is because they have a lower basal metabolic rate. 'Basal metabolic rate' is the amount of energy we need to keep all our bodily systems functioning properly while we are at rest or asleep. The heart still beats, breathing still takes place, urine is formed, the brain still functions and body temperature is maintained – but to do this requires energy. It is worth noting that infants and young children have a higher basal metabolic rate than adults, and this is why they need a higher proportion of energy per kilogram of their body weight than adults. Females have less muscle than males but more fat. This again reduces their need for energy.

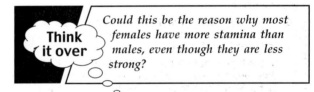

Think it over

Could this be the reason why most females have more stamina than males, even though they are less strong?

Physical activity

We have already noted the relationship between energy and activity. Our muscles use a lot of energy, so any activity that involves considerable muscular work will require us to eat more food. Sitting and standing use up approximately 6 or 7 kJ per minute (for an average 25-year-old male weighing 65 kg) but playing football raises this consumption to over 30 kJ per minute. Moderately hard work (such as gardening or cycling) uses up between 20 and 30 kJ per minute, whereas light work (such as driving or playing golf) only requires 10–20 kJ per minute.

Religion, race and culture

As we have seen throughout this book, the UK is a multicultural society. An individual's food preferences will vary depending on the individual's race, religion or culture. Examples of the differing food customs people in our society follow are listed on the following page:

- No animal products at all (the Hindu religion).
- No pig products or food containing blood (the Jewish and Muslim religions).
- Meat and dairy products not to be eaten at the same time (the Jewish religion).
- No alcohol (the Muslim religion).

Socio-economic factors

Many people in the Western world (Europe and America) and the majority of people in other countries have very little money to spend on food, due to their social conditions and lack of money. As a result they can only afford cheap staple foods such as bread, rice, maize and potatoes. The diets of these families are likely to be deficient in protein and some types of fat because protein foods tend to be expensive and are therefore difficult to buy. Different countries have different supplies of fruit and vegetables depending on their climates, so sometimes these can also be in short supply, and this means that many people's diets have vitamin and mineral shortages.

Affluent people (those with money) can afford to buy lean meat, out-of-season fruit and vegetables and exotic foods. Sometimes they overeat and do not take in enough complex carbohydrate and fibre-containing food.

People in poor housing conditions may not have electricity and gas to cook with and they would be even less likely to have microwaves, steamers or pressure cookers.

Without the right equipment to store and cook food or the money to buy all the components of a diet, it is impossible to follow guidelines for a balanced diet – simply trying to get enough food to survive is the main concern.

You need to take account of your client's social and economic conditions when designing a diet for him or her; otherwise it will simply be ignored as being unrealistic and impractical to operate.

Personal preference
State of health

Someone in a poor state of health may not eat very much and may need to be coaxed into eating at all. It is therefore important to present the food well and not to pile heaps of food on to the plate. Such a person may also need his or her food to be cut up into small pieces. The food might also have to be fairly soft as eating is an energy-consuming activity and a frail person may soon tire if a meal requires a lot of chewing.

Clients who require special diets

Diabetes mellitus is a disease where the body's ability to produce insulin is impaired. Insulin is a hormone secreted by the pancreas, and our bodies need insulin to break down carbohydrates, protein and fat into a form our bodies can use.

Someone with diabetes mellitus, therefore, will have to be very careful about the content of the food he or she eats. Most diabetics must avoid foods containing sugar. As their bodies cannot break sugar down, it is absorbed quickly into the blood stream. This makes their blood sugar levels too high. To get rid of this excess of sugar in the blood stream, the body tries to excrete it in the urine. This causes the diabetic to urinate frequently, which means they use up a great deal of the water contained in their bodies. This in its turn leads to intense feelings of thirst.

Other symptoms of diabetes mellitus include an increased appetite, muscle wasting (because the

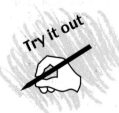
Try it out

In groups of three or four, make lists of those foods you do not like. Some people will have only a few dislikes but others may have many! The following is a list of some of the more common 'dislikes':

white of egg	tripe	liver	kidney
dates	figs	cucumber	cabbage
kippers	watermelon	squid	prunes

Would you like it if you were served your 'pet hates' time after time? Hence it is important when planning meals for clients to ask them for their preferences first.

body cannot obtain sufficient energy from the food eaten) or obesity (because of the excessive stored energy retained in the body) and susceptibility to infections (sugar is a good medium for bacteria and other organisms to live in!).

Complex carbohydrates (such as wholemeal bread) are therefore much better for diabetics as the sugar is released slowly during the digestive process. Carbohydrates have to be spaced out regularly, and meals should not be missed. If so, a diabetic's blood sugar level will fall too *low*, making the person feel dizzy and confused. Diabetics are taught to recognise these symptoms and often carry some sugar lumps to reverse falls in their blood sugar levels. They are also taught how to change their intake of carbohydrate in order to stabilise their blood sugar.

Food hygiene and storage

The basic rules of food hygiene and food storage

Figure 5.14 lists those things we must remember when preparing and serving food. Figure 5.15 lists guidelines for the safe storage of food. The right types of foods are important to health, as

- Always wash your hands before touching food, particularly after visiting the toilet, after touching animals, your own skin and hair, and after touching raw food.
- Always cover any break in the skin of your hands, or sores or spots, with a waterproof adhesive dressing (preferably a highly coloured one so you notice it if it comes off).
- No smoking during the preparation of food.
- Avoid preparing food if you have any illness (particularly skin, nose or throat infections and sickness or diarrhoea).
- Do not allow animals into the food preparation area.
- Cover food to protect it from flies and other insects.
- Wrap all food waste and dispose of it in a covered waste bin.
- Clean as you go. Wash surfaces down with hot water and detergent.
- Wipe spills up immediately with kitchen tissue and place this in a covered bin.
- Serve food as soon as possible after preparing it.
- Never allow raw food to come into contact with cooked food; common ways in which cooked food is contaminated from raw food are through the hands, knives and working surfaces.
- Wear clean clothing and be clean yourself.
- Do not cough or sneeze over food.

Figure 5.14 The basic rules of food hygiene

- Do not leave food at room temperature for longer than necessary.
- Bacteria can breed at room temperature.
- Store food either in a refrigerator or freezer.
- Label and date food stored in a freezer.
- Store frozen food according to the star ratings printed on the packet.
- Check refrigeration temperatures regularly.
- Place raw food below cooked food so that no drips can reach the cooked food.
- Cover all food when stored.
- Ensure no chemicals (such as cleaning fluids) are stored near to food.
- Use older food first – rotate the stock.
- Check sell-by dates and do not use food that is out of date.
- When dried food has been reconstituted with water, treat it as fresh food.
- Thaw food thoroughly after freezing, according to the instructions.
- Ensure dried food is stored in sealed, waterproof containers.

Figure 5.15 The basic rules of food storage

you have learned. However, if the food you eat makes you ill because it has not been prepared or stored safely, then having a balanced diet becomes less important. Older people and young babies are particularly vulnerable to food poisoning and may even die from it.

The main sources of food contamination

The main contaminants of food are bacteria and viruses. The most common of these are as follows:

- **Salmonella** The Salmonella bacteria lives in the intestines of humans, animals and poultry. If we eat food that contains salmonella this can make us violently sick, and it may also cause diarrhoea, stomach cramps and fever. However, the bacteria is destroyed by adequate cooking and safe food-handling procedures.
- **Campylobacter** also live inside animals and cause an illness similar to salmonella.
- **Listeria** are bacteria that can thrive in poorly prepared cook-chill food products. Pregnant women and people who have immuno compromised conditions (e.g. HIV/AIDS) are particularly prone to Listeria.

◇ **Staphylococci** are bacteria that live on the skin and in the upper respiratory tract. These bacteria can cause numerous illnesses and are controlled by safe food-handling procedures.

◇ **Escherichia coli** (usually known as E.coli) is a bacteria found in the faeces of humans and animals. It can cause a wide range of digestive illnesses, particularly in children. Contamination is controlled through hygienic food-handling procedures.

◇ **Norwalk virus** is a virus we can ingest from contaminated shellfish. It can cause gastroenteritis.

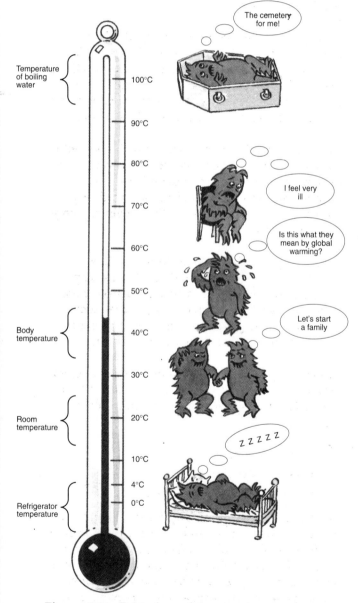

Figure 5.16 Bacteria and temperature

Other ways food can become contaminated are through incorrect storage near poisonous chemicals, the deliberate contamination of food by pressure groups and through poisonous fungi.

As we can see from the list on the previous page, cows, pigs, poultry, eggs, fish and shellfish are common sources of infection. Bacteria thrive particularly well in high-protein, moist foods. Raw food is always contaminated with bacteria. However, thorough cooking at high temperatures destroys most types of bacteria (see Figure 5.16), so it is important we do not allow raw food to come into contact with cooked food so that the cooked food is reinfected.

The planning, preparation, cooking and serving of food
Planning menus

What are the important things we must bear in mind when planning a menu?

Try it out

In small groups, discuss those things you need to consider when planning a menu for a specific client. It would help if you first decided exactly who the client is. Look back at the case studies earlier in this unit. These may give you some ideas about the types of things you must bear in mind when deciding on your client and in planning the menu. The following are a few ideas to start you off:

◇ personal preferences

◇ the equipment you have at your disposal

◇ the client's age, gender and current state of health.

Remember – healthy eating means a balanced diet.

Preparing and serving a meal

After covering yourself in clean, protective clothing and having washed your hands thoroughly, collect together all the ingredients you need for the meal. (You should keep your nails short and scrub under them with a brush.) Prepare the raw food first and then wash your hands before dealing with any cooked food. Remember, you may need to heat the oven to the correct temperature.

When the food is cooked, serve it in an appetising way: garnish it, perhaps with a small sprig of parsley on the potatoes or with a slice of tomato or lemon, which adds colour. Take care not to have drips or runs on the dish, as this looks unsightly. Put the plate on a tray that is covered with a cloth or paper mat. Do not forget to add appropriate, clean cutlery and salt and pepper. A small posy of flowers always makes a meal look more attractive.

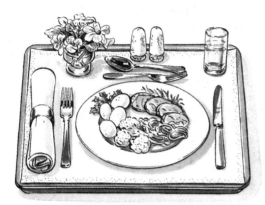

A well-laid table setting will make a meal far more appetising

Cooking food

If you have not yet learned to cook, borrow books from the library or ask a friend or relative to show you how. You should learn how to use cooking appliances safely and correctly to boil, simmer, steam, grill, bake and microwave food.

Supporting clients who need assistance with eating

It is important we maintain and respect our clients' independence and dignity as far as this is possible within the practicalities of the setting we work in. This principle applies equally if we are called upon to help clients with their eating. Do not force people to eat food they do not like. If you know someone does not like the fruit he or she is provided with, offer a drink of blackcurrant or fresh orange juice instead to supplement his or her vitamin C intake. Make sure the table is laid attractively and allow people to sit near companions of their choice. If you have to help clients who behave noisily or anti-socially at meal times, position them carefully at the table so that other people are not offended or put off their food. Provide napkins for those who are used to them and attractive crockery and cutlery. Make sure people who require dentures are wearing them.

Sitting at a table is the most comfortable position for eating, but some older people may need special support to be able to do this. Anyone with a weak arm (perhaps as a result of a stroke) will need his or her arm supporting. A client who uses a wheelchair will probably need a wider space at the table, or a table of their own specially adjusted for height. Some people may need chairs with arms for support, and others may need a cushion for padding and support.

A baby or toddler should be strapped in a high chair that has attached to it an easily washable tray. Plastic, washable floor mats are now available that can be laid down when a baby tries to feed him or herself. Progression to sit at the table may be accomplished through the use of a cushion.

Anyone who is bedridden should be helped into as near a sitting position as possible because it is extremely difficult to eat while lying down. Feeding cups (which are rather like small teapots with spouts) are available for those who can only lift their heads.

When people find it difficult to use cutlery, specially designed large-handled utensils may help, and rubber grips can be placed over these. Non-slip mats beneath plates stop plates sliding on the table, and guards on the edges of plates enable the food to be 'trapped' more easily.

Visually impaired people will usually have learnt how to recognise the positioning of the food on their plates through the following conventions (see Figure 5.17):

- meat at 12 o'clock
- potatoes at 6 o'clock
- vegetables at 3 and 9 o'clock.

Remember to tell the visually impaired person that the food is served and what it is. You should ask if he or she would prefer anything cut up or if he or she would like help with anything. Never overfill cups or glasses. Some visually impaired people prefer a dish with a rim to prevent their food sliding off the plate.

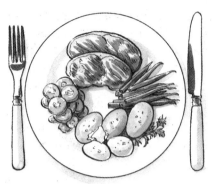

Figure 5.17 The conventional arrangement of food on a plate for a visually impaired person

If you do need to help an adult client to eat, try to sit alongside him or her. If you are working with very young children you might need to sit opposite in order to keep eye contact. Provide small, easily managed mouthfuls, allowing rests in between for swallowing. Offer the foods separately so that each taste can be appreciated. Many clients like to sip a drink with their meals as it helps them to swallow. You should take care with the temperature of both food and drink – make sure they are acceptable.

Safety first

Throughout this unit and throughout all the units in this book, the safety aspects of the procedures

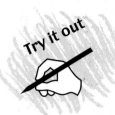

Try it out

Working in pairs, experience for yourself the problems clients might have while eating. Practise feeding yourself and your partner (you could use a snack for this or, preferably, a cooked meal). You might, for example, use a blindfold, tie rubber bands around two or three of your fingers, put your hands in cardboard splints to simulate arthritis, tie one hand behind your back and so on.

How did it feel?

How would you feel if the disability was permanent?

Discuss with each other how it felt to be fed by someone else. Also discuss the strengths and weaknesses of your partner's approach.

and jobs you may be called upon to undertake have been emphasised.

Focusing for the time being on the safety aspects involved in food handling and preparation, complete the following exercise. This should help you to check whether you have appreciated all the dangers and safety issues involved when handling food.

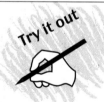

Try it out

On a large piece of paper (A3), write down the heading 'Safety'. Draw six columns down the paper and label these columns with the headings shown below. Write down appropriate safety points under each heading. Use this in your assessment. Some have been done for you to get you going.

Safety

Preparing myself safely	Using kitchen utensils safely	Cleaning food preparation areas	Using cookers safely	Serving food safely	Feeding clients safely
Tie long hair back	Always pass a sharp utensil to another person handle first	Use hot water containing detergent for washing	The handles of saucepans should not overhang the cooker	Don't pass hot food or drink over a client's head	Check the food or drink is not too hot or cold
Wash your hands with hot, soapy water and scrub under the fingernails			Never leave chip pans unattended		

Unit 5 Assessment

Obtaining a Pass grade

You will need to show that you have understood the components of a balanced diet including the correct proportions of the main nutrients that supply energy and raw materials for growth and repair. You can do this by planning a weekly balanced diet for a client that you know, taking into account his or her choice of food, economic circumstances, religion, culture, level of activity, age and gender. Include the time of year in your planning and provide food that is available in the shops at reasonable prices. Make sure that you give the reasons behind your selection of dishes so that you can demonstrate that the meals meet your client's needs. If your client has a medical condition that requires a special diet, such as diabetes, then you must show the importance of following a prescribed diet. You might ask to visit a dietician to get specific information relating to the client's condition.

You should be able to show your understanding of the causes of an unbalanced diet. These might include lack of money, illness, unsuitable false teeth, temper tantrums, inadequate facilities for preparing or cooking food, lack of time, poor cooking skills, a client living on their own, lack of education or depression. You will be able to think of several more potential causes.

The second part of your evidence collection relates to preparing, cooking and serving food and assisting clients with eating.

You need to produce a description of the safe practices you would use in preparing, cooking and serving food. Choose a two-course meal from your weekly plan and describe how you would make these meals and which safety points would be important. You could prepare a chart that included the key safety features or a flow diagram and annotations in colour with safety points. Remember to include protective clothing, appropriate storage, safe disposal of waste, handling of sharp tools such as knives and above all good personal and kitchen hygiene.

When you are describing the procedures for assisting a client with eating, you could compile a table with 3 columns like the one below.

Client's needs	Special aids available	Points of good practice
Client has had a stroke and has a weak right arm	Cutlery with thick, easy-grip handles	Allow the client to manage on his or her own as much as possible
	Self-tipping teapot	Ask if assistance is required with cutting of meat as client is right-handed
Client has visual impairment	No aids required	Place meat at 12 o'clock, potatoes at 6 o'clock, vegetables at 3 and 9 o'clock Explain to client the components of the meal and observe for difficulties
Client has difficulty chewing	Client manages best with a spoon and fork	Food is served in small pieces

You will find excellent free leaflets to help you with your assessment from:

* The Health Education Authority
* Local Health Promotion unit
* Family doctor's surgeries or health centres
* Supermarkets
* Ministry of Agriculture, Food and Fisheries: 'Healthy eating for older people', 'Healthy diets for infants and young children'.

Obtaining a Merit grade

You need to be more specific if you are trying to achieve a *Merit* grade and you must explain how one of the meals from your weekly plan meets the nutritional needs of your client. In other words, you need to analyse the food content of a meal and state the function of that food in the client's diet. Once again, a table would make the analysis clear and concise. You need to add the possible effects of an unbalanced diet. Describe the effects of eating an unbalanced diet over a period of time, using your client as your example. For instance, a young child who consumes many sugary foods and sweets is likely to be overweight and prone to dental decay. Alternatively, if he or she does not eat enough protein because of a dislike of meat and fish this may influence growth and the child might be shorter in height than others of the same age.

As well as showing that you understand the key features of health and safety during the preparation, cooking and serving of the two-course meal, you will need to explain how these safety measures prevent risks to clients and others. For example, thoroughly thawing poultry and then cooking it at a high enough temperature for the prescribed length of time will ensure that all harmful bacteria are killed and cannot cause food poisoning – particularly Salmonella bacteria. This protects any poultry consumers but also others who might develop the disease from poor

personal hygiene of the poisoned victims and others using the same facilities.

You need to provide evidence of ways you might encourage clients to greater independence with eating. For example, if Mrs Frith has her meat cut into small pieces, do it behind the scenes rather than cutting it up at the table where everyone can see. This will preserve her dignity and mean that she can eat her meal independently. Arranging the parts of the meal in the standard way before presenting it to a visually impaired client will increase the person's self-respect, but make sure that he or she knows what the meal consists of. It can be upsetting for someone who cannot see the food to start eating something that he or she does not like.

Obtaining a Distinction grade

To develop your work for this grade you will need to discuss some ways to improve your client's diet, giving reasons for your suggestions. For instance, you might substitute an apple for stewed apple if your client has no problems eating fresh fruit. This would provide more vitamin C (because it has not been cooked which reduces the quantity of water-soluble vitamin C) and provide more fibre to help with bowel action. You might add watercress to a salad dish to provide iron or add a spoonful of bran to a breakfast cereal of crisped rice to give more fibre. Try wholemeal bread for toast or sandwiches instead of white bread, brown rice instead of boiled white rice, and think about different cooking methods such as steaming fish to reduce fat (if it was usually fried) and retain more vitamins. Providing a glass of water might be beneficial to clients who have difficulties eating drier foods.

There are lots of ways to improve a person's diet and it is worth bearing this in mind when you construct the main weekly plan.

Secondly, you need to explore ways of improving the whole eating experience for your client. This might involve using special aids to assist certain clients, playing soft music, enhancing colour on the plate and improving the surroundings such as by putting small posies of flowers on the tables and by using brightly coloured paper napkins for a change. Some clients may eat noisily or have table manners which offend other clients –

you might think about moving one or two table settings with an invitation such as, 'Would you like to sit nearer the window?'.

Take care not to move people without giving them a choice, as you might end up upsetting clients who will then not eat their meals!

Unit 5 Test

1   Name the 7 major components of food.

2   Which component provides the most energy per gram eaten?

3   If you ate a meal comprising fish, chips and peas, which part of the meal would provide you with the material you need for the growth and repair of body tissues?

4   Mrs Smith requires more Vitamin D and calcium in her diet. Which of the following is a good source of these substances?

    a   Cheese on toast.
    b   Spaghetti on toast.
    c   Chicken salad.

5   Which of the following would help to maintain a client's independence?

    a   Providing him or her with a balanced diet.
    b   Making the food look attractive.
    c   Asking the client about his or her food preferences.

6   Vitamin C helps wounds to heal more quickly. Is this true or false?

7   State three basic rules concerning hygiene when handling and preparing food.

8   Name three types of bacteria that can cause food poisoning.

9   Your client has diabetes. How will this affect his or diet?

10   Describe how you should place food on a plate for a visually impaired client.

Meeting the needs of individuals in care settings

This unit covers the knowledge you will need in order to meet the assessment requirements for Unit 6. It is written in five sections.

The first section discusses the care value base and how this relates to the law, policies, procedures and care practice. The second section looks at the various ways we can assess our clients' needs. Section three explores the ways care plans can support our work with clients. How we can monitor the effectiveness of care plans is discussed in section four. Finally, section five outlines those factors that can influence the delivery of care services.

Advice and ideas for meeting the assessment requirements for the unit and for achieving Merit and Distinction grades are at the end of the unit.

Also at the end of the unit is a quick test to check your understanding.

Values in care settings

People receive care because they have physical, intellectual, social or emotional needs that make them vulnerable. Young children are vulnerable because their intellectual, social and emotional development depends on the care they receive. People with learning disabilities may not achieve their full potential unless they are given the right support. Older people may be socially isolated and emotionally vulnerable. People receiving medical treatment may face threats to their self-esteem.

Because clients are vulnerable, care workers must work within a set of values. These values are described in Chapter 1 of this book. The NVQ standards, published in 1998, emphasise the importance of valuing the diversity of people, their rights, responsibilities and confidentiality.

The three principles of the value base are to:

1   foster the equality and diversity of people;

2   foster people's rights and responsibilities; and

3   maintain the confidentiality of information.

To foster diversity, care workers must check they do not label, stereotype or make assumptions about people. Care workers should regard differences between people as a positive thing to be celebrated. Differences in race, sexuality, customs, age and gender should not be seen as a problem but as things that enrich our experience of life. People have a right to be different.

How to reduce the effects of discrimination

The two main reasons why discrimination occurs are as follows:

1   People have prejudices or have stereotyped views about others.

2   People assume that everyone should be the same as they are. They treat everyone the same way – the way they would like to be treated.

Many people are not sensitive to differences in other people. Being a good care worker requires you to learn about differences and to value differences. Some ways in which people are different are shown in Figure 6.1.

Some general ways to try reduce discrimination are as follows:

•   Learn about the different cultures and communities individual clients come from and about their beliefs.

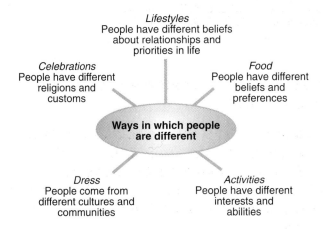

Figure 6.1 Some of the ways in which people are different

- Try to value the differences between people and to meet their different needs.

- Check you do not 'treat everyone the same' by doing the same routines and by giving everyone the same food. People are individuals and their needs are different.

- Use your listening skills to build an understanding of other people's needs – this may help to overcome stereotyped thinking and mistaken assumptions about other people.

You could try the exercise below to help with this.

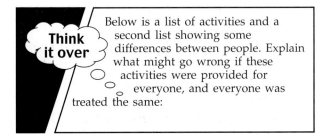

Think it over

Below is a list of activities and a second list showing some differences between people. Explain what might go wrong if these activities were provided for everyone, and everyone was treated the same:

Activities

- Learn how to cook bacon.

- Take turns in washing up.

- Sing Christmas carols.

- Play bingo.

- Go to a sherry or drinks party.

- Play cards, gambling for pennies.

- Learn to paint.

- Do old-time dancing.

- Talk about photographs of England in the 1920s.

Differences

- Religion.

- Beliefs about what it is right to eat.

- Beliefs about alcohol.

- Countries of origin.

- Ethnic groups.

- Gender and gender roles.

- Social class.

- Levels of practical ability and disability.

Clients' rights

Clients' rights are very important. For example, clients have a right to choose how to live. People have a right to practise their own religion but they have a responsibility not to impose their views on other people. People have a right to their own cultural beliefs and habits, but they have a responsibility to respect the different cultural beliefs and habits of others.

Figure 6.2 lists key rights and some of the ways of maintaining them.

Confidentiality and the boundaries of confidentiality

Confidentiality is an important right for all clients. But while clients have a right to confidentiality, they also have a responsibility in relation to the rights of others. Confidentiality may even have to be broken when the rights of others are affected.

Keeping confidentiality within boundaries means that a carer may need to tell his or her manager about something learnt in confidence. However, the information is not made public, so it is still partly confidential. Information may need to be passed on to managers when:

Figure 6.2 Key rights and ways of maintaining them

Clients have a right to	Ideas for maintaining these rights
Be different	Try to learn about different customs and lifestyles – be positive and interested in differences
Be free from discrimination	Understand different forms of discrimination. Be careful not to make assumptions about people. Watch for labelling and stereotyping. Identify your own beliefs and prejudices, and challenge your own prejudices
Confidentiality	Understand and follow policies and procedures on confidentiality. Never pass on information about clients to people unless they have a need to know.
Choice	Always ask clients what they would like – offer choices in the food, routines and help you can provide.
Dignity	Develop conversation and interpersonal skills that demonstrate respect for the people you work with
Safety and security	Watch for safety hazards and for risks to clients' property
Independence and the development of personal potential (sometimes called self-determination)	Use communication skills to understand each person. Ensure the rights to choice and dignity are maintained. Develop skills and approaches to support intellectual, social and emotional development

- there is a significant risk of harm to a client;

- a client might be abused;

- there is a significant risk of harm to others; and

- there is a risk to the carer's health or well-being.

Some examples of such situations are given below:

- An old person in the community refuses to put her heating on in winter; she may be at risk of harm from the cold.

- A person explains that his son takes his money – he might be suffering financial abuse.

- A person lives in a very dirty house infested with mice and rats. This may be creating a public health risk.

- A person is very aggressive, placing the carer at risk.

Confidentiality and legislation

The Data Protection Act 1984 was passed to protect people's rights about the way information about them can be stored. The Act originally covered only information stored on computer, but the Access to Personal Files Act 1987 extended the law to cover manual (paper-based) records kept by local authorities. The Access to Health Records Act 1990 further extended the law to manual records kept by health providers.

A new Data Protection Act was passed in 1998 which updates the law on confidentiality of information. This Act states that all records about clients that are filed will be considered as data, whether they are held electronically or on paper. The Act provides individuals with a range of rights, including the following:

- The right to know what information is held and to see and correct the information if necessary.

- The right to refuse to provide information.

- The right that data should be accurate and up to date.

- The right that information should not be kept for longer than necessary.

- The right to confidentiality – that the information should not be accessible to unauthorised people.

Care workers should always keep to the following principles regarding information:

- Keep information confidential, and only pass information on to people who have a right and a need to know it.

- Record information accurately.

- Keep records safely so that they cannot be altered or lost, or seen by people who do not have a need to use them.

Access to records

Not all care staff have access to all the information about clients. For instance, regulations under the Registered Homes Act 1984 require that residential homes keep a case record for each resident. Some homes maintain personal files on residents to which all permanent staff have access, although some sections may be restricted to senior staff.

The information available to all permanent staff may include personal details, such as the person's doctor, next of kin, age and religion. Details about personal finance, action to be taken after a resident's death and legal arrangements may be restricted to managers because other staff do not need this information in order to care for residents.

Personal files must be kept for at least three years after a client leaves care. Each home or service will have its own policies on recording information and on who has a need to know it.

Giving information

When information is passed to other professionals it should be passed on with the understanding that they keep it confidential. It is important to check that other people are who they say they are. For example, if you answer the telephone and someone says he is a social worker or other professional, you should explain that you must phone him back before giving any information. Phoning back enables you to be sure you are talking to someone at a particular number, or within a particular organisation. If you meet a person you don't know, you should ask for proof of identity before passing on any information.

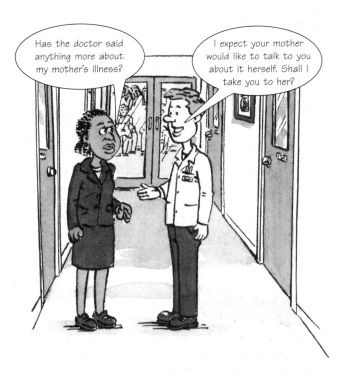

Figure 6.3 It is sometimes better if relatives discuss things directly with clients

Relatives will often say they have a right to know about clients. Sometimes it is possible to ask relatives to discuss issues directly with the client rather than giving information yourself (Figure 6.3). Remember, it is important to explain that you cannot share confidential information without the client's consent.

Legislation

The law establishes legal rights for people. The Sex Discrimination Act 1975, the Race Relations Act 1976 and the Disability Act 1995 explain people's rights not to be discriminated against. Other laws contained in the Health and Safety at Work Act 1974, the Registered Homes Act 1984 and the Children Act 1989 also create legal rights for people. Further details about the main Acts of Parliament that influence care are set out below.

Sex Discrimination Act 1975

This Act made it unlawful to discriminate between men and women in respect of employment, goods and facilities. The Act also made it illegal to discriminate on the grounds of marital status. It identified two forms of discrimination: direct and indirect discrimination.

The Act tries to ensure equal opportunities for both men and women to get jobs and promotion. To make sure that people's right are protected, the government set up the Equal Opportunities Commission to monitor, advise and provide information on men and women's rights under the law. Individuals can ask the Equal Opportunities Commission for help and advice if they believe they have been discriminated against because of their gender.

Race Relations Act 1976

This Act makes it unlawful to discriminate on racial grounds in employment, housing or services. Racial grounds include colour, race, nationality and ethnic or national origins. The Act makes it an offence to incite or encourage racial hatred. As with the Sex Discrimination Act, both direct and indirect discrimination are made unlawful. The Commission for Racial Equality was set up in 1976 to make sure the law against racial discrimination is enforced. The commission can investigate cases of discrimination and give advice to people who wish to take legal action because of discrimination.

Disability Discrimination Act 1995

This Act is designed to prevent discrimination against people with disabilities, in matters of employment, access to education and transport, housing and obtaining goods and services. Employers and landlords must not treat disabled people less favourably than non-disabled people. Services must ensure they meet the needs of disabled people.

The Children Act 1989

This Act established children's rights to be protected from significant harm. The Act also established the principle that children's needs should take priority when situations are assessed.

The National Health Service and Community Care Act 1990

This Act established the right that people who are in need of community care should have their needs assessed and have services to meet their needs, provided they meet certain criteria.

The Registered Homes Act 1984

This Act controls the setting up and running of residential care homes. It also sets out the conditions for registration and inspection of all residential homes. It lays down the rules covering staffing levels, facilities, record-keeping and safety. The records the home must keep must include the following information:

- A list of clients being cared for, their names, addresses, dates of birth and their GPs' details, as well as other personal information.

- A daily comment on the well-being of the client.

- Details of all staff employed by the home.

- Details of the practices agreed for health and safety, including fire practice arrangements and fire alarms.

- A record of the maintenance of equipment, such as cookers, heaters and lifts.

The Act also states the home must ensure there are adequate:

- levels of staffing;

- space, furnishings and lighting;

- kitchen and laundry facilities;

- arrangements for clients' medical and dental needs;

- arrangements for recording, safekeeping, handling and disposal of drugs;

- arrangements for the disposal of clinical waste; and

- arrangements for clients' occupation, recreation and privacy.

The Act states that homes must be registered with the local authority. Nursing homes are also covered by the Act and by the registration and inspection arrangements laid down within it.

The Health and Safety at Work Act 1974

The Health and Safety at Work Act 1974 is a piece of legislation that impacts on the running of homes as well as on other organisations where people are employed or clients dealt with. This Act details the responsibilities of both employers and employees with the aim of ensuring a safe working environment.

It states the employers' responsibilities as:

- preparing and publishing a written policy on health and safety;

- taking steps to minimise the risks of accidents;

- training staff in safe working practices; and

- providing equipment to support the health and safety of both staff and clients.

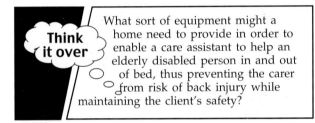

Think it over

What sort of equipment might a home need to provide in order to enable a care assistant to help an elderly disabled person in and out of bed, thus preventing the carer from risk of back injury while maintaining the client's safety?

Employees must:

- follow the organisation's health and safety policy on health and safety at all times; and

- report potential hazardous situations to senior staff.

The Health and Safety at Work Act and the Manual Handling Regulations 1992 both deal with the issues of moving and handling people. This is very relevant to homes where people are often being helped in and out of their beds or the bath. The employer is responsible for assessing the risk of injury when help with moving someone is needed. They also have the duty to take steps to reduce any risk. This may include providing adequate training for staff in safe techniques and providing adequate equipment.

Although the law can create rights, it does not create good-quality care. Because there are laws against discrimination and laws that give people rights to confidentiality, managers and professionals will be very careful to make sure that policies and guidelines for practical work

respect these rights. Guidelines for practical work are called **procedures**. Professional bodies, such as the British Association of Social Workers (BASW) and the United Kingdom Central Council (UKCC) for nurses, midwives and health visitors, design codes of conduct. These codes of conduct for social workers and nurses are designed to protect client rights. *Home Life* is a code of practice for residential care workers produced in 1986. Details may be found on pages 50–51.

Laws provide the background to policy-making, and policies and standards guide managers when they design procedures (Figure 6.4). Staff will be given set procedures to follow to ensure that clients' rights are respected.

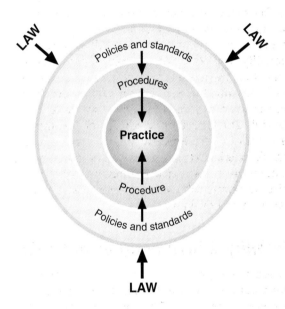

Figure 6.4   Laws, policies and procedures influence practice

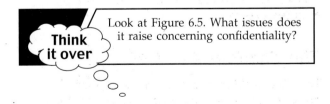

Think it over

Look at Figure 6.5. What issues does it raise concerning confidentiality?

Assessing the care needs of clients in care settings

Assessments should not be done 'on' clients – assessments should be **negotiated** with clients.

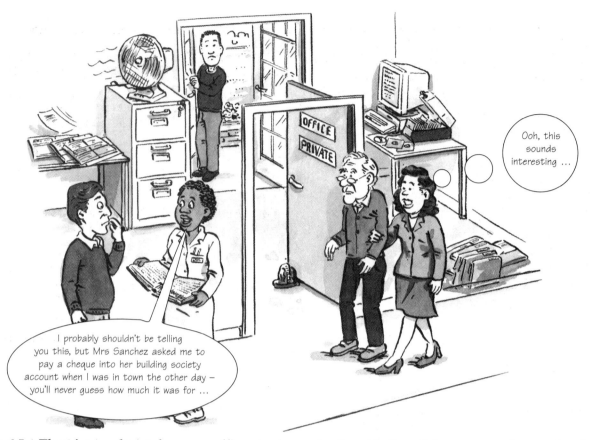

Figure 6.5   The picture above shows an office at a home for the elderly – it is not a good example of how to maintain confidentiality! If you were in charge, what suggestions would you make to ensure that information about the clients in your care was kept confidential?

CASE STUDY – Mrs Wilken

Look at this record of a conversation between Mrs Wilken and an interviewer. Mrs Wilken is 86 and lives alone:

Interviewer: So you are finding it difficult to work in the kitchen nowadays. Perhaps we could reorganise the kitchen and use some aids and adaptations to make life easier?

Mrs Wilken: No, I don't think so, it is too difficult nowadays.

Interviewer: Would you rather have Meals on Wheels, or perhaps your home care worker could make you a sandwich?

Mrs Wilken: Yes, I'm 86 and I just want to be waited on – I've spent all my life cooking and looking after others, and I don't want to be bothered any more.

Interviewer: But won't you lose your feeling of independence?

Mrs Wilken: No – as long as I've got my phone and TV and my family around me – that's the independence I want. I don't mind giving up the housework. Giving it up is the one thing I'm looking forward to.

Question

Do you think this assessment was handled well? If so, why?

Clients have a right to make choices about their care. The people assessing the client and other care staff should always show respect towards the client and should support the client when making choices.

Sometimes carers try to get people to be more independent – aids and other equipment can help. Mrs Wilken is very clear she doesn't want this type of independence. Because she has a right to choose, and because she has been consulted about their views, she can have the service she wants.

If people feel that care is being 'done to them' rather than agreed with them, they may feel powerless and helpless. When people become powerless they may experience:

- frustration
- anger
- withdrawal
- depression
- anxiety.

The problems listed above can make illness or disability much worse. The right to be consulted and to choose how you would like to be cared for is an important part of care work. No form of treatment or care should ever be given without the consent of the individual receiving it, unless there is a legally justifiable reason to impose it (such as in serious cases of mental illness).

Advocacy

Sometimes a client may use the help of an **advocate**. An advocate is someone who speaks for someone else. When a lawyer speaks for a client in a court room, he or she is working as an advocate. An advocate argues the case for clients. In care work, a volunteer might try to get to know a person with dementia or with a learning disability, then argue the case for that person.

The process of assessing clients' needs

The National Health Service and Community Care Act 1990 gave people the right to have their needs assessed. It is important to find out what people need before suggesting they might go into a home, a day centre or have home care. The needs that might lead into a care service are shown in Figure 6.6.

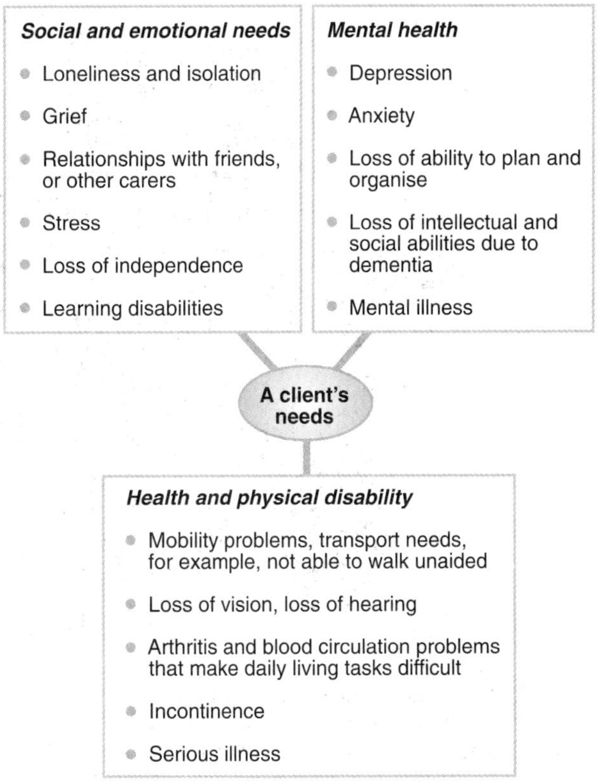

Social and emotional needs
- Loneliness and isolation
- Grief
- Relationships with friends, or other carers
- Stress
- Loss of independence
- Learning disabilities

Mental health
- Depression
- Anxiety
- Loss of ability to plan and organise
- Loss of intellectual and social abilities due to dementia
- Mental illness

A client's needs

Health and physical disability
- Mobility problems, transport needs, for example, not able to walk unaided
- Loss of vision, loss of hearing
- Arthritis and blood circulation problems that make daily living tasks difficult
- Incontinence
- Serious illness

Figure 6.6 Factors that may cause a person to need care

People do not usually have just one need. People who lose their mobility may become depressed and they may become lonely because they can't get out. People can have complicated needs. The NHS and Community Care Act established the concept of assessment because people should not 'just' have home care. People need a service that will meet their individual needs.

Develop care plans in a care setting

Before a care plan to meet a person's needs can be developed, the person will have to be assessed. The methods of assessment are explained below.

The first step is to explain to the person which services can be made available. This information is necessary so that individuals can be sure they are treated fairly. Many social services departments have very limited funding, and cannot meet every kind of need in the community.

The next step is that people are **referred** – they begin to enquire about receiving a service. A person might be referred by a doctor to social services or nursing services. Relatives might phone social services to make an enquiry, or the person concerned might enquire. Some assessments can be simple, because the enquiry is straightforward. Other assessments can be complex and might involve a team of specialists.

Care plans should not be decided only by professionals (such as social workers or district nurses) – they should be developed after discussion with clients and relatives.

A care plan might suggest the provision of a service, such as home care. But the plan will clearly state what needs have to be met, i.e. the goals of the programme. After the plan is put into practice, clients, carers and relatives will need to check how well it is working. This stage is called **monitoring**. After a set time, the plan will need to be reviewed and evaluated by everyone concerned. The **review** may lead to a new plan being made.

The process of assessment and designing care for people therefore goes round in a circle or 'cycle' (see Figure 6.7). A person's needs are assessed and a plan devised. The plan is later monitored to see if it is working and assessed again when the review takes place. Each stage of assessment can lead to changes in the plan.

The care planning cycle explains the process of providing a plan to meet clients' needs. For example, a social worker will talk with an older man and his relatives and agree that the client needs help with shopping and cleaning the home. The care plan may just state the services needed and who will provide these services. Perhaps a private care business will do the shopping and cleaning. This private company may design a more detailed plan of what is needed. This detailed plan may state which days the shopping will be done, which shops will be used, what areas will be cleaned, when the named home carer will visit and so on. Detailed plans are sometimes called **micro-care plans** or **care action plans** to tell them apart from the major assessment and care management process. These detailed plans are the documents that care assistants are most likely to see and work with.

We should always remember, however, that clients should feel in control of their own lives, both when care plans are being drawn up and when day-to-day care is delivered.

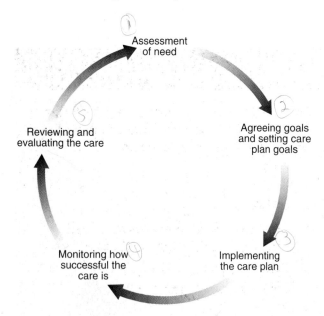

Figure 6.7   The care plan cycle

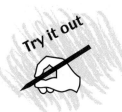

Try it out

Think about the practical care task of helping someone to eat. You could try this exercise in pairs. Wear a blindfold or use glasses that limit your vision so that you can play the role of a client with a visual disability. Work with another student who will act as your 'carer' and who will help you to choose and prepare a sandwich, or feed you with yoghurt or some other form of food. You could swap over, so each of you has a chance to experience being on the receiving end of care. Follow safety rules. You do not necessarily have to eat the food at the end!

At the end of the exercise write notes on how it might feel to be cared for. In particular, did your carer:

• Check your beliefs and preferences – or just tell you what to do?

• Talk you through things?

• Respect and value you?

• Try to find out what you could do for yourself?

• Give you choices?

• Help you to do things for yourself?

Meeting individual needs

If you went on holiday and were injured in a road accident, you might feel left alone, a long way away from friends and family. Your needs could be understood using the following headings (see also Unit 10).

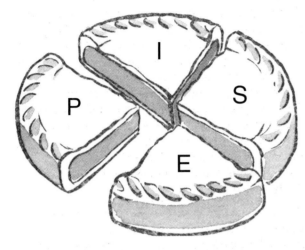

Physical needs   You would need medical treatment, food, shelter and warmth.

Intellectual needs   You would probably want to understand what had happened and what was likely to happen to you – how long would it take to get better?

Emotional needs   You might feel lonely, or not feel safe being away from home. You would want to feel the staff cared for you.

Social needs   You would probably want to phone friends and family – you would want to belong with other people and not feel isolated.

You might feel your physical health was the most important issue; it is sometimes easy to go without social contact for a few days. But if you were ill for a long time your social and emotional needs might seem more important.

Physical needs are often important, but it would be a mistake to see physical needs as the main issue for every client. Each person's needs are different. Intellectual, social and emotional needs can be very important. The psychologist, Abraham Maslow, believed there were different levels of need people experience as they grow and develop. The most basic human needs are physiological or physical. After this, people have a need for physical and emotional safety, and then a social need to belong. If our physical, safety and social needs are met, we have an emotional need for self-esteem. Finally, the purpose of life is to fulfil our physical, intellectual, social and emotional potential.

CASE STUDY – Mr Collins

Mr Collins is 79 and has lived alone since his wife died last year. His children manage to visit only once every two weeks. Mr Collins has a heart problem, which limits his ability to collect shopping. He is also being treated for depression.

His physical needs include help with daily living activities and shopping. Intellectual needs include a need for conversation – someone to talk to. Emotional needs include a sense of grief and loss. Social needs are for company and conversation. Mr Collins would say that his social and emotional needs were his main concern.

Questions

1   Think of some ways in which care services could meet Mr Collins' needs.

2   How will Mr Collins feel if only his physical needs are met?

Care plans and care settings

Care plans need to focus on the full range of human needs and not just physical care needs. Settings that work with people in the community include the following:

- Community nursing and therapy services.

- Mental health services.

- Child protection and family support services.

- Residential care (including rest and nursing homes).

- Day care.

- Sheltered housing.

- Home care.

Meeting individual care needs in different care settings

Each care service must understand a person's physical, intellectual, emotional and social needs. For instance, think back to the exercise you did earlier in this unit about helping a visually impaired person to eat. The person's physical needs for nutrition could be met if a care worker simply spooned food into his or her mouth. But care work is more than this. Most people would have an intellectual need to know what food they were eating. A carer could meet this need by describing the food on the plate and asking for the person's views on what should be eaten and in what order. Most people would have an emotional need for self-esteem, respect and dignity. A carer might meet this need by using conversational skills that make the person feel valued and that offered choice. Most people would have social needs, and this may mean they would not wish to eat in silence. Meals should be an enjoyable social occasion, and not just about receiving nutrition. You may have already experienced this yourself from doing the exercise.

Every care activity must take into account a range of physical, intellectual, emotional and social needs. Some care needs in different care settings are listed below; issues linked with PIES are described for each one.

Aids and adaptations to assist in a person's own home

Physical needs: Is the equipment right for the person – does it need adjustment?

Intellectual needs: Does the person understand the equipment and how to use it?

Emotional and social needs: How does the person feel about the equipment? Some people lose self-esteem or feel less dignified when they use walking frames or other aids.

An occupational therapist might assess individual needs but might also teach a person how to use the equipment and try to meet needs for dignity and self-esteem.

A reminiscence discussion group in a day centre for older people

Physical needs: People often feel more relaxed if food and drink are provided (perhaps tea/coffee and biscuits). Seating must be comfortable.

Intellectual needs: Topics for discussion must be relevant and interesting. Photos and material from the past must be relevant to the people in the group.

Emotional and social needs: The meeting should be enjoyable – everyone should feel included.

A care assistant might lead this meeting but would need to organise a room, food and drink. The care assistant would also need good communication and groupwork skills.

Some groups might be led by volunteers. Spiritual leaders might lead discussions in groups that share the same religion.

Dressing a leg ulcer in a residential home

Physical needs: To improve the physical health of the person.

Intellectual needs: The person may wish to understand why the ulcer has developed and what he or she could do to help it 'get better'.

Emotional and social needs: The person may be worried about his or her health and may seek emotional reassurance and help.

A district nurse might undertake this work, which has an intellectual, social and emotional aspect as well as a physical care aspect to it.

Cutting out shapes for a picture in a nursery setting

Physical needs: To feel comfortable and to use scissors safely.

Intellectual needs: Learning hand-eye co-ordination – learning about shape and colour.

Emotional and social needs: Learning to co-operate with others; learning to feel safe with other children. Enjoying practical activities

An early years instructor or nursery nurse might undertake this work. He or she would need to consider safety and emotional issues as well as the intellectual needs of the children.

The roles of care workers

It is important to remember that care workers usually work with others when assessing client need and when giving care. For example, a social worker may assess the needs of an older person living in his or her own home, but may ask for information from a GP or for an assessment by an occupational therapist. A home care manager may check a person's needs before a home care worker (similar to a care assistant) is allocated to work with that person. The client's medical needs might be met through the services of a district or practice nurse. Counselling might be provided at the doctor's surgery. The social worker might be responsible for organising reviews of the client's care plan and for checking that the services provided are meeting the person's needs.

Monitor the effectiveness of care plans

The only way to be sure a care plan is right for a client is to check it is working in practice. A care manager (who might be a social worker, occupational therapist or home care manager) will need to check the following:

- That services are actually being provided as planned.
- That different agencies who are working with a client understand the work each agency is doing, and that they communicate with each other.
- That detailed needs are understood – that clients are being given a practical service that meets their needs and that clients are not being discriminated against.
- That there is still enough money available to pay for services.
- That friends' and relatives' ideas are taken into account.
- To see if the clients' needs have changed or if any changes are needed to improve the service.

Monitoring may lead to a full review of the care plan if:

- There is a possibility that care is no longer needed.
- The client's needs have changed.
- The client or his or her friends and relatives are not happy with the plan.
- There are difficulties between care services working with a client.

- It is time to review the plan formally in line with agency policy.

Monitoring is about checking a plan is working. Monitoring leads on to a review if the plan needs to be redesigned.

Who monitors care plans?

Formal monitoring should be done by the care manager who designed the plan.

Very often, care assistants, home carers and other care workers are the people who really know what is happening because they are in daily contact with the client and his or her relatives. Care workers who have a day-to-day contact can use listening and communication skills to build a relationship with clients and to develop a deep understanding of clients' thoughts and feelings. Care workers may be able to discuss the detail of the care plans with clients and relatives. Care workers can also notice changes in a client's behaviour or health. They can help to monitor plans because they may understand clients better than managers.

CASE STUDY
— Sonia

Sonia is a residential care worker. She is a 'key worker' or special worker for Mr Boud. The care plan includes the daily duties of helping Mr Boud to get up, wash, dress and to go to breakfast.

One morning Sonia notices that Mr Boud seems withdrawn and is not speaking clearly. This is different from the way he normally behaves. Sonia reports this change to the officer in charge of the home who decides to call a doctor. Mr Boud may have had a small stroke or have an infection.

Sonia 'monitors' or checks the behaviour and health of the people she works with.

Question

1 What health risks might Mr Boud have been exposed to if Sonia had failed to monitor his behaviour?

CASE STUDY
— Douglas

Douglas is a home carer. He works with a client whose detailed care plan includes shopping from a local supermarket. One day the client says: 'I used to like the cereal from that other supermarket. I didn't want to say anything when that home care manager came, but do you think you could go there instead?'. Douglas agrees to ask his manager if he can do this.

Douglas is monitoring his client's satisfaction and may change the detail of what he does to meet the client's wishes.

Questions

1 If Douglas did not monitor his client's wishes, he would not be working within the value base for care. How would this affect the client?

2 Which client rights would be ignored if a care worker failed to talk with a client?

In theory, care plan managers should check how care plans are working with carers on a regular basis. In practice, care workers may often notice or be told about key issues before social workers or other care plan managers know. Care workers have a vital role to report and discuss what they know with managers.

Factors which influence the delivery of care

The type of place we live in can influence our emotions. A home that has plenty of space, and is attractive and comfortable, will feel better than a crowded, unattractive or poorly equipped home. The quality of furniture, the size of rooms and the type of facilities in a care setting may influence the self-esteem of people who live or go there.

One reason some people prefer care in their own home is they have chosen the furniture, bedding, appliances, etc. In your own home you can also choose how to live, when to get up, how to set out your room and so on. When you use health care facilities or attend a day centre, you will be influenced by how good the facilities look. If a health centre or day centre looks run down, you may feel you are not very important but at least you can go back to your own home.

When a person goes into a rest or nursing home, however, he or she may be there for life. The quality of the facilities may strongly influence the residents' emotions. Because of this, most registration authorities set standards that must be met before a rest or nursing home can be registered. Residential care homes must usually have at least 80% of bedrooms as single rooms. Single-bed rooms usually have to have a minimum of 10 square metres in floor area. There might be a minimum of 2–3 square metres per resident in the lounge area, and 1–4 square metres per resident of dining area. There will be recommendations about window areas in residents' rooms and about minimum standards of furniture and equipment.

Recommendations may suggest that each resident's bedroom contains, as well as a bed, at least:

- an armchair;
- a separate wardrobe for each resident;
- a lockable cupboard; and
- a table.

Registration criteria are designed to ensure that people in residential care are not crowded and that they have reasonable surroundings and equipment. As well as emotional needs, officers will check safety, toilet and hygiene facilities, and security and comfort in the home. Homes will need a call system, an adequate heating system, adequate security and a minimum of one toilet for every four or five residents and one bath or shower room for every eight to ten residents. Many homes will have *en suite* toilet and washbasin facilities in bedrooms. Inspection of homes will include laundry and kitchen facilities and access for wheelchair users.

Different people have different needs. A wheelchair user may need sinks and basins to be set low so they can be used from a wheelchair. A person with arthritis in the spine might find it painful to have to bend to use a low sink, and may need the height of washing facilities to be raised. Wheelchair users may find sliding doors more appropriate than doors with hinges, but some people with memory impairment may experience difficulty in using sliding doors. There is no simple, ideal specification for the equipment and facilities every room should have. Rooms and facilities may need to be adjusted to meet the needs of specific individuals or groups of clients.

Resources

Good facilities and staff who work within the value base for care are not enough to ensure quality care is provided. There also needs to be enough staff time, enough equipment, transport facilities, aids to daily living, training, supervision – and money to pay for these resources (Figure 6.8).

Staff levels

The number of staff available to work with clients in day or residential care may vary depending on the needs of the clients. Where clients are relatively independent, fewer care staff might be needed compared with the situation where clients are very dependent or have challenging behaviour. Generally, the more staff there are to

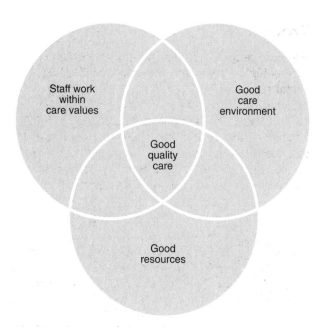

Figure 6.8 Quality care depends on care values, a good care environment, and suitable resources

the number of clients, the more chance there is for staff to know, understand and monitor the individual needs of each person. Poor staffing levels can result in staff who are stressed, and have inadequate time to communicate with clients or properly understand their needs.

Time is a very important issue in domiciliary care. Where home care and other workers have very limited time, it can be difficult to understand and meet the needs of clients. Staff time is expensive, however. When organisations have to save money, they may cut the amount they spend on staff hours, and therefore staff ratios.

Skills

Clients may often need services from a range of different people, such as occupational therapists, GPs, nurses, social workers, care staff and so on. Being able to see these people quickly and when needed (maintaining a continuity of care) will depend on staff resources and whether there is sufficient finance to pay for a high level of service.

The development of care skills will be influenced by the availability of staff training and staff supervision. Training and supervision also depend heavily on financial resources.

Equipment

Some people may require specific equipment to assist them with daily living tasks. Some examples are shown in Figures 6.9, 6.10 and 6.11.

Communication aids: Many people use glasses to correct impaired vision, or hearing aids to assist with poor hearing. Other communication aids, such as fax machines, email and 'mini-com' services, are useful to some people with hearing difficulties. Ideally, equipment needs should be assessed by an appropriately qualified person. Many clients may be able to select their own equipment from catalogues, following appropriate advice from health or care staff.

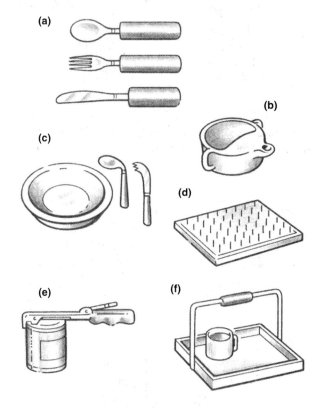

Figure 6.9 Aids for eating and drinking: a light thick-handled cutlery; b a feeding cup; c deep bowl with combined knife and fork and a pusher spoon; d spiked board (helps when buttering bread or peeling potatoes); e a gadget to help take lids off jars: f a non-slip tray with a handle will enable someone who can only use one arm to carry several items at once

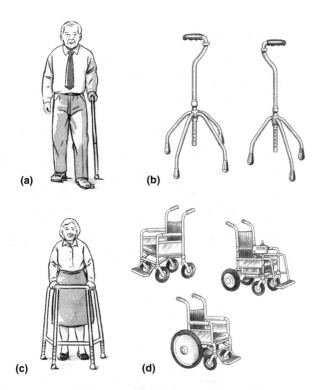

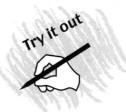

Figure 6.10 Aids to mobility: a walking stick; b a quadruped and a tripod; c a walking frame; d different types of wheelchair

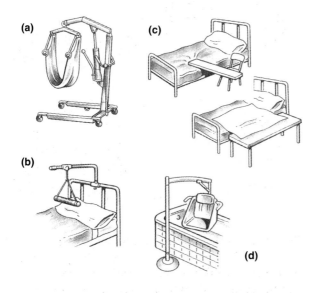

Figure 6.11 Equipment for moving and lifting: a a hoist; b lifting handle; c a transfer board and table; d a bath lift

Transport

Attendance for outpatient treatment and for day care is highly dependent on transport facilities. Social services usually provide some transport facilities, while hospitals may use ambulance or car services to bring patients in for therapy or treatment. The availability of suitable transport can vary from area to area, and is dependent on financial resources. 'Dial a Ride' services provide a special bus service for disabled people.

Try it out

> Find out about transport facilities in your area and their cost.
>
> You could use this as an example in your assignment.

Finance

Social services departments have a duty to assess people's needs for services under the Community Care Act. If a person needs a place in a residential or nursing home, the local authority will carry out a financial assessment to work out how much that person should contribute to the cost of his or her care. If a person owns property above a certain level (£16,000 in 1999), they have to pay the costs of his or her care. People still have to pay towards the cost of their care out of their income and also from their savings, if they have more than £10,000 in savings.

The state will give money towards the cost of care when a person owns less than £16,000 (1999 figures). The costs of residential care can quickly use up the savings a person may have had.

Legislation

Legislation also influences care. For details of the main legislation in care settings, see pages 205–207 earlier in this unit.

Unit 6 Assessment

You will undertake an internally marked assignment for this unit. Some issues to explore in detail for a *Merit* or *Distinction* grade include:

- clients' rights in relation to assessment and care planning
- the role of legislation in influencing practice
- influences on the delivery of care.

Clients' rights

People need care plans because they need help and support of some kind. People may have physical or learning disabilities which mean they cannot look after themselves or perform daily living activities. Helping people means more than just doing things for them. People who have difficulty looking after themselves do not simply need food, shelter and warmth. People have emotional and social needs as well as physical needs. When people are assessed and a care plan is written, it is very important that the person's social and emotional needs are understood. It is not good enough just to meet physical needs.

A key question in developing a care plan and providing care is, 'Who has the power?'. In the past, some care workers may have thought of themselves as 'experts' or as important or official people who had the right to study and make choices for their clients. They may have said things like, 'Oh, Mrs Biggs would be better off in a home, then she could get used to care before her condition becomes worse'.

If other people don't consult you or discuss your needs with you then you will get the feeling that you don't matter; your emotional needs will not be met.

Carers should always try to 'empower' or give power to clients, rather than trying to control or manipulate others. The client is

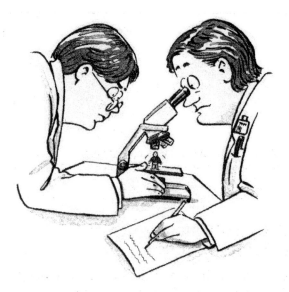

Experts who examine people can make them feel small!

the expert on his or her own needs and clients have a right to be involved and to make decisions about their care plans. Empowerment means that clients should be in control of their daily lives and should not be dependent on a carer who tries to control them.

Care workers should encourage clients to express their own needs and wishes and should offer choices wherever possible.

When working with clients it is important that:

- workers use effective communication and listening skills to understand clients' needs
- workers are careful to value differences in other people
- workers offer choices and encourage clients to control their own lives as much as is possible
- workers maintain confidentiality.

Clients should be empowered and be in control of their own lives, both when care plans are designed and when day-to-day care is delivered.

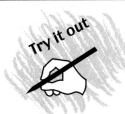

Merit grade

Explain how you can empower clients and promote their independence while helping them with food or mobility.

Distinction grade

Discuss how rights and empowerment are taken into account in assessing client needs and delivery of care.

The role of legislation in influencing practice

Law has an important influence on practice. Two areas which illustrate this are the law on Equal Opportunities and the law on Confidentiality. Three main Acts of Parliament make up the law on Equal Opportunity:

* the Sex Discrimination Act 1975
* the Race Relations Act 1976
* the Disability Discrimination Act 1995.

Details of this legislation can be found on pages 205–206. These laws are designed to ensure that men and women, people of different races and abilities all have equal opportunities in life. In the area of Confidentiality, three main Acts of Parliament make up the law:

* the Data Protection Act 1984 and 1998
* the Access to Personal Files Act 1987
* the Access to Health Records Act 1990.

Details of the legislation can be found on pages 204–205. These laws mean that care workers must keep information confidential, record information accurately, keep records safely, and make sure that information is only given to people who have a right to know it.

On their own, laws cannot make sure that discrimination doesn't happen or that people's rights are always respected. Laws are important because:

* they make employers design policies
* employers will usually provide training to make sure staff understand policy and law
* people may be able to take legal action if their rights are not respected.

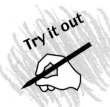

Merit/Distinction grade

Visit a care service provided by a large employer. Ask if you can have a copy of the agency's policies on equal opportunities or confidentiality. Look at the detailed rights and ask what training staff might receive to help them with equal opportunities and confidentiality. List the problems that clients might face if there were no laws on confidentiality or equal opportunities (look back to pages 204–206 to help you with this). At *Distinction* level you should discuss the specific benefits that one area of legislation (perhaps Equal Opportunities or Confidentiality) provides for clients.

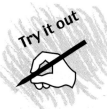

Merit/Distinction grade

Visit a care home, day centre or nursery and make your own list of advantages and disadvantages. At *Distinction* level you will need to explain how advantages and disadvantages could be maximised and minimised.

Influences on the delivery of care

Some advantages in a local care environment might be:	These advantages could be maximised by:
Easy travel to local shops, restaurants and entertainment.	Care staff arranging visits, arranging transport to help people use facilities.
Various religious and community groups available.	Care staff knowing where these facilities are and putting clients in touch with community groups.
Easy travel for friends and relatives.	Care staff knowing clients' relatives and helping relatives to stay in touch.
Good equipment and facilities such as bathrooms and kitchens.	Care staff having appropriate training to use equipment. Care staff being able to explain equipment to clients.
A good staff to client ratio.	Care staff spending time listening and communicating with clients.

Some disadvantages might be:	These disadvantages could be minimised by:
An isolated care environment.	Care staff assisting clients with transport and with telephone contact with relatives.
Few voluntary or community groups nearby.	Care staff checking services that may be further away and trying to arrange transport out to temples, churches, etc.
Poor staff to client ratios.	Trying to encourage voluntary workers to talk with clients or lead voluntary activities.
Staff who are stressed.	Training and support for staff.

Unit 6 Test

Complete the following sentences.

1   Before a care plan can be written for a person, that person should be assessed. This assessment should always be:

    a   done by skilled medical doctors
    b   done by expert social workers who can tell the client what they need
    c   based on a shared understanding between client, carers and assessors
    d   provided by a client's relatives.

2   Interviews during care planning should always feel like:

    a   an exchange of views between client and assessor
    b   an expert professional asking clever questions
    c   being put under a microscope
    d   the client getting everything they want.

3 The law on reports means that:

a anything you know about a client is secret and can never be told to anyone else

b anything you know about a client can only be passed on to people who have a right and a need to know it

c anything you know about a client can only be passed on to relatives or managers connected with the client

d anything you know can be passed on to others as long as the client doen't find out.

4 Monitoring procedures are important because:

a monitoring may help to save money

b it is important to check that services are meeting people's needs. People can be put at physical or emotional risk if care is not monitored

c accurate records of everything that happens must be kept for inspectors to see

d the law says that care plans must be monitored.

5 Advocacy means:

a going to a court of law
b hiring a solicitor to take legal action
c acting on behalf of another person
d believing that an argument is right.

6 Clients should be involved with the delivery of their care services. Which of the following is not likely to be an effective way of involving clients?

a Informal conversation with staff.
b Residents' or members' committees.
c Asking for signed, written evaluations of individual experiences.
d Discussion groups.

7 Reasonable, good quality, day or residential care is when a care service:

a gives people everything they want

b meets people's emotional, social and intellectual needs as well as physical needs

c just caters for people's needs for food, shelter and warmth

d leaves people to sort out their own problems.

8 Care values mean that:

a carers always have to do what clients want

b carers have to work in a way that values clients and their rights

c carers must never make mistakes or forget things

d carers have to work in a way that pleases most people.

9 The quality of the physical conditions in which people live is important because:

a furniture, decoration, room size, equipment and facilities can influence people's sense of self-esteem and being valued

b people need lots of space around them

c good furniture, decoration, room size, equipment and facilities make people happy

d people need good physical conditions to watch TV.

10 When providing equipment to help a person's daily living routine it is important to:

a just assess the person's physical needs – such as whether the equipment is the right type and height

b just ask the person what they want

c get an expert to decide what a person needs and make them use the equipment properly

d work with the person and take their physical, intellectual, social and emotional needs into account.

UNIT 6 ASSESSMENT

Dealing with hazards and emergencies

This unit covers the knowledge you will need in order to meet the assessment requirements for Unit 7. It is written in five sections.

Section one outlines those common hazards that are often encountered in the home and in care settings. Section two discusses those things we must do in order to minimise risk to ourselves and others. Section three summarises the major legislation concerning health and safety and how this legislation applies to care settings. Section four provides an overview of those things we must do if we find ourselves at the scene of an accident or emergency. Finally, section five explains the principles and procedures involved in common health emergencies.

Advice and ideas for meeting the assessment requirements for the unit and for achieving Merit and Distinction grades are at the end of the unit.

Also at the end of the unit is a quick test to check your understanding.

Hazards in the home and in care settings

> **Think it over**
>
> Imagine you have arthritis which means walking is very painful for you. You visit a health centre for advice about your arthritis and you fall over some rubbish bags left carelessly in a corridor. As a result you break a leg.
>
> How would you feel about the health centre and about the staff who work there? You would be very angry at the extra pain and immobilisation you now suffer, and would perhaps not trust the people at the health centre any longer – after all, it was their negligence that caused your extra suffering.
>
> But accidents can be worse than this. They can be fatal. Vulnerable people recover less well, and are more prone to accidents, than healthy people.

The home is not a safe place. People are more likely to have accidents that need medical treatment when they are in the home than anywhere else. The Royal Society for the Prevention of Accidents (RoSPA) have said: 'Every year in the UK more than 4000 people die in accidents in the home and nearly 3 million turn up at accident and emergency departments seeking treatment.' (Source: www.rospa.co.uk/rsfacts.htm.)

Of course, this is only the tip of the iceberg: for every accident that needs medical treatment, there are probably dozens more that are treated at home. When we work in a care environment (be it someone's home or a more formal setting) we must know what action we must take to reduce the number of potential accidents and also what to do when things do go wrong and there is an accident.

You will have noticed that the word 'hazard' is used in the title of this unit. A **hazard** is a danger. We are all too well aware of the dangers of roads, rail tracks, rivers and canals but we tend to think of our homes and gardens as safe places. However, in 1995, RoSPA reported that 37% of all accidents requiring hospital treatment happened in the home. And all areas of the home caused accidents: the kitchen, living areas, stairs, bathroom and bedrooms. Perhaps because we feel safe at home we often act without thinking, or we take short cuts not thinking about how safe or not this short cut might be.

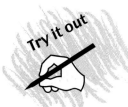

Working alone or in pairs, complete the following list on the possible causes of accidents. Apart from the headings already given in the list, you might also like to consider:

- substance abuse
- lack of knowledge of safety issues
- curiosity (about things unknown or about what things can do)
- a person's size, strength and so on.

Do not forget to include the practical reasons why accidents happen (e.g. faulty wiring, worn-out parts, etc.).

The first few entries have been done for you to get you going.

A person's mental state

- Under stress (other worries mean he or she does not stop to think).
- Forgetful (perhaps because of his or her age).
- Tired (overworking, not enough sleep the night before).

A person's personality

- Careless (can't be bothered to read the instructions).
- Negligent (doesn't care about the consequences of what he or she does).
- Impatient (in a hurry to finish and go home).

In the garden

- Not taking the plug out before cleaning, adjusting, etc., electrical gardening equipment.
- Standing on chairs, stools, etc., to prune tall-growing trees and bushes.
-
-

Outside

- Slipping on ice or snow that has not been cleared from paths, steps, etc.
-
-
-

Over half the accidents in the home are as a result of falls, falling objects and bumping into things. Older people and children are at particular risk of this type of accident. Also, people often climb on to chairs, stools or tables to reach high objects instead of using a properly designed stepladder. In our eagerness to reach something, we either do not think about, or are not aware of, the possible dangers (Figure 7.1).

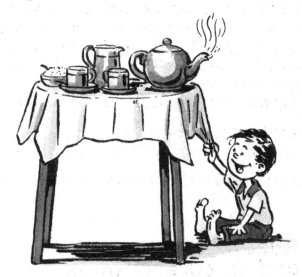

Figure 7.1 In our eagerness to reach something, we may not be aware of the possible dangers

Older people are often unsteady on their feet and may suffer giddy or dizzy spells. They cannot turn quickly and, when they do, often momentarily lose their balance. They are hence particularly prone to falls. Babies and young children pull themselves up on anything within their reach (see Figure 7.1). Young children and older people's sense of balance is not so well developed, and they are less likely to be able to save themselves if they trip over an obstacle in their path. While young children tend not to injure themselves when they have accidents such as these, older people are more likely to suffer injury (particularly fractures) as their bones are more brittle (see the section on fractures later in this unit).

Stairs, slippery floors, loose rugs and light coverings of frost, snow or ice on garden paths are the chief areas where people fall.

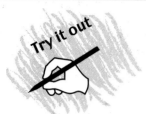

Working in small groups, identify the hazards that may occur in each room of the house. Each member of the group should take one particular room and list all the hazards he or she can think of that may be present in that room.

When you have finished, share your thoughts with each other. Add to the lists any other ideas that arise. A list of the possible hazards that may occur on the stairs has been done for you to give you an idea of the sorts of things you could include:

Possible hazards on the stairs

* Loose or worn carpets; carpets not fitted but held with grips on each step.
* Polished, slippery stairs.
* Dark, badly lit at night; lights not working properly.
* Objects left on the stairs (toys, hand-held sweeping brushes, shoes, etc.).
* Pets (especially cats) that curl up to sleep on the stairs at night.
* Electric cables (e.g. for a vacuum cleaner) left trailing across the top of the stairs.
* Loose or broken banisters.
* Slippery carpets (especially those consisting of a lot of nylon fibres – people in stocking feet may slip on these).
* Stairs that rise too steeply are difficult to climb and are easy to fall down.
* Bedrooms or bathrooms that open directly on to the stairs (a sleepy person at night may forget and tumble straight down the stairs).
* An unprotected glass door at the foot of the stairs.
* No gate at the top/bottom of the stairs to prevent babies or toddlers gaining access to the stairs.

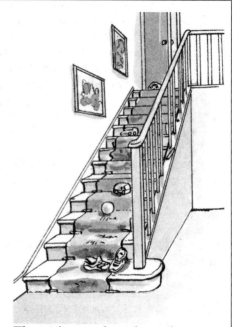

The stairs can be a hazardous place

Did you think there could be so many hazards on the stairs?

Use and misuse of appliances

Many of the accidents caused by faulty electrical or gas equipment are the result of the equipment not having been serviced or maintained regularly. For example, carbon monoxide is a gas that can be given off by faulty gas heaters and fires. It has practically no smell and so people may not be aware a faulty gas appliance is emitting this substance. When someone breathes in carbon monoxide, it passes into his or her blood stream. Here it is taken in to the haemoglobin (which normally takes in oxygen). Because the carbon monoxide has now replaced most of the oxygen in the person's blood stream, the person's vital organs do not receive sufficient oxygen, and the person effectively suffocates. Carbon monoxide poisoning can be fatal. It particularly occurs in rented flats and caravans, where neither the owner nor the tenant carry out regular maintenance checks.

The overloading of electrical adapters, poor connections and frayed wiring are frequent causes of electrical fires and electric shocks. Other equipment can also cause accidents. Chairs can collapse, shelves can fall down and insecure or rickety stepladders can topple over. Rotating machinery (machines with parts that go round and round) of any type is dangerous if used by people who have long, loose hair, loose clothing or who are wearing dangling jewellery (bangles, etc.).

It is extremely dangerous to poke electrical equipment (e.g. with a knife or screwdriver) to try to free it of obstructions (such as to free a fan heater of accumulated dust or to dislodge a piece of burnt toast from the bottom of a toaster). Even though we may have disconnected the equipment from the mains by removing the plug, we may have unwittingly damaged the equipment. When we plug it in again, it could overheat. The element could burn out or, at the least, it could blow the fuse. If we did not take the plug out before we poked around inside it, it could be ourselves that overheats!

All electrical equipment should be checked regularly by a qualified electrician (this is a legal requirement in most care settings). All electrical equipment that runs off the mains should be protected by a fuse of the correct amperage. If a 13 A fuse is fitted into the plug of a piece of equipment that should be protected by a 5 A fuse, the fuse may not blow (and hence not stop the equipment from working) if something goes wrong with it. This could mean the equipment has become unsafe and a potential hazard.

If this is an outline of how vigilant we must be at home, you might by now have realised how extra vigilant we must be in care settings, where many different people will come into contact with, and will use, equipment of all kinds without thinking about the hazards involved in their use.

Finally, we should not forget to consider toys. These days, good-quality toys that have been tested and approved for their safety *should* be safe as long as they are used only according to the manufacturer's instruction (and this includes for which age group they are appropriate).

However, we can never be 100% sure a child is using a toy safely. In some settings (such as a play group) toys may be shared among many children of differing abilities and temperaments. In such settings we must be absolutely sure *all* the toys the children might play with are safe for *all* the children.

Second-hand toys present even more problems as they will probably no longer have their original instructions for safe use (if they ever had any in

the first place). These must be checked thoroughly by a responsible person who can assess any dangers the toys may present for the children (small parts that might be swallowed, sharp edges that could cut, toys that might easily break and become dangerous and so on).

We need to be equally vigilant when children play with toys as when an elderly or disabled person uses a piece of equipment that might have potential hazards.

Dangerous substances

There are many substances found in the home and in care settings that have the potential to harm. Perhaps chief among these are cleaning substances (e.g. bleach, detergents, polish, etc.). These must be handled with great care as they contain harmful chemicals that can corrode, burn or irritate body tissues. Most people keep such materials in the cupboard under the sink – exactly where young children can get at them. Cupboards such as these should have extra childproof locks (Figure 7.2) or, better still, dangerous substances should be kept where they are not within the reach of children.

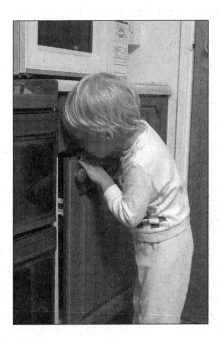

Figure 7.2 A childproof lock

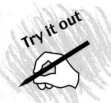

Try it out

Take a look in your own sink cupboard at home. List the materials you keep there, and read the labels on the containers. How many of these labels contain warnings, and what do these warnings tell us?

Do any contain advice about what to do in case of accidents? Did you know what to do should there have been an accident with any of these substances *before* you read the label?

On no account should cleaning substances be removed from their original containers – e.g. bottles of bleach poured into empty lemonade bottles. What is a young child to think about such a bottle should he or she find it, say, on the kitchen table?

Now you have looked at the cleaning materials you have at home and have realised the importance of the warnings and emergency procedures printed on their labels should accidents happen, the dangers inherent in removing cleaning substances from their original containers should be very apparent. Would you know what to do if someone swallowed bleach by mistake *without* reading the advice printed on the original bleach container?

Apart from cleaning fluids, other hazardous substances are:

* pet droppings (they contain bacteria and parasites)

* spilled liquids (on to the floor – can cause people to slip)

* inflammable liquids left near to heat sources

* liquids that are being heated (in pans, kettles, etc.).

Finally, we must not forget medicines. These should similarly be kept in a locked cabinet (in most homes, this is in the bathroom). However, people often leave medicines on the kitchen table or by the kettle to remind themselves to take them, but this can be a hazard, particularly to children who may think they are sweets or to elderly, confused people who may think the medicines are for them.

As for cleaning materials (and for the same reasons given for cleaning materials) *never* remove medicines from their original containers. Apart from the reasons given for cleaning substances outlined above, in the case of medicines bought over the counter you will also be throwing away the dosage instructions, the medicine's batch number (which allows the medicine's manufacturer to identify precisely when the medicine was made should something be wrong with it) and the manufacturer's name itself!

Think it over

Would you allow a small child to take his or her medicine out of the cupboard, count out the correct number of tablets, decide this was the correct time to take the medicine and then take the medicine – either with a glass of water, dissolved in water, while standing, etc.? But we sometimes leave elderly people to do this on their own.

Is this always the right course of action? What else could we do to help an older person take the medicine safely and as prescribed on the label?

Fire hazards

Fire is a hazard anywhere. It spreads rapidly, injures and kills people through flame or smoke and causes great devastation. Chip pans, misused or faulty appliances, frayed or incorrect wiring and smoking materials are the main causes of home fires.

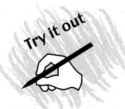

Try it out

Examine Figure 7.3. Can you identify any fire hazards? Make a list of these.

What would you do to get rid of these risks?

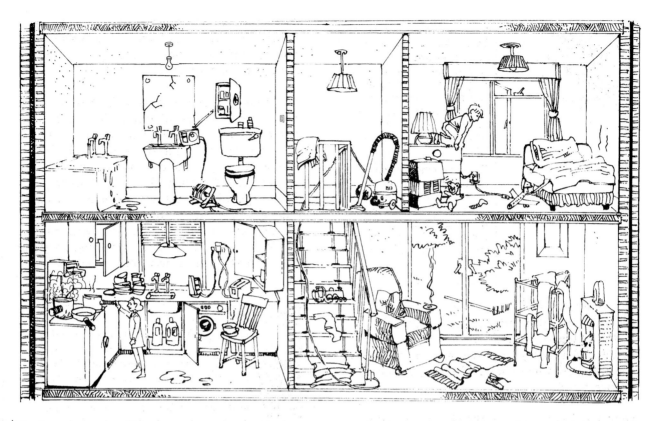

Figure 7.3 Potential hazards in the home

Hazards in the garden

The garden is normally a happy place where adults and children play and relax but there are dangers too. You may have already listed some of these hazards in the activity you did at the start of this unit, but here we will look at a few of these dangers in more detail.

Just a few centimetres of water in a pond have been known to be fatal to small, curious toddlers. It is all too easy for a child to fall, strike his or her head (which makes the child unconscious), and then roll into a pond, or trip and fall directly into a pond where he or she similarly strikes his or her head and becomes unconscious. Hence it is possible to drown in a relatively small amount of water. Garden pond drownings comprise 2% of all drownings and, in the UK in 1997, there were 440 cases of death by drowning.

Garden equipment is often sharp, dirty and heavy and, as a result, it is capable of causing serious injury. Pruning knives and secateurs are sharp and should be used with great care. They should

never be left lying around and secateurs should be closed after use and secured with a clip. All garden tools that come into contact with the soil are dirty, and soil is a source of **tetanus** infection. Overloaded wheel-barrows are heavy and can easily topple over.

Chemicals are sometimes used in the garden to kill weeds and pests. These chemicals contain toxic substances that are harmful to humans, even in small doses. Many garden chemicals can be absorbed through the skin and can cause serious, even fatal, illness.

You may have already listed some of these yourself earlier, but other hazards include electrical equipment (such as hedge cutters and lawn mowers) whose flex is accidentally cut through, garden rubbish, broken glass and plant pots, forgotten tools and poisonous plants (e.g. extremely toxic plants – foxgloves, laburnums – plants that may be harmful if eaten – poppies, sweet peas, lupins – and plants that may irritate the skin – primulas, bluebells, tulips).

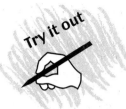

Have another look at Figure 7.3. List all the hazards you can find in the picture.

Can you think of yet more?

Poor maintenance of buildings

If a well maintained home can be a dangerous place, imagine how dangerous a badly maintained home can be! We have already looked at some of the hazards in the home. Can you think of hazards that might arise as a result of not keeping the building *itself* in good repair?

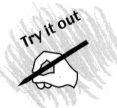

Either working in pairs or in small groups, study Figure 7.4. Make a list of all the hazards you can find in the figure, and say what dangers to health (either through accidents or as possible sources of illnesses or diseases) these hazards pose.

Can you think of any more? Add them to your list.

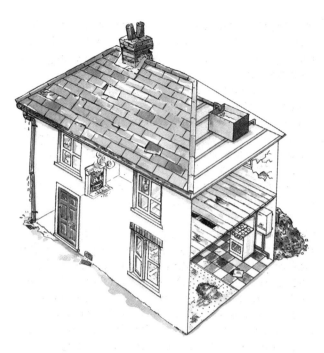

Figure 7.4 Potential hazards in a poorly maintained house

Traffic

In the UK, on average, 16 people are killed every day and over 900 are injured on our roads. The victims of traffic accidents are of all ages, but young children are most vulnerable (one victim in seven is a child under the age of 15 years).

There are even more hazards outside (you may have already listed some of those in the activity above):

- uneven paths

- over-hanging tree branches

- large stones, plant pots or discarded rubbish hidden in long grass

- slippery, moss-lined walkways

- rusty fences or gate posts with nails exposed

- broken glass or roof slates scattered everywhere

- missing or broken gates – children could easily run into the road.

Think it over

Study the following statistics:

- Most pedestrian accidents occur to children in the 5-9 age group, with elderly people coming second (60% of children under 5 years of age are injured within 100 metres of their home).

- Most bicycle accidents occur to children and young people in the 12-15 age group.

- Most motor bike accidents occur to young people in the 16-20 age group.

- Most car accidents occur to people in the 17-25 age group (75% of drivers involved in collisions are within 10 miles of home).

Why do you think the age group 5-9 years is at most risk of pedestrian accidents? How important do you think experience of driving a vehicle is? Why do most bicycle accidents happen to people in the 12-15 age group?

In 1999, the National Road Safety Conference said that by 2020, traffic accidents would represent the third greatest hazard to world health – beating wars and the spread of HIV infection! This increase in traffic accidents is perhaps understandable. People everywhere want the independence being able to drive can bring. In the UK, the loss of so many railway lines in the 1960s has meant people have come to rely on cars and buses. This has choked our roads with traffic to such an extent that the government is now encouraging people to use other forms of transport.

One such means of transport is the bicycle. However, cyclists generally wear very little in the way of protective clothing – only serious cyclists and children tend to use safety helmets. The same conference stated that, although more bicycles were sold than cars in 1997, only 2% of road users were cyclists. People like the idea of cycling as a mode of transport, but are discouraged from using their bicycles on congested roads.

For cycling to become a safe alternative to the car, more money must be spent on cycle lanes and other means of making the roads safer for cyclists (e.g. persuading people to wear protective clothing and helmets, improving road junctions and roundabouts – which are the most common danger spots for cyclists – and in educating cyclists to be safe road users).

National statistics also show that riding a motor bike is more hazardous than driving a car. This is so even though in the UK it is compulsory to wear a crash helmet when riding a motor bike, as either the driver or passenger.

> **Think it over**
>
> *Why do you think it is more dangerous to ride a motor bike than to drive a car?*
>
> *Look back at the statistics about motor bike accidents given in the activity earlier in this section. Do these help to explain this fact?*

Infectious diseases

Infectious diseases are those diseases that are passed on from one person to another. We have all experienced (or know of people who have experienced) the situation where there is one person at home who has contracted an infectious disease and nearly all the other people in the household fall victim to it. It is well recognised that all the members of a household, one after the other, can 'go down with' flu or a heavy cold. Food poisoning, although not infectious, is also likely to affect more than one person if the food was cooked at home or if food hygiene precautions somewhere down the line in preparing the food were not adequate.

Most adults are immune to childhood infectious diseases except chicken pox, which can be transmitted to adults in the form of shingles.

Minimising the risks
Ensuring others are aware of risks

If you recognise a hazard you cannot deal with yourself, then you need to inform people about it. If other people do not know about a hazard, then the chances of an accident occurring are much greater. You can inform people by telling them about the hazard or by placing a notice close to the hazard. Notices are much better because it is nearly always impossible to tell everyone who needs to know about the hazard.

(*Note:* In some settings you cannot expect everyone to be able to read notices – settings involving old people, young children, people with learning disabilities, etc. In such cases you must make sure the hazard is dealt with immediately, or that no one who may not understand the hazard can possibly come into contact with it.)

However, many **risks** can be minimised by people being careful in the way they work. The following is a checklist of simple actions that can minimise risks:

- Always put equipment away immediately after use.

- Keep things tidy. If you see things lying around, put them away.

- Keep cupboards closed and locked.

- Always throw rubbish away immediately.

- Read instructions for equipment before use.

◦ Always wash your hands after going to the toilet, after handling toxic substances, after handling pets and before preparing or serving food.

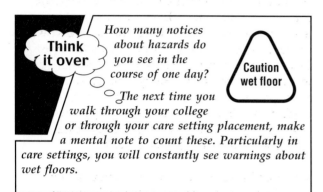

> **Think it over**
>
> *How many notices about hazards do you see in the course of one day? The next time you walk through your college or through your care setting placement, make a mental note to count these. Particularly in care settings, you will constantly see warnings about wet floors.*

Caution wet floor

Allocating responsibility for health and safety

In most medium to large-scale organisations there will be employees who have special responsibility for health and safety. These are people from all levels of the organisation, and they will have regular health and safety meetings. At these meetings, the number of reported accidents will be discussed and new ways to minimise risks to people's health put forward.

Most organisations also have a special budget for addressing health and safety issues and priorities, and the health and safety committee will decide on how this budget is to be spent. If the organisation is too small to have a special committee (for example, a small residential home), the management will take responsibility for health and safety.

Using and maintaining equipment

If people learn to use equipment safely and correctly, then the potential risks of accidents will be reduced. Manuals and handbooks are issued with most equipment, and people should read these carefully and follow them. With more complex equipment, regular staff training should be undertaken into its correct use and fault checks (routine maintenance) should be carried out and the dates of these checks recorded.

In the home, such checks are rarely carried out – most people wait until a fault occurs before seeking help.

Public and personal alarms

You will find public alarm systems in most care settings, particularly for fire. Everyone should know where these alarms are situated. Fire drills should be practised regularly and training given so each person knows his or her role in an emergency.

Violence is, regrettably, a fact of modern life hospital workers have to cope with, and emergency alarms exist just in case a worker is attacked. Some hospitals even have police stations on their premises. You should make sure you know how to contact the security personnel or the police in any care setting you work in.

Particularly on night shifts, many care workers are supplied with (or purchase for themselves) personal alarm systems that emit piercing sirens or whistles when pressed.

As well as fire alarms and personal alarm systems, organisations will have other security systems specific to that particular organisation. Find out what these are in your care setting.

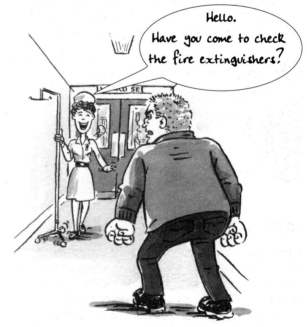

Always check people are who they say they are

Personal hygiene

The spread of infection will be minimised if a high standard of personal hygiene is maintained in both the home and in care settings (see Unit 5).

Storing medicines and harmful substances

Care settings have strict rules about the storage and dispensing of medicines. Most drugs have to be signed out by competent practitioners and checked by another person to ensure the correct drug is given in the correct dosage to the correct client. Even so, the newspapers and TV and radio news regularly report cases where mistakes have happened in the storing and dispensing of drugs, and such incidents have even formed the basis of story lines in TV plays and soap operas.

Furnishings

Some furnishings (including such things as curtains, settees and their covers, carpets, mattresses, etc.) are not only highly flammable but, when they do catch fire, also give off highly toxic fumes. Regulations brought in recently now control those things that can be sold and used for furnishings, and so the older, more dangerous furnishing materials can now no longer be used to cover settees, etc. However, this does not mean the older furnishings have disappeared: plentiful amounts of these furnishings are still to be found.

> **Think it over**
>
> In what settings do you think you are most likely to come across these older, dangerous furnishing materials?
>
> What extra hazards do they present in such settings?
>
> How could you minimise these hazards?

Road safety training

Road safety training is essential if children are to cross roads safely. With the increase in car travel (25% more cars over the last 10 years), fewer parents now walk any distance with their children. This means that the opportunities parents have to train their children about road safety – particularly the safety issues involved in

being a pedestrian – have been drastically reduced.

Hence some parents now think that road safety training is the responsibility of the school, road safety officers or the police, but these institutions and people have very limited time to spend with children on such issues. As our roads become busier, *everyone* must share the responsibility of looking after children's safety though, sadly, you have only to stand and observe adults crossing roads to see that few people act as good role models. Good road sense taught to children would also serve we adults as well!

We should take the time to cross roads safely, using subways, pedestrian lights and crossing patrols whenever possible. Even when there is no traffic in sight, we should show children the right way to cross roads and explain the reasons why. For children aged about 7 years, there is the *Green Cross Code*. For younger children there is the three-finger code – I must stop, I must look, I must listen.

The Green Cross Code

Repeat these steps EVERY time you cross the road.

- **Find a safe place to cross the road.**

  A zebra crossing, a pelican crossing, or a clear stretch of road with NO parked cars or obstacles in the way of your view.

- **Stop, look and listen for traffic.**

  Remember, all the different types of traffic to look out for. Even bicycles can do damage.

- **If there is any traffic, let it pass.**

- **Look in both directions, and when the road is completely clear, walk across. Keep looking and listening as you cross the road.**

Car driver and motor cyclist training have also improved in recent years, and the *Highway Code* is an important part of such training. All new drivers should be expertly trained, even though the cost of expert tuition may be high. Although not obliged by law to take a test, cyclists should take a course in road safety and be familiar with the *Highway Code*, road signs and the rules of the highway.

Cycling proficiency tests are good at motivating children to learn about road safety, and these can easily be arranged through road safety officers.

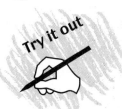

Try it out

How many parents are good role models to their children and how many not, when it comes to road safety?

Stand at a busy intersection controlled by pedestrian lights for about 15 minutes. Record how many adults 'jump' the green man. How many adults with children give their children road safety training while waiting at the lights?

Try doing this on a Saturday when children are out shopping with adults.

We often see adults out cycling with children. The next time you notice an adult with children on bicycles like this, observe the adult carefully:

Is he or she wearing a crash helmet and/or protective clothing? Are all the bicycles well maintained (lights, brakes, etc.)? Is the adult demonstrating good road sense (not cycling on pavements, making clear hand signals, looking behind him or her when making a manoeuvre)?

Similarly, observe an adult who has a small child in a seat attached to the adult's bicycle. How safe is the child?

First aid

In a perfect world, first aid training would be part of everyone's normal school curriculum, topped up with regular refresher courses. However, this is not the case: it is left up to individuals to decide whether they wish to undertake training or not. Hence only a small number of people in this country have received first aid training, and an even smaller number take refresher courses every three years. This is very unfortunate as more lives would be saved if everyone knew the correct things to do in an emergency.

As a care worker, you will be encouraged to take a first aid course and to keep your qualifications up to date. Part of this training involves checking that the first aid equipment in any establishment is readily accessible and complete. This means that someone must be responsible for checking the contents of the first aid box regularly, and for maintaining the equipment in good order.

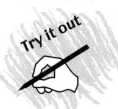

Try it out

In both your college and your care setting placement, make sure you know where the first aid supplies are kept. You may find there is more than one first aid box. Find out where *all* the first aid boxes are located.

Examine the contents of one or two of the boxes. Bring any deficiencies to the notice of the appropriate responsible person and recheck the boxes in a week's time. Repeat this reporting procedure if the contents have not been updated.

Legal requirements for health and safety

You need to know the key features of the legislation concerning health and safety matters.

Health and Safety at Work Act 1974

The key features of the Health and Safety at Work Act 1974 (HASAW) can be found in Unit 2.

COSHH legislation

The key features of the Control of Substances Hazardous to Health (COSHH) Regulations 1994 can be found in Unit 2.

Fire Precautions (Workplace) Regulations 1997

The key features of the Fire Precautions regulations are given in Figure 7.5.

- Both employers and employees must comply with the fire regulations.
- Workplaces should possess a current fire certificate.
- Workplaces must be equipped with appropriate fire fighting equipment, alarms and fire detectors.
- Such equipment must be easily accessible, simple to use and indicated by signs.
- The appropriate equipment, alarms and detectors will be determined by the size of the building, the physical and chemical substances used on the premises and the number of people likely to be present in the building at any one time.
- Some of the employees must be trained in the correct use of the equipment.
- Emergency exits and all other exits must be kept clear at all times. Emergency exits must be unfastened, labelled and must lead directly to a place of safety.
- In an emergency, it must be possible to evacuate employees quickly and safely.
- The number of exits must be compatible with the number of people likely to be present at any one time.
- Emergency doors must open out in the direction of escape and must be supplied with emergency lighting if these exits are illuminated in normal working circumstances.
- The workplace, equipment and devices must be kept in good working order and in good repair.

Figure 7.5   The key features of the Fire Precautions (Workplace) Regulations 1997

At the scene of an accident/emergency

Use the chart in Figure 7.6 to help you decide what to do if you are the first person at the scene of an accident or an emergency.

Accidents

Road traffic accidents can be very frightening. The blood, broken glass, bent and twisted metal and, possibly, fire all serve to increase the horror of the situation.

One of the simplest things anyone can do is turn off the car's ignition switch to reduce fire risk. Leave any trapped casualties where they are (unless they need urgent resuscitation) because of the risk of neck and spinal injury. Even if you

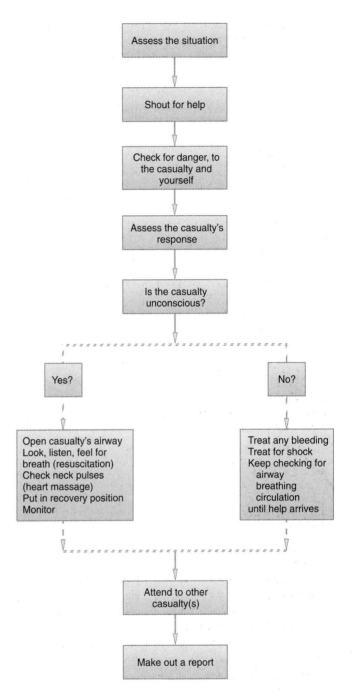

Figure 7.6   What to do if you are the first person at the scene of an accident

cannot move a trapped casualty you can still protect the airway *by lifting the head gently and pulling the chin forward and up.*

Shout for help as loudly as you can.

Approach carefully, look around and be sure you will not put yourself in danger and increase the number of people who are ill or injured.

Assess the situation carefully. Can you see all the people who are hurt? Sometimes people are thrown quite some distance from moving vehicles. Are there any hedges, fences, etc., people could have been thrown over?

Do you need the emergency services? You certainly will need to call the fire brigade if there is any danger of fire or if anyone is trapped. This service has all the equipment for such jobs. The police will usually be informed in cases of road traffic accidents, where the circumstances are suspicious and where there is injury or death. However, this is not your responsibility as a first-aider. Any problems associated with the sea and boats will involve the coast guard and lifeboat services.

You will definitely need to call the ambulance service in cases of:

- unconsciousness
- absence of (or difficulties with) breathing
- absence of pulses
- haemorrhage (serious bleeding)
- suspected heart attack
- severe burns or scalds
- fractures of the skull, back or legs (other fractures need hospital treatment but do not necessarily need an ambulance)
- poisoning
- shock.

Sometimes it may be more appropriate to call the local doctor if you know he or she is much closer (such as in a small village).

Having assessed the situation you should **act**. Who will you help first if several people have been injured? Give about 30 seconds to each one, while quickly assessing his or her condition. Go to the quiet ones first – if someone is screaming, groaning or crying you can be sure he or she is at least breathing.

Now you will need to find out if there are other people around (bystanders) who can help you or who are more experienced than you – in other words people *you* could assist. Try shouting for help as you work because there may be someone within hearing distance whom you cannot see.

But don't wait. The most serious cases cannot be left while you go to get help. You need to be there to keep the airway open, carry out resuscitation and external chest compression if required.

This poses a very difficult problem if the first-aider is on his or her own. In cases of serious heart attack, for example, the longer the delay in getting the person to hospital the smaller the chance of survival. However, you must not leave a patient in a condition which seems likely to change for the worse (an **unstable condition**). If the patient is conscious, breathing well, has controlled bleeding if any, is in the **recovery position** and appears unlikely to change, it may be possible to seek help. Otherwise, stay with the patient until help arrives.

Calling for an ambulance

If you are going to call for an ambulance, you must know what to do and say. If you are taking charge and sending someone else, you must be capable of telling *that person* what to say. Make sure the person can give the message and ask him or her to return to let you know how long the ambulance is likely to be, and whether there are any special instructions to follow.

Find a place where you can use a telephone (if you have a mobile phone, obviously you should use this; someone else at the scene of the accident may also have a mobile phone, but make sure he or she is in a fit state to use it – a shocked or injured person may not be able to remember his or her password, etc.). Otherwise, you will have to find a telephone. Do not look only for public call-boxes; use common sense. Houses, shops and public houses usually have telephones.

This is what happens:
1 The operator asks you which service you require.
2 Ask for 'ambulance'.
3 The operator then asks for the phone number you are calling from. This can be found on the phone itself or on a notice in the box.

4 The ambulance control officer will then come on to the line and ask for:

* the location of the accident
* the nature of the accident
* how many people are hurt
* what their condition is (for example, unconscious, bleeding)
* what other risks there are (for example, fire, fumes).

Give your answers as clearly as you can. If necessary, provide landmarks to help the ambulance crew. Put lights on and post lookouts if you have assistance.

5 Sometimes, first aid instructions are given by the ambulance controller. Listen carefully.

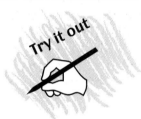

Try it out

Contact the local ambulance depot to see whether a speaker can come to talk to your group.

Find out how many calls a day the service has, and the main reasons for the calls. Display the information in the form of a bar chart.

Find out how much an ambulance costs to buy, to maintain and to staff for 24 hours.

Ask the ambulance officer what, if his or her opinion, is the most useful first aid measure people can do and what is the most harmful thing people can do, thinking they are helping.

Assessing an emergency

First, make sure your own emotions are under control: take a few deep breaths and stop to think. Are you in danger, is anybody else in danger and is there anyone present with more experience and knowledge then yourself? It is not brave to be careless about your own safety. You may increase the number of casualties and put more lives at risk.

If you do not know how to deal with the emergency, recognise this fact and use common sense to carry out tasks that you *can* do, such as making the area safe and sending for help. Other useful things to do are to talk to the casualty to make him or her feel safe and secure or, if a child is involved, talk to the parent or guardian first.

Explain any treatment you might be going to carry out and answer questions as truthfully as you can.

Do not leave the casualty except under the most serious of circumstances. Avoid asking irrelevant questions and try to obtain essential information from the casualty (such as his or her name, address, who needs to be informed and so on). Hold the casualty's hands while you talk to him or her. Always act in a calm manner to give the casualty confidence, even if you are frightened.

You may need to give physical support to the casualty, for example, control bleeding, cushion or splint broken limbs, or in more serious cases, resuscitate or place the casualty in the recovery position.

Conscious casualties do not like to be stared at, so try to make the area private by asking people to form a screen, for example by turning their backs to create a wall. Make sure the casualty's clothing is not awry so that he or she is not caused embarrassment. Cover with a light blanket if available.

When the emergency services arrive, make sure they have accurate information, written down if possible. Tell them all you know about the emergency and the support you have given. If the casualty's condition has altered, make sure they know this. Give your name and address and encourage others who have witnessed the accident to do so.

Opening and maintaining the airway

An unconscious person is usually showing all these three features. He or she is

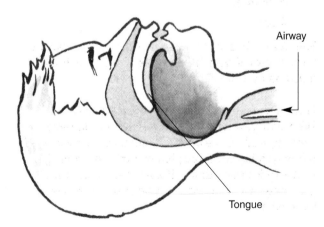

Airway

Tongue

Figure 7.7 The tongue may block the airway

⋄   not awake

⋄   not attentive

⋄   not aware

In addition, the person may or may not be breathing and may or may not have a pulse. In this case the person is at risk of dying because no oxygen is being carried around the body.

Ordinary sleep can be said to be a lower or reduced form of the normal wakeful state (which is full consciousness). When you lift a sleeping person's arm, it feels loose and floppy, but it still has some firmness to the touch because a few muscles are still contracting. In an *unconscious* person the limb is very soft and loose, like a rag doll's, because no muscles are contracting. This is very important to understand because it is the chief reason why, in unconscious people, the *tongue* tends to fall *backwards and block* off the air passages (see Figure 7.7). This obviously does not happen in ordinary sleep. An unconscious person may need immediate first aid to unblock his or her air passage.

Reflexes are automatic muscular movements that occur as a result of some nerve stimulus (such as in response to a speck of dust in the eye).

Remember

Do not try to give an unconscious person anything to eat or drink.

Your first aim is therefore to **keep the person's airway open**.

To do this, first put one hand underneath the person's neck and the other on his or her forehead. Then *gently* tilt the forehead backwards so that the chin moves upwards. Moving your hand from the neck, gently lift the chin upwards and forwards – the mouth will stay slightly open and the nostrils should be directly upwards. This position will pull the tongue away from the back of the throat, and straighten out the air passages.

Even if you suspect there are injuries to the head, neck or spine **you must still clear the airway**.

Remember

Many people die unnecessarily each year because they have been left face-up in an unconscious state.

Your next important job is to check **breathing and pulse.**

Is the person **breathing?** Put your ear close to the person's mouth and nose for five seconds and:

⋄   *Look* for evidence of the chest and abdomen moving.

⋄   *Listen* for sounds of breathing.

⋄   *Feel* for the touch of breath on your cheek.

This sounds like the road safety drill you may have learned as a child (see earlier in this unit). Perhaps you could learn it by repeating it over and over, just as you did with the road safety code.

If you find that the casualty is breathing, place the unconscious person in the **recovery position**. Stay with the person and regularly check breathing until emergency medical help arrives.

If the casualty is *not* breathing, check and quickly remove any obvious blockage from the airway. 'Look, listen and feel' again and, if there is still no breathing, start **resuscitation** techniques immediately (see below).

Reflexes are missing in unconsciousness, so any fluid or material in the throat cannot be cleared and may be breathed into the lungs, causing **asphyxiation** (suffocation). This serious condition is most often the result of bringing up the stomach contents (vomiting). When this happens the delicate linings of the lungs are intensely irritated. Watery fluids ooze out to fill the lungs, so stopping the oxygen in the air from reaching the blood stream.

Resuscitation: artificial ventilation

When any casualty has stopped breathing and is turning bluish-grey, you must get some oxygen from your own breath into his or her chest as soon as possible.

Approximately 20% of the air around us is oxygen and, even when we have breathed this in and used some of the oxygen, there is still 16% oxygen left. This is enough to support another person and is the reason why *mouth-to-mouth resuscitation* works.

You cannot try this with another breathing person, so technology has provided us with dummies (more correctly called 'manikins') on which to practise. Manikins usually have inflatable chests and compressible hearts. They are quite expensive so you will probably have to join a first aid class to gain access to one.

Procedure

1   With the casualty flat on his or her back, open the airway as described above, taking care to remove any obstruction by sweeping your finger around the casualty's mouth.
2   Close the casualty's nose by pinching the nostrils with the thumb and forefinger (see Figure 7.8).
3   Take a breath for yourself and seal your mouth around the casualty's mouth. Barrier devices (such as face shields) are available to help with this but in an emergency you could use a handkerchief or a piece of clothing to help you achieve a seal.

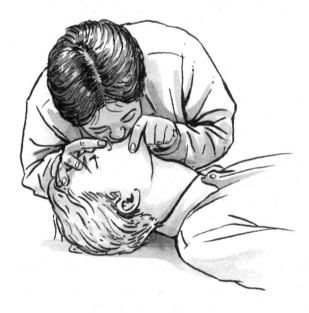

Figure 7.8   Mouth-to-mouth resuscitation

4   As you blow gently but firmly into the casualty's mouth, watch to see if the chest rises. Take your mouth away to breathe for yourself and watch the chest fall. Repeat the process 10 times to load up the casualty's lungs with oxygen. The rate should be approximately 10 breaths each minute: two seconds to inflate followed by four seconds of rest each time.
5   Check the pulse is still there. If you can, call or telephone for help between series of 10 breaths, checking the pulse at these intervals as well.
6   If you are doing it properly you should begin to see a change in skin colour, particularly in the lips and tongue. If the colour does not improve, double-check your technique – especially the open airway and the pulse.
7   If the chest is failing to rise, check the airway position and your mouth seal. Is the nose blocked off and any obstruction cleared? Use your fingers to hook out any obstruction you can see in the airway.
8   Continue until the casualty begins to breathe unaided. Then place him or her in the recovery position (see pages 239–240).

Mouth-to-nose ventilation

This is a variation which can be used if there is damage to the mouth or possible poisoning, or if the resuscitation is taking place in water.

Clearly, it is important to close the mouth with one hand. You are less likely to meet vomit or saliva using this method, but it is often more difficult to do.

Young children and babies

The procedure is slightly different for babies and children up to about 4 years of age.

Place the child on the floor or along your arm and seal your mouth around the child's mouth and nose. Give short, gentle breaths at about 20 per minute.

Resuscitation: blood circulation

If a person's heart stops pumping blood around the body, you will have to be an artificial pump until the heart restarts or until expert help arrives. The casualty's blood has to carry oxygen around the body, and to the brain in particular.

The place to feel for a blood pulse is in the neck – the **carotid pulse** (see Unit 2 for more details about taking a person's pulse). Do not try to feel the wrist pulses, because the casualty's body systems are likely to have closed down the blood flow in the outlying blood vessels to save the more important blood flow to the so-called vital centres – brain, heart and lungs (see Unit 4).

A casualty's heart may be pumping blood but the person may have stopped breathing. In this case the heart will soon stop owing to lack of oxygen (see Unit 4 for details about the functions and structure of the heart).

Chest compression (heart massage)

First, as mentioned above, check the carotid pulse (not the wrist pulse) in one of the two large arteries lying at the side of the windpipe in the neck. Feel with two fingers pressed deep into the side of the neck.

If the carotid pulse is absent you must call an ambulance then start chest compression immediately.

External chest compressions, if correctly performed, will artificially pump about one third of the body's blood around the circulation and, if this blood contains oxygen, it will keep the casualty alive for the time being.

The technique squashes the heart between the vertebral column at the back and the rib cage/breastbone at the front. This action expels

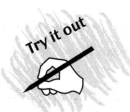

Take your own carotid pulse by counting it for 15 seconds and multiplying the number by 4 to get the beats per minute.

Now take a friend's or a relative's carotid pulse to practise feeling for it.

blood from the heart, towards the lungs and into the main artery (aorta). As you release the pressure, more blood is sucked into the heart from the big veins supplying it. You are therefore making the heart pump blood.

Method of chest compression

To be successful, the pressure must be applied to the correct place.

1 Locate the base of the breastbone where the ribs meet in the centre at the bottom of the rib cage (see Figure 7.10). Establish a baseline of two fingers' width up from that point.

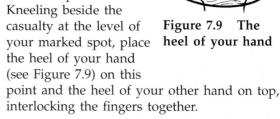

Figure 7.9 The heel of your hand

2 Kneeling beside the casualty at the level of your marked spot, place the heel of your hand (see Figure 7.9) on this point and the heel of your other hand on top, interlocking the fingers together.

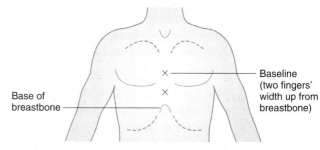

Base of breastbone

Baseline (two fingers' width up from breastbone)

Figure 7.10 Finding where to apply compression

3 Lean forwards over the casualty with arms straight. Push firmly down until the chest is compressed at least 4-5 centimetres and then release. Keep your fingers off the chest, using only the heel of the lowest hand. Do not move the hands in between compressions (see Figure 7.11).

4 You must aim for at least 80 pumps per minute. Experts agree that to help you keep to time, it is useful to say 'one and two and three and four' up to 15, and then begin counting again.

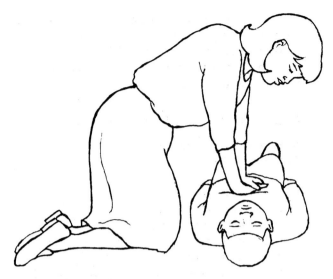

Figure 7.11   Applying compression

Cardio-pulmonary resuscitation (CPR)

Cardio-pulmonary resuscitation (CPR) is exhausting and, if you are on your own, you may not be able to continue for long. Therefore, before you start, shout or phone for help.

While you are on your own carry out two breaths followed by 15 chest compressions, followed by two breaths, 15 compressions and so on. Do not stop to check pulses until you see some sign of blood circulation. If the heart restarts, check the breathing – if it is absent continue resuscitation. If there is breathing, place the casualty in the recovery position (see below) and recheck every ten minutes.

If you have a helper, one of you can be at the head doing mouth-to-mouth resuscitation while the other one is doing chest compressions. In this case

Remember

⬥   *Do not practise on a living person!*

⬥   Join a class so that you are properly trained in the techniques. The best way to learn is to practise.

⬥   The ideas in this section will be easier to remember if you have tried them out in first aid training.

one breath is given after every five compressions of the chest. Monitor the casualty's response as above. Exchange tasks every few minutes so that you can both keep it up for longer.

An unconscious patient who is breathing and whose blood is circulating must now be placed in the recovery position.

If the person is semi-conscious (only half conscious) or worse, always put him or her in the recovery position and check **airway, breathing** and **circulation** (pulse). You should monitor these vital signs every ten minutes.

This is known to first-aiders as the **ABC rule,** and it provides you with the three important things to check for – and in the right order! Add to this (for an unconscious person) **monitoring** the levels of response, and you are well on the way to coping with serious emergencies.

The recovery position

Experts agree that if more people knew how to put an unconscious person into the correct position, many more lives would be saved.

There is really no substitute for a trained person demonstrating the technique to you, who then watches you practise several times. You should try to do this with all first aid procedures. So, if necessary, join a local first aid class. Your local library will be able to tell you where to find one.

The **recovery position** is a steady position which keeps the airway open, allowing fluid (particularly vomit) to drain out of the mouth so that it does not enter the lungs. It also prevents the tongue from falling back and blocking the back of the throat.

Putting a casualty into the recovery position

The procedure is the same for a woman or a man.

1   Tilt the chin to open the airway.
2   Kneel alongside the casualty and straighten his or her legs.
3   Place the arm nearest to you at right angles to the casualty's body with the elbow bent and the palm facing skyward.
4   Lift the knee furthest from you and hold it. Take the furthest arm across the casualty's chest

and tuck his hand palm downwards under his or her cheek to cushion the head. Cradle the head from this point on.

5   Draw the bent knee towards you and the casualty will roll on to his or her side with remarkably little effort.

6   Re-extend the casualty's airway then make a ninety-degree angle of the bent knee.

7   Adjust the casualty's head to lie on the hand so that it remains tilted backwards and the lower bent arm gives stability.

> ### Remember
>
> It is best not to leave the casualty alone. If you have to go to get help, then return as soon as possible.

Dealing with common health emergencies

Situations that can be dealt with in a care setting

The types of emergencies you would be able to deal with in a care setting would depend on the nature of the care setting itself – you would obviously be able to deal with far more emergencies in a well equipped old people's home than if you were working in an older person's own flat or house.

If you look back to page 234 you will find a list of situations where you would definitely call for one of the emergency services – usually the ambulance service. However, there will be situations *when you just don't know* whether you should call for the emergency services or not. In such situations, err on the side of caution and seek expert medical advice. For example, the condition of children who contract certain infectious diseases can worsen very quickly, and such children need hospitalisation (e.g. very young children with urine infections need close monitoring in a hospital).

The role of care assistants in preventing accidents

Care assistants get to know the clients they work with very well, and they come to know their

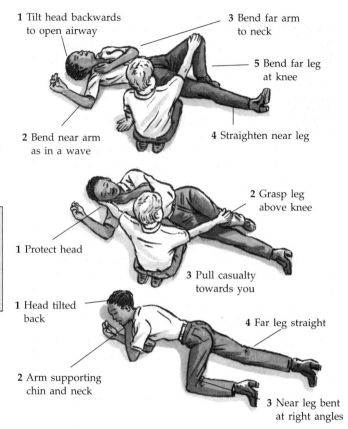

> ### Warning
>
> *If you suspect fractured bones, neck or spinal injury, do not attempt this but protect the airway.*

Figure 7.12   Placing an unconscious person in the recovery position (numbered labels indicate order of placing)

clients' individual strengths and weaknesses. For example, they will recognize occasions or events that might make certain clients become overexcited, or they will spot times when a client may have become confused or preoccupied. It is the ability to recognize these changes in mood that can help prevent accidents. An overexcited or preoccupied client may not take that little bit of extra care needed to negotiate the stairs or may not remember to switch off the fire when going to bed.

A care assistant's intimate knowledge of his or her clients, coupled with the ability to observe events and to act appropriately, will prevent innumerable accidents from happening in the first place.

What are the potential hazards in the following situations? What would you do to minimise the risks of accidents?

1   You visit an elderly, frail client who lives on his own. The client is very quiet and seems preoccupied – all the time you are talking to him his thoughts seem to be elsewhere. He suddenly asks you to read a letter he has just received while he goes to the kitchen to make you a cup of tea.

2   A group of young children at a playgroup are very excited: it's getting near to Christmas and has just started to snow heavily while they are outside in the playground. The carer and yourself decide to get the children back inside. Some go in readily; others are more difficult to persuade and become upset at having to go in out of the snow.

You notice as the children go slowly back inside that they are trailing in on their shoes melting snow and mud.

The role of the care assistant in dealing with accidents and emergencies

When care assistants are called upon to administer first aid they are usually in the company of other carers – some of whom may be more qualified to deal with emergencies. In such situations, the care assistant's role will be to assist the more qualified carer.

The first thing the care assistant should do is to call for that person's help quickly by raising the alarm or by shouting for help. In the mean time, the care assistant should not delay in taking action. If working with other care assistants, he or she may take charge until the more qualified carer arrives.

A care assistant's intimate knowledge of his or her clients will again be of great value in such situations. He or she may know about the client's past medical history and so will have important information to pass on to the more qualified carer when he or she arrives.

Care assistants will be generally experienced in dealing with emergencies and will therefore be able to handle any unpleasant sights more easily, and to keep their feelings under control, than a person not experienced in dealing with emergencies.

Maintaining the dignity of casualties of health emergency situations

We have already looked at those things we can do to help maintain the dignity of casualties of road traffic accidents (see page 235). In care settings, care assistants should call for help to remove other clients from the scene of the emergency, if this is at all possible. They should also pull screens around the client who has had the emergency, if appropriate, and, if necessary, close all doors as soon as this is practically possible.

Procedures for recording and reporting accidents

It is a legal requirement that, within a very short time-span, work-related accidents and some diseases must be reported to the Health and Safety Executive, according to the Reporting of Injuries, Diseases and Dangerous Occurrences Regulations (RIDDOR) 1985.

Care establishments should also keep their own records of accidents and emergencies, either as completed accident forms or as an accident book. The names of witnesses should be entered as well as the name of the casualty, the nature of the injury, the cause and, if appropriate, the environmental conditions at the date and time of the accident. It is also necessary to record how the casualty was treated in the care setting and to record any subsequent action that was taken, such as being sent to the accident and emergency department by ambulance. The details should be completed as soon as possible, and certainly within 24 hours. The appropriate relatives should be informed, particularly guardians or parents if the casualty is a child.

The reasons why so much paperwork is required are as follows:

◦   It may provide other carers with valuable information about the client's past medical history.

- There may be delayed reactions to the accident/emergency. Records will help others understand why these reactions have occurred.

- Records help to monitor the number, type and frequency of accidents.

- The client may become eligible for compensation or industrial injury benefits at a later date.

- Records are invaluable when devising accident prevention schemes.

- There may be a possibility of legal action being taken by the client or the client's relatives. Accurate, correctly recorded accident details may help decide who was responsible for the accident occurring in the first place – or if indeed the accident *was* the result of anyone's lack of care or negligence.

Common health emergencies

The training you would receive while undertaking a first aid qualification would equip you with the relevant knowledge you need to be able to fulfil the requirements of this part of the unit. However, general guidelines and summaries for emergencies are provided here, but if you need more extensive details you should use a good first aid manual such as *The First Aid Manual* (Dorling Kindersley, 1999).

Asthma (Figure 7.13)

People who suffer from asthma have difficulty in breathing, particularly breathing out. Asthma can affect anyone, but children and young people are particularly prone to asthma attacks.

Bone, joint or muscle injuries

Fractures (Figure 7.14)

Young children's bones are more 'bendy' or elastic than adults and, hence, when their bones fracture these fractures are often incomplete breaks ('greenstick fractures'). The bones of older people are more brittle and so fracture more easily (usually into complete breaks).

Figure 7.13 Asthma

Signs and symptoms	Procedures
Difficulty in breathing out, often accompanied with wheezing	Try to calm and reassure the person
There may be a bluish tinge to the lips and skin	Sit the person at a table (preferably near fresh air) and get him or her to lean forward
Watch out for signs of improvement or deterioration	Assist with medication, if available. This is likely to be an inhaler (as in the photograph). Younger children often use a diffuser with their inhaler – the diffuser helps them to breathe in the required amount of medication. Monitor pulse and respiration every 10 minutes. Send for a doctor or call an ambulance if there is no improvement.

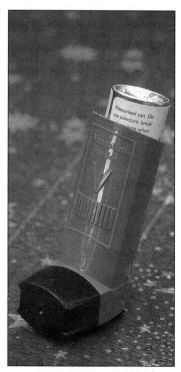

An inhaler

Figure 7.14 Fractures

Signs and symptoms	Procedures
Recent fall or knock	Support and hold the injured body part
Pain at the site of injury	Tie the injured part to another rigid part of the body. Tie from a joint below the injury to a joint above the injury to prevent movement. Pad bony bumps with soft padding
Swelling and bruising	Control the bleeding by direct pressure. Pad well with cotton wool and a bandage
Deformity (the limb looks the wrong shape)	Send for the emergency services
Possible signs of shock (see page 247)	Keep the client still (but move the person if remaining where he or she is would put him or her in danger). Do not give the person food or drink

Sprains

Sprains are injuries to the ligaments that reinforce a joint. They are usually caused by an over-extension of the joint. The treatment of sprains is the same as that for strains (see below).

Strains (Figure 7.15)

Strains are injuries to a muscle or to a tendon that joins a muscle to a bone. They are treated using the RICE procedure (Rest, Ice, Compress, Elevate) – see Figure 7.15.

Dislocations

A dislocation occurs when a bone becomes displaced from a joint. They are treated in the same way as fractures, but you must *not* try to reposition the bone into the joint.

Circulatory disorders

Heart attacks (coronary thrombosis)

Figure 7.16 outlines the signs and symptoms of a heart attack.

Let the victim settle into the most comfortable position, which is usually half-lying and half-

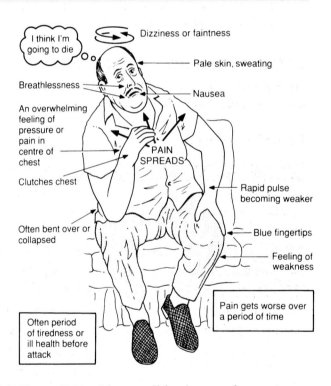

Figure 7.16   The possible signs and symptoms of a heart attack

I think I'm going to die

Dizziness or faintness

Pale skin, sweating

Breathlessness

Nausea

An overwhelming feeling of pressure or pain in centre of chest

PAIN SPREADS

Clutches chest

Rapid pulse becoming weaker

Often bent over or collapsed

Blue fingertips

Feeling of weakness

Pain gets worse over a period of time

Often period of tiredness or ill health before attack

Figure 7.15   Strains and sprains (the RICE procedure)

Signs and symptoms	Procedures
Pain at the site of injury	Rest the injured body part
Bruising	Cool the injured body part with Ice wrapped in cloth
Swelling	Compress the injured body part with wool or plastic foam rubber, and bandage it Elevate the injured part

sitting. Support him or her with cushions, rolled-up coats or something similar, under the knees and at his or her back. Monitor consciousness, breathing and pulses, and be prepared to resuscitate if this becomes necessary while you are waiting for the emergency services to arrive. If the victim is conscious, an aspirin chewed slowly will often ease the effects of a heart attack.

Angina

Angina is often the forerunner of a heart attack. It is characterised by severe chest pain that often runs down the back, down the hands or up to the jaw. It is accompanied by shortness of breath and sudden weakness.

Angina patients often carry medicines (such as tablets or a puffer spray) to ease their attacks. Ask the victim if he or she has such medicine and help him or her to take it. The symptoms should ease within a few minutes, but monitor the victim and call the emergency services if the pain persists.

Stroke (Figure 7.17)

There are several causes of a stroke but they all involve interruption of the blood supply to the brain.

Choking (Figure 7.18)

Choking tends to occur in care settings where there are very young children or elderly people. It is caused by objects becoming stuck in the throat which block the airways.

Concussion (Figure 7.19)

Concussion is caused by a blow of some type which shakes the soft brain inside the hard,

bony skull. This results in a brief loss of consciousness.

Epileptic fits (sometimes called seizures or convulsions)

Febrile convulsions or seizures

'Febrile' means feverish – when you are running a high body temperature. Febrile convulsions or fits are quite common in babies and young children, and these occur when body temperature is raised above normal. Febrile convulsions can be quite alarming: when parents or carers meet them for the first time they may need reassurance that they can cope with the situation.

A child who is having a febrile convulsion may look hot, and his or her skin may appear pink. There may also be some sweating. The child may also hold his or her breath and, consequently, his or her face may go red or acquire a bluish tone. Dribbling at the mouth may also often occur, together with muscle twitching, an arched back and clenched fists.

Cushion the child to prevent injury, and remove bedding to cool the child's body. Sponge the child's body with tepid water, beginning at the head and working downwards. Place the child in the recovery position and observe him or her.

As soon as you can, get medical assistance to help you find the cause of the seizure.

Major fits (grand mal) (Figure 7.20)

Grand mal fits may signify an electrical disturbance to the brain – they are not an illness in themselves. The normal way to suppress such fits is by medication (the brain suffers poor oxygenation during a fit). Fits experienced over a long period of time could lead to brain damage and, hence, more fits: a vicious circle of disability.

Figure 7.17 Stroke

Signs and symptoms	Procedures
Sudden severe headache	If conscious, lie the person down with his or her head and shoulders supported. Turn his or her head to one side
Confusion and stress	Loosen belts and tight clothing to ease breathing
Weakness or paralysis, slurred speech, incontinence, dribbling of the mouth	Monitor the client's breathing, pulse and consciousness

Note: In all cases of suspected stroke, call the emergency services immediately. The effects of stroke vary, depending on the part of the brain affected. A stroke may affect one side of the body only.

Figure 7.18 Choking

Signs and symptoms	Procedures
The person grasps his or her throat or coughs violently	Bend the person over until his or head is lower than his or her chest. Slap the person hard between the shoulder blades, about 5 times
Difficulty with breathing – gasping	If the symptoms persist, stand behind the person, put your arms round the person and lock your hands together just below the breastbone (one hand should be in a fist and the other should be holding it). Sharply thrust your joined hands in and up towards the chest, 4 or 5 times
The skin and lips turn bluish	Repeat the back-slapping and the thrust procedures (as above) 5 times each
Difficulty with speaking	If the obstruction is still present, monitor the person's breathing and pulses. Call the emergency services

Note: Do not use thrusts on a baby or young child. Also, use less force when back-slapping.

Figure 7.19 Concussion

Signs and symptoms	Procedures
Brief loss of consciousness and possibly:	If the person is still unconscious after about 3 minutes, place him or her in the recovery position and call the emergency services
Mild headache Dizzy or feeling sick Cannot remember the event happening	Watch the person closely and insist that he or she sees a doctor

Anyone can have a fit, but people who have suffered brain damage or head injury are more prone to fits than others.

Fainting

Fainting is a brief loss of consciousness caused by a temporary loss of blood flow to the brain. A person who is fainting falls to the floor, looks pale and has a slower pulse than normal. Straighten the person out and raise his or her legs above the level of the heart. This will improve blood flow to the brain, and recovery will take place in a minute or so.

When someone says he or she feels faint, but has not yet fainted, try to prevent the faint by bending the person over at the waist until his or her head hangs lower than the heart. A few minutes in this position will normally do the trick. If you can do this while the person is sitting down, this will be more comfortable.

Foreign bodies

In the ear

Children may push small objects into their ears, and older people may leave cotton wool balls in their ears out of forgetfulness.

Never attempt to dislodge an object embedded in someone's ear – always seek expert help.

In the nose

As before, always seek expert help and encourage the client to breathe through his or her mouth.

In the eye

Two situations occur when a foreign object becomes lodged in the eye. If the body is embedded in the eye, cover the eye with a pad and a bandage and take the person to hospital.

Figure 7.20 Major fits (grand mal)

Signs and symptoms	Procedures
Loss of consciousness, resulting in a fall to the ground	Cushion the fall if possible. Create a space, prevent injury to the person and try to maintain his or her dignity
Arched back and stiff muscles, followed by spasms	Unless the person is in physical danger, leave the client alone but observe him or her closely. Loosen tight clothing, especially around the neck
Breathing stops and the lips and skin look bluish	Place the person in the recovery position as consciousness returns
Urine may be passed or the bowels opened	If one fit follows another or lasts more than a few minutes, call the emergency services
After a few minutes, breathing commences, the muscles relax and the person becomes conscious. He or she may be either dazed or sleepy	Insist on the person seeing a doctor if this is his or her first fit ever

If the foreign body is not embedded, seat the casualty down facing good light and stand behind him or her. Gently open the eyelid and irrigate the area with a stream of *cold* (previously boiled) water. If the object does not come out, try lifting it off with a moist swab or piece of clean linen. If you are still unsuccessful, take the person to hospital, to an ophthalmic opticians or to a GP's surgery.

In the skin
If a foreign body is firmly or deeply embedded in the skin, you may cause further injury by trying to remove it. Instead, pad the area around the foreign object with sterile pads (such as gauze), bandage the injury and take the person to a GP's surgery or to hospital.

If the foreign body is protruding and you are likely to remove it easily, clean the area around the object, take a pair of tweezers and, grasping the object firmly, pull it out in the same direction as it went in. Afterwards, encourage some bleeding to clean the area and then dress the wound. Check whether the client has had a tetanus booster recently; otherwise, advise the person to consult a GP.

Heatstroke
Heatstroke must not be confused with sunstroke – heatstroke is a more serious condition that can be fatal.

Heatstroke is a failure of the brain to control body temperature. The casualty collapses after a period of feeling unwell and can quickly become unconscious. The skin becomes hot and dry, which is an indication the casualty is not sweating. The person may feel restless, confused and dizzy. His or her pulse is full and appears to bound.

Take the casualty to a cool place and remove as much outer clothing as you can. Wrap the person in a wet sheet, and keep the sheet wet by spraying it with water. Call the emergency services immediately. If the casualty becomes unconscious, place him or her in the recovery position. Monitor body temperature if you can and, when it decreases, wrap the person in a dry sheet and monitor him or her closely.

Hypothermia
(See Unit 4 for full details of hypothermia.) Anyone can be affected by hypothermia, not just elderly people who are trying to save on expensive bills: younger people can become immersed in cold water or can be exposed to extreme cold weather conditions. Similarly, babies may suffer a temperature drop in a room that is too cold. In all cases, medical help must be called for immediately.

In hypothermia, the casualty's skin is cold and dry and the casualty has no will to help him or herself at all. Breathing is shallow and the pulse is slow and weak. There may also be a slow drift into unconsciousness and the casualty may be confused mentally.

Remove any wet clothing and replace this with dry, warm clothing. Put the casualty to bed if possible and, remembering that a lot of heat is lost from the head, put a woolly hat on the casualty's head. Give the casualty hot, sweet drinks to sip, or hot soup. If the casualty is able to get into a hot bath, this will warm his or her body better. However, if there is any measure of loss of consciousness, do not put the casualty into a hot bath.

If the casualty becomes unconscious, place him or her in the recovery position and watch him or her closely – be prepared to resuscitate the casualty while waiting for the emergency services to arrive.

Poisoning (Figure 7.22)

Treating a case of poisoning is a complex procedure (see Figure 7.22).

To assist the emergency services identify the poison, keep safe any vomit or empty containers, and tell the emergency services about any circumstances you know of that may have caused the poisoning (e.g. a fume-filled room, etc.). See Figure 7.22 for general guidelines about how to treat a casualty of poisoning.

Electric shock

Never forget to protect yourself: do not touch someone with bare hands if he or she is connected to the electricity supply. Switch off the supply if you can, then remove the person from the supply with a wooden broom handle or chair (or something similar – but something *not* made of metal) as in Figure 7.21. Take particular care if there is water or dampness about, because this will increase your chances of receiving a shock yourself.

The signs of shock vary: from the person appearing shaken up to unconsciousness where

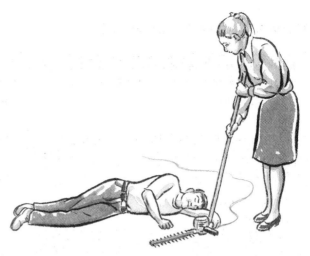

Figure 7.21 Move the casualty away from the electric current

the heart stops beating and the casualty stops breathing. The casualty appears grey and clammy; the pulse is rapid, breathing is shallow and fast, and the person may complain of thirst or nausea. There are often burns where the electricity has entered the body, and these may be deep.

Check breathing and circulation. Lay the victim down on a blanket and cover him or her with another blanket. Raise the legs above the rest of the body. Loosen any tight clothing to assist breathing, and wait for the emergency services to arrive. If the person is unconscious, put him or her in the recovery person and, if his or her heart has stopped beating, be prepared to resuscitate.

Shock (generally)

Apart from electric shock, people can suffer shocks for a number of reasons (e.g. fright, pain, as a response to substances someone may be allergic to, stings from insects, etc.). Shock is dangerous for whatever reason as the vital organs could stop functioning at any time. Do not let the casualty move about, eat, drink or smoke – but you may moisten his or her lips if there is repeated complaint about thirst.

The condition of shock can develop in any person who has lost significant body fluids through such things as blood loss, burns, severe diarrhoea and vomiting.

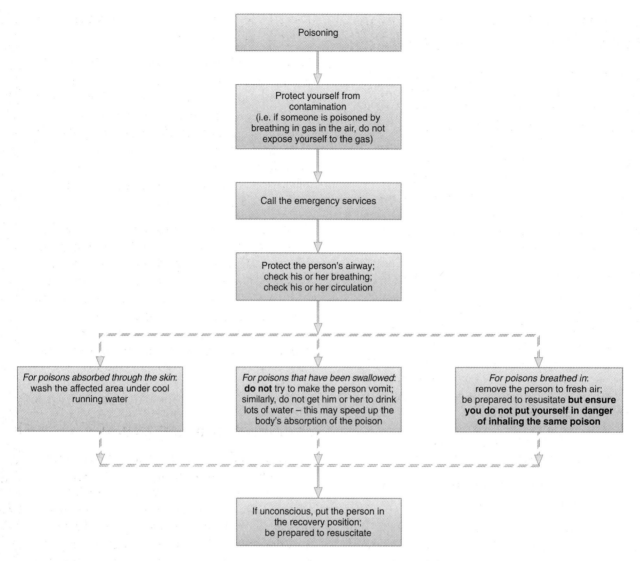

Figure 7.22   The steps involved in dealing with a case of poisoning

Wounds and bleeding

There are many types of wounds and bleeding. The following are some general guidelines:

- Protect yourself against body fluids of any sort (but particularly blood) by wearing disposable gloves.

- Raise the bleeding part if this is possible (this is often easier to achieve if the person lies down). Then apply direct pressure to the wound with your fingers (preferably over a clean or sterile dressing).

- When the bleeding subsides, apply a firm dressing (if the blood seeps through this, add another dressing on top). If anything is

sticking out of the wound, apply pressure to the nearest pulse or pressure point for a few minutes – but for no more than 10 minutes. Build up dressings either side of the object until it is above the wound, and then bandage firmly. Take the victim to the nearest surgery or hospital.

- If the wound or blood loss is extensive, call the emergency services immediately.

- Blood loss may be followed by shock, so be prepared for this.

Unit 7 Assessment

You are required to investigate the possible health hazards and emergencies that might occur in two care settings. One setting might be your placement, voluntary or paid care work, or you might choose to use a client's own home. Your other might be a grandparent, relative or friend who is receiving care of some kind. Alternatively, you could make several visits to a local residential home or nursery (after seeking permission, of course!).

You must relate the hazards to the clients' age and ability, so choose carefully to give yourself plenty of scope. Having described the hazards accurately, you must then say how these might pose risks to everyone (including clients, visitors and employees/care workers). It might help if you revise the difference in meaning between the two words 'hazard' and 'risk':

* A **hazard** is anything that has the potential to harm someone in some way.

* A **risk** is a measure of how likely the hazard is to cause harm.

You might like to devise a scale of 1 to 5, where 1 represents a highly unlikely hazard and 5 represents a positively dangerous hazard. You could score the hazards for each group of people who might come into contact with it.

Your next task is to examine critically how each care setting meets the legal requirements of HASAW, COSHH and the Fire Precautions Act. You might do this by compiling a chart.

The home is not expected to comply with legal requirements, and in most instances it will not! So you will have rather an unbalanced chart or report. Make sure the settings you choose have the potential to come under the requirements of all three

pieces of legislation, and decide which items you are going to monitor.

For your third task, you will probably need to talk to a manager to find out which policies or procedures he or she implements to reduce the hazards in the particular setting. You must then describe this policy in detail (it might include, for example, procedures to prevent cross-infection or to minimise the dangers inherent in clinical waste or soiled bed linen).

Finally, you must demonstrate you know how to give resuscitation and cardiac massage to a client who has stopped breathing and has no pulse. You will need access to a manikin to do this, as you cannot practise on a living person. Joining a first aid class is a worthwhile activity, and you could be assessed on this part of the unit at the same time as you are studying for your first aid qualification.

Obtaining a Merit grade

You will need to demonstrate you can link the action to minimise hazards to legal requirements. For instance, if one of the substances used for cleaning is particularly hazardous and the risk from spilled liquid is considerable to the cleaners, then changing the substance to one less toxic will meet the requirement of the COSHH legislation. You could also set up a short training session to induct the cleaners into the use of the new substance so that its use complies with COSHH requirements.

You will also need to write a short report explaining why it is necessary to record accidents in a care setting, and to show how this is done. You will have to demonstrate, practically, that you can deal with a casualty who has more than one problem. Once again, this is within the scope of a first aid class but remember, if you are providing written evidence of this, you should deal with the most life-threatening problem first.

Do not forget to protect yourself, to shout for help and to maintain the client's dignity as far as this is possible.

Obtaining a Distinction grade

You are required to identify the strengths and weaknesses of any actions taken to minimise hazards in each care setting, and to suggest one improvement for each course of action. You must also compare the ways in which the two care settings deal with these hazards. A chart would once again prove useful here, with the hazards common to both in the left-hand column and your comments for each care setting in the right-hand column. Remember, you are not just listing the hazards but comparing them.

Also, remember that, if you have chosen to study someone's home, your chart may not cover all the legal requirements.

Your final task is to demonstrate how you would deal with an emergency involving more than one person. Your tutor will probably arrange for a simulation to take place, as you will not be expected to be caught in a multiple emergency. Once again, remember to protect yourself, to shout for help to maintain the person's dignity, etc. In this role play, remember to go to the quiet casualties first, as people who are making a noise must be breathing and must have pulses! Organise others to assess the other casualties and to look around in case someone has been missed.

Unit 7 Test

1   Who is responsible for health and safety in the workplace?

2   What are the signs and symptoms of a fractured limb?

3   Which legislation states that emergency exit doors must open outwards?

4   What would you do if an elderly client suffered concussion as a result of a fall?

5   What would you do if a small child in your care had an epileptic fit?

6   A powerful, new cleaner has just been announced. You think it would be ideal for your nursery floor. However, it is a hazardous substance. What do you do next?

7   Maisie is 86 years old. She lives alone in a flat with only her state pension to live on. She has painful arthritis and finds it difficult to move around. It is a very cold winter so you tell her you will collect her pension for her each week until the spring. Actually, you are calling regularly to ensure she doesn't develop … What is the missing word?

8   Working as a care assistant at Freshfields, you notice that Milly rises from her bed very quickly and is very dizzy for about 5 minutes afterwards. You are fearful she might fall at this time. What advice would you give Milly and other care assistants to prevent her falling?

9   One of your male residents has started to spill drops of urine on the floor before going to the toilet first thing in the morning. What are the dangers of this?

10 How would you prevent this from happening in the future?

This unit covers the knowledge you will need in order to meet the assessment requirements for Unit 8. It is written in five sections.

The first section explores all aspects of child development (physical, intellectual, emotional and social). The second section discusses those things that can influence a child's development. Section three looks at those people whose job it is to look after children and what these jobs entail. Section four discusses the reasons children may need care and the causes of those needs. Finally, section five looks at the legislation concerning the care of children.

Advice and ideas for meeting the assessment requirements for the Unit and for achieving Merit and Distinction grades are at the end of the Unit.

Also at the end of the unit is a quick test to check your understanding.

Child development

In this first section, all aspects of child development are investigated. However, you may find that growth tables, information from health visitors and clinics and from early years settings will also be useful in your work. If you wish to investigate the area of child development even further, biology and psychology books will help you.

Child development is rather like a jigsaw puzzle. The whole picture contains lots of smaller pieces that work together to build the finished object. When looking at child development, two important concepts are recognised: growth (which is an increase in size) and development (which is an increase in complexity, ability and control). Many child care professionals have studied the way children develop in order to find patterns in these stages of development and to set benchmarks for all areas of development. These areas are as follows (you might also find it useful here to look back at Unit 3 and Unit 6):

 Physical development

 Intellectual and language development

Emotional development.

Social development.

Sometimes you will also find another area, that of spiritual development, mentioned. You will recall from Unit 6 that a useful way of remembering these different areas is by their initials – PIES.

The purpose of learning about developmental stages is to be able to ensure a child is developing in a healthy way and to check when there may be a problem. It is important to recognise that children differ in the rate at which they pass through these stages and, hence, to use them as guidelines rather than rules of stone.

Physical growth
Development milestones

Reflexes Reflexes are the instant reactions babies have. These reflexes usually vanish quite soon after birth, in most cases, and always by the time a baby is 3 months old. After this time, a baby is able to control its reactions. Examples of some of the simple reflexes a baby is born with are rooting, swallowing and sucking (see Figure 8.1).

Motor skills Motor skills (our ability to co-ordinate the actions we make with our limbs) can be divided into two areas. Gross motor skills are large limb movements (such as waving or standing). Fine motor skill are such things as

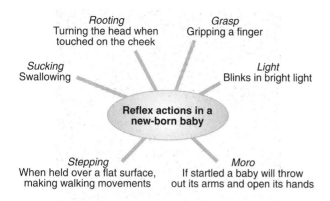

Rooting
Turning the head when touched on the cheek

Grasp
Gripping a finger

Sucking
Swallowing

Light
Blinks in bright light

Reflex actions in a new-born baby

Stepping
When held over a flat surface, making walking movements

Moro
If startled a baby will throw out its arms and open its hands

Figure 8.1 Simple reflexes in a new-born baby

drawing a line with a pencil or picking a hair off someone's jumper.

Development follows a pattern because one stage of development usually relies on another (think of the old saying: 'You have to learn to walk before you can run'). This saying is, in practice, quite true. Babies first learn to roll, then to crawl; they then manage to get on to their feet and to walk. Running comes later.

Babies develop from head to toe. They start off learning how to turn their heads to follow their carers' movements; then they control their arms and their backs before finally getting as far as their legs. They also develop from the outer to the inner. They first learn how to wave their arms, then to clap and, finally, to pick up a bead or a brick. Development similarly evolves from the general to the specific. An 8-month-old baby will crow with delight or scream with displeasure whereas a 7-year-old will smile or frown.

Ways of observing and measuring growth and development

Before a child reaches school age, many checks will have been carried out on his or her growth and development. A new-born baby is examined one minute after birth by the midwife and a paediatrician to check that the basic reflexes are present. This test is known as the Apgar score and it assesses the five vital signs: respiratory effort, heart rate, skin colour, muscle tone and response to stimuli. For each of these, the baby is given a score of 2, 1 or 0, and the total is a score out of ten. A score of between 8 and 10 indicates the baby is in good condition.

As the child grows, health visitors continue to make basic checks on the child's needs. These take place at about 6–8 weeks, between 6 and 9 months, at 18–24 months, somewhere between 3 and 4 years and on school entry. Any child who seems to have a problem or a delay may have more frequent checks.

Children are weighed and measured to ensure they are growing properly and they are assessed for their control of both gross and fine motor skills. Speech is also checked. The reason for these checks is to make sure the baby or child is developing correctly and at the right speed. By undertaking these checks, any extra help the child needs can be supplied so that the child might attain his or her full potential.

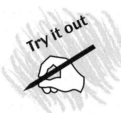

Try it out

Ask an under-8s setting you know if you can visit to measure the height of the children in one year group. You may have to produce a letter to be sent home with the children first, explaining what you want to do and why. (If the children do not want to participate, do not force them; remember that the care values encourage freedom of choice.)

When you have your results, write them up as a graph and look at the **mean**, **mode** and **median** heights within the group (this will give you evidence for both IT and application of number). You should find a cluster of similar heights in the middle of your chart with a few scattered at each end.

What does this tell you about the way children grow?

An important way of checking and measuring the changes a child progresses through is by observation. When we work with older people, a good way of finding out about them is by talking with them and questioning them, but this isn't always possible with children. Depending how young they are, they may not have the ability or the vocabulary to help you out with your questions. By developing good observational skills, it is possible to measure and check the way a child is developing and, hence, to help him or her achieve his or her full potential.

The development of motor skills

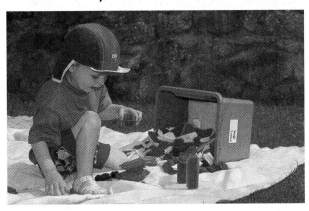

Fine motor skills

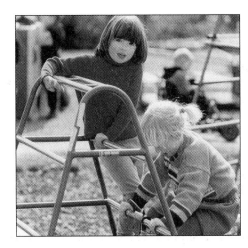

Gross motor skills

Figure 8.2 The development of motor skills

Age	Gross manipulative skills	Fine manipulative skills
6 months	Can roll from front to back. If held in a standing position, bounces up and down. Can put his or her feet into his or her mouth. Sits with support	Stretches out with both hands for interesting small objects within grasp. Passes large objects from one hand to the other, occasionally dropping objects
12 months	Can sit from lying down. Walks with both hands held by another; some may walk alone. Can sit up unsupported. May attempt to climb the stairs	Has a 'pincer grip' and can pick up tiny objects , such as beads, with finger and thumb. Points well. Drinks from a cup and is starting to feed him or herself. Still turns a spoon upside down to get it into his or her mouth occasionally
18 months	Walks and runs safely. Can kneel and bend without wobbling. He or she can climb the stairs, but comes down backwards, facing the treads. Pushes toys along	Scribbles with crayons, pulls off shoes, hats, gloves. Can stack a tower of three cubes. Turns pages well, and is beginning to show a preference for one hand over the other
2 years	Walks upstairs and downstairs holding the banister. Runs and climbs. He or she can stand on tiptoe, and jump off a low step. Riding wheeled toys is possible	Can unwrap a sweet. Can help get him or herself dressed and builds towers of more than seven bricks. He or she feeds him or herself well and can draw circles and dots with accuracy
3 years	Climbs stairs like an adult, but may still come down more cautiously. Throws and kicks a ball strongly; may be able to catch a large ball with two hands. Riding a three-wheeled bike is possible	Can draw a recognisable, if odd, human form. Builds a high tower and a simple bridge with bricks. Some may use scissors with help
4 years	Climbs ladders, hops and jumps with ease. Can avoid things when running and walk down a line	Can do simple jigsaw puzzles and shape puzzles. Eats tidily and drinks from a tumbler. Buttons are no longer difficult, although zips may be a problem. Draws well
6–8 years	Rides a two-wheeled bike, balances and has control of general locomotion. Plays ball games with accuracy. Skips. Can stand on one leg for about ten seconds without wobbling	Writes and draws neatly. Uses construction toys with ease, can sew, cut and most can tie their shoelaces. Could make a sandwich or cut a slice of cake. Eats neatly (mostly!)

As we have already seen, a child's ability to control movement is known as motor skill development. Mastering these motor skills will enable a child to have full control over his or her body. These skills develop in a certain order (see Figure 8.2).

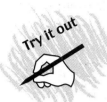

If possible, arrange to visit your health visitor during a baby and toddler clinic. If you do, you may have the opportunity to interview primary carers and to observe the children, as well as to talk with the health visitor about the way he or she checks the children's development.

The development of hearing and sight

Hearing Babies are able to follow sounds and, later, enjoy making noises of their own. At birth a loud noise will startle a baby and make it cry. A baby learns very quickly how to pinpoint where a sound comes from, and will look in familiar places for familiar noises. Babies sometimes stop feeding if they are disturbed by an unexpected noise, and will often become still if a person enters the room.

By 3 months a baby will turn to try to locate the sound of a familiar voice and may smile. At 6 months the location is much more accurate: whisper behind a child of this age and he or she will turn his or her head the right way to look at you. By 1 year, not only are noises located but also their meaning can be understood by the child. He or she may even be able to reply.

Children learn about language by listening and imitating, so it is important that any hearing impediments are discovered and treated as quickly as possible in order for the child to be able to learn to communicate without difficulty.

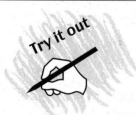

Watch a group of carers who are looking after babies of less than 1 year old.

What differences do you notice in the way the carers speak to the babies? Do they use the same methods of communication with older children? Why do you think communication is used in different ways?

One of the differences you may have noticed in the way carers speak to babies is in their facial expression. Because it is important to keep the baby's attention when speaking, the carer may use exaggerated gestures and expressions. What did the baby do?

Babies are capable of hearing noises from inside the womb as early as three months before birth.

Sight New-born babies have a fixed focus of about 25 cm. They are aware of darkness and light and of still and moving shapes, but anything outside their field of focus is fuzzy and without meaning (see Figure 8.3).

Figure 8.3   The development of vision

Age of baby	Development
3 months	Short-sighted, but with a greater range. Good eye control. Watches activities
6 months	Eyes now work together nearly all the time; this is known as binocular vision. Turns head to watch and to look at interesting things
1 year	Can follow the progress of an object that moves quite quickly, such as a toy car or an animal. Recognises faces of people, and can focus over quite a distance
2 years	Has total vision, within biological ability
3 years +	Is able to recognise colours (about 8% of boys may have some degree of colour blindness)

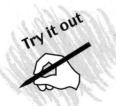

Put a brightly coloured sticky shape on a ruler at the 25 cm mark. Then place the ruler on the bridge of your nose. That's about as far as a new-born baby can focus! If you can make a 'cradle' with your arms and look down at an imaginary baby, that is about the same distance.

Within a few days of birth, a baby has learnt to recognise the face of his or her primary carer.

Talk it over

Desmond Morris believes that a short field of focus is 'The height of efficiency. [The baby's] blurred, long-distance vision is a valuable anti-anxiety device. Since the infant is physically more or less helpless, there is no advantage in knowing what is happening far away from its body. Its blissful ignorance of the long-distance world leaves it snugly relaxed and contented' (*Babywatching*, published by Cape).

Discuss this extract. How true do you think it is?

Intellectual development

Language

Communication is all about language, be it spoken, signed or inferred by body posture. We learn to communicate by watching and imitating those around us. A baby soon learns that smiling faces are nicer to have around than frowning ones, and it will imitate these. Language and learning are closely linked: the child who has good language skills can express him or herself and can talk about all the things he or she sees and does.

The prelinguistic stage   Even before a young child develops a vocabulary, he or she can communicate his or her thoughts and needs. A crying baby demands attention, whether this is for food, warmth or affection. New parents soon learn to associate particular cries with particular needs. They can spot the difference between a hungry cry and a tired cry. Responding to these in an appropriate way reinforces the communication that is taking place. Linguists call this stage of development the 'prelinguistic stage'.

The linguistic stage   It would be very strange if babies woke up one morning and started to speak like adults. Instead, they develop a *pattern* that later becomes language. A baby of about 8 weeks will happily babble to itself; by about 5 months this may have developed into recognisable syllables such as 'Da-da-da'. Babies are good mimics – they can copy 'Atishoo' and 'Yum-yum' noises easily. All babies have the desire to communicate with, and to get a reaction from, adults.

Around the age of 12 months, babies say their first words. They have learnt enough language to understand simple commands and requests, such as 'Show me your feet', 'Wave bye-bye' and 'Give me the car'. By 2–3 years, most children know many words. They can ask questions and can put three to four words into sentences. From 4–8 years of age, children develop quickly. They use language to socialise and can tell jokes. The average 5-year-old has a vocabulary of 5,000 words.

CASE STUDY – Tanya

Some children are difficult to understand

Tanya is babysitting when 2-year-old Jack wakes up. He is cross and upset. Tanya gives him a cuddle and tries to find out what is wrong. He keeps saying the same word, which sounds like 'kurka'. Tanya hasn't got a clue what he means and tries to find out, largely by a process of elimination: 'Shall I open the curtains? Is it too dark?'

This seems to make Jack angrier. 'No!' he yells, wriggling furiously, 'kurka!' Tanya tries a drink, a cuddle, a tape and a story book. Jack is very frustrated that Tanya doesn't understand him. Finally she offers him a soft toy tortoise that has fallen on to the floor by his bed.

He beams at her: 'kurka!'

Finally she realises what he has been telling her: 'Yes, it's a lovely *turtle*, Jack'.

Jack soon settles down to sleep.

Question

Could this situation have been avoided, or do you think that misunderstanding helps the process of learning language?

Memory

Babies are born without the ability to file things into their brains for later use. Adults, on the other hand, can use this filing and storage facility and call it 'memory'. Babies learn to imitate – first movements and then sounds. This imitation is filed away.

Think it over

If you smile at a new-born baby, the only chance you have of him or her smiling back at you is if he or she has wind! A baby will start to smile back properly in the first month to six weeks of life and, as he or she gets older, the child will smile more readily. This is because the child has memorised the response needed to get positive feedback from the people around him or her. First smiles, first 'words' and first achievements – recognised in a positive way with affection or praise – encourage the child to remember and to move on to the next stage of development.

As children reach toddlerhood, they are able to remember more and more. This can help them with planning and with handling unfamiliar situations. They remember similar situations and are able to predict, with some accuracy, the likely outcome.

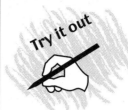

Try it out

Watch a child with a new toy (for instance, a 'pull-back' train). The child might have had a push-along train and so he or she 'drives' it down the carpet with his or her hand. If the child pulls the train backwards by accident and then lets go, the train will rush forward.

The child may be surprised at first but the action is funny, so he or she tries to repeat the situation. If the child manages to do this, the information is stored. Now he or she knows that trains all move forward, and some might go backwards as well.

If the child is presented with a pull-back car, he or she will automatically try out the action that worked with the train. The child is using his or her memory to predict the action.

Perception (the way we see the world)

It takes time for children to become aware of themselves and how they fit into the world around them. Gradually in the first year, a child will become aware of his or her own name and, slightly later, of the names of the members of his or her family and own home.

A small child will soon be able to tell people who he or she is and how old he or she is. Children are keen to tell you about the things they sense 'belong' to them (brothers and sisters, adult

CASE STUDY – Ahmed

Ahmed is 10 months old. He stands at a coffee table and bangs a biscuit on it. His mother comes in. He perceives his mother (i.e. he is aware that she has come into the room). Ahmed then links the prior experience he has of his mother with this present one. He also has a concept she will come to talk to him – she has always done this in the past.

This is an early concept of Ahmed's mother and of the sorts of things she does.

Questions

1 Might Ahmed think that banging a biscuit on the table summons his mother into the room?

2 How and when will he know this is not true?

relatives, pets, playmates and so on). They want to explain how they fit in with the world around them.

A child's perception of him or herself also runs to capabilities and shortfalls: 'I'm nearly 5 now, and so I can ride a bike with two wheels. My sister can't, but she's only little, she's not even 3 yet.'

Perception is linked to memory, which is in turn a key part of planning ahead and coping with the different experiences in life. This helps with the formation of concepts or fixed ideas. **Concepts** help with the organisation of thinking, with idea formation, organising previous experiences and perceptions and also with the prediction of the future.

Piaget and children's learning

A Swiss psychologist, Jean Piaget, studied children's cognition and learning. He thought that, although a child's understanding of the world was first based on the visible features of life, that understanding changed with experience. Hence a child would come to recognise not only that other people might see things differently from him or herself but the child would also understand why. Piaget suggested that children think in a different way from adults, and that their understanding went through four distinct stages.

The first stage is the **sensori-motor stage**, which occurs from birth until about 18 months of age. This is where a child's understanding of the world around him or her is limited by the client's own senses and movement. Children are *egocentric* at this stage (i.e. they see the world as revolving around themselves). At this stage, a child usually understands the idea of *object permanence*. Children recognise that objects and people still exist even if they are out of sight.

Stage two is known as the **preoperational** stage, and this occurs between 18 months and 7 years of age. Preoperational children do not always understand how meaning works in language, and do not use logic in the same way as adults.

> **Think it over**
>
> Suppose you had a litre of water. When it is in a measuring jug, you can see by the markings on the jug there is one litre. Pour the water into a bath, and there appears to be very little water. But an adult knows there is still a litre because he or she can *conserve* the volume.
>
> A small child, on the other hand, might think there is much less water because it is hardly visible in the bath as it covers a greater area and is much shallower. If you asked the child which container held more water, he or she would tell you there was more in the jug. To the child it would seem full, so there must be more there. The child has not learnt to conserve the volume.

Animism also occurs at this stage. The children give thoughts and feelings to objects. For instance, they might think that 'The car is much happier now we've washed it' or 'The naughty door bumped my head'. This vanishes when a child is about 5 years old. Children at this stage are still egocentric and cannot see another person's point of view.

In the third stage, the **concrete operational**, children are between 7 and 11 years old. They think logically and can take account of more than one aspect of a situation (this is known as decentring). They are aware of conversation and are no longer egocentric. Children at this stage are able to use symbols to represent words, directions, music or any other concept that demands them, and they are aware of the reasons behind the rules. At this stage the child is moving towards logical, abstract thinking, where he or she can work out ideas in his or her head rather than needing to see the concept in reality.

The final stage is known as the **formal operational** stage. At this stage, adolescents can imagine the impossible and can manipulate ideas in their heads. They can also test different hypotheses. This can prove useful when something mechanical goes wrong – it gives an individual the ability to think: 'Well, if the car won't start, it might be out of petrol, or it could be . . .' This stage of development also gives an individual the ability to challenge ideas and concepts, which often leads to conflict between adolescents and adults!

These four stages are all part of the learning or intellectual development an individual undergoes.

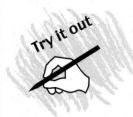

Fill two jars with water. Put six fat pebbles in the first jar and ask a small child which jar has more water in it. (Most children will say the jar with pebbles in it, as the water level appears higher.)

Pour the water from each jar into a measuring jug to show the child that the same amount is in each container. The next time you do this, you could let the children drop the pebbles in.

Emotional development

How a child bonds with his or her primary carer

Bonding is the word used to describe the way a child and his or her primary carer develop an emotional attachment. Bonding starts at birth, but develops through a child's life right into adulthood and old age. A bond is something that ties you to something else, in this case an emotional reaction that makes you feel close to another person. It is reinforced every time the two people with a bond are together.

Bonding occurs when a child feels he or she is safe and secure in the company of his or her carer. The child develops an emotional need and attachment for that carer, whether the carer is the child's mother or father or another adult responsible for the child's day-to-day welfare (see Figure 8.4).

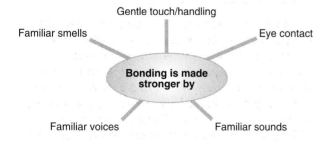

Figure 8.4 Bonding

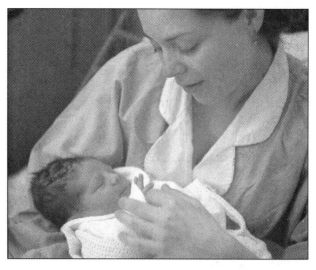

Figure 8.5 The process of bonding

The first bond a baby makes is with its mother (see Figure 8.5). A researcher into this area, John Bowlby, studied the effects bonding and attachment have on adolescents and juveniles. He thought that the first bonds were very important, that they happened instinctively and were caused by a biological need. He considered that, if a child had not formed a secure attachment by 3 years old, he or she would have problems making attachments in later years. Other studies have shown that even when a child is raised in institutional care, good secure attachments are formed in childhood, certainly by the time a child is 8 years old.

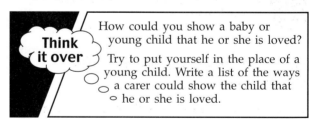

How could you show a baby or young child that he or she is loved? Try to put yourself in the place of a young child. Write a list of the ways a carer could show the child that he or she is loved.

How attachments develop

Babies respond to any carer with the same degree of attachment until they are about 3 months old. After this age they become aware of familiar faces and are pleased to see people they know. A baby as young as 3 months will be able to recognise and show delight at the arrival of a parent at the end of the day. At around 6 months, a baby not only prefers people around who are familiar but will also begin to show fear of strangers and distress at being separated from the person who cares for the baby. By about 9 months the baby has usually formed a secure attachment.

An attachment develops when a baby or child feels safe and secure. They look for comfort and protection from a person who is special to them, and they are confident they are safe with that person. One of the most important aspects of forming a secure attachment is for the baby to be treated consistently by the person who looks after it. If a carer reacts the same way all the time, the baby or child can gauge the way the carer will behave. Equally, if the carer is not consistent or is unpredictable in the way he or she responds, the baby is uncertain of the reaction it may get and so feels insecure.

Attachments help children in later life. They help the child to:

- learn how to get on with others;
- be confident and develop self-esteem;
- learn how to talk, think and understand the world around him or her.

Think it over

Many young children have a special comforter, such as a blanket or teddy they use to make them feel safe.

Did you have one of these or do you know someone who had one? At what age did you/they give it up? How would you feel if someone took it away from you?

How children develop self-awareness

By comparing themselves with other children, and by asking questions, children start to develop an idea of who they are. A very small child might define him or herself by whom he or she 'belongs' to: 'My name is Chan and my brother is called Li.' Gradually, physical characteristics become obvious to children: 'I'm as tall as Noriko and not as tall as Damien.' Often, small children do not notice racial differences. They see everyone as being different and do not see patterns of difference as being anything special. Gender differences are often reinforced from an early age: 'Clever girl! Good boy!'

Children gradually learn the differences between themselves and others through the way other people react to them. This helps them to develop their own self-image. A positive self-image is important for a child to feel secure. If you were constantly told you were stupid, eventually you might believe it. Would that encourage you to try to do something new? What if you were praised for trying, even if you didn't succeed? Would you try again? If your self-image is reinforced by the people around you, it becomes stronger. If you are happy with your self-image, you become more confident in life.

Think it over

Why do you think the following situation might occur?

Peter (aged 3 years) is giving his teddy some 'medicine'. He tucks the teddy into a shoe box and says: 'Good boy, Edward, now if you have a sleep, you'll soon feel just fine again!'

Sacha (aged 6 years) is 'teaching' her little brother Leo: 'Leo, if you wriggle around like that you'll fall off the chair and hurt yourself. Sit still and listen and you'll soon be clever like me.'

Children often reinforce the ideas they have about their own self-image and the images of others. They imagine what it must be like to be a doctor or a teacher and, by putting themselves into someone else's shoes, they start to recognise the differences between people.

Social development
How children start to make relationships with others

As individuals become older, they become part of a larger and larger society. This might sound strange, but think about a new-born baby. Although many people may visit to admire the baby in the first few weeks of his or her life, the main people in that baby's social circle are his or her parents and siblings. Later on this circle widens to include friends of the people who care for the child and perhaps their children as well. Once a child joins a toddler group, that circle widens again, with the important difference that

Figure 8.6 Social development

Age	Development
6 months	Friendly with strangers, but occasionally shy. Touches and pats familiar people and objects. 'Kisses'
12 months	Is affectionate to familiar people, but distressed when they are absent. Waves and may say 'Hello' or 'Bye'. Is often upset when seeing or hearing another person upset. Babies of this age often look for the owner of a howling voice in a supermarket and appear worried for them
18 months	Alternates between being clingy and resisting adults. Doesn't like to be alone with unfamiliar people. Plays alone or in tandem with others
2 years	Demands carer's attention ('Why') and is urgent with demands. Plays with other children. May share, but unwillingly. Is quite prepared to throw a tantrum if thwarted
3 years	Likes to help, joins in with songs and stories, plays games with adults and children. Shares and shows affection
4 years	Argues but hits less often. He or she will be competitive and takes turns in a game, and can understand the need for rules. Often appears adult in his or her concern for others
6–8 years	Has a circle of friends whom he or she is determined to keep. Has a strong sense of who he or she is and where he or she belongs in society

other adults are in control, rather than mummy or daddy or the person who normally looks after the child during the day. This circle could alter again, at preschool, and again when the child starts to attend school at around the age of 5 years (see Figure 8.6).

During these changes, a child starts to develop friendships and relationships with the adults and children he or she meets frequently. If a stable relationship is formed, the child will feel more secure and happy to be in the company of someone other than his or her primary carer.

The influences on developing relationships

The first relationships children make are within their own families, with the people they see and live with day to day. As they grow and have more experience of life, their circle of relationships widens. Some people may be friends, some might be family, some might be in a position of authority, but they are all relationships.

Growing children learn to make relationships with the people around them, and to respond in the correct manner to people according to the type of relationship they have. Often there is

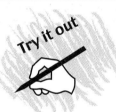

Try it out

On a sheet of paper, write down the names of all the people you have spoken with this week, even if all you said was as brief as 'hello' or 'thank you'. Use red to underline your family, blue to underline your friends, black to underline anyone you have spoken to who is in a position of authority and green to underline people you have come across generally, such as bus drivers, shop assistants, canteen assistants and so on.

Now draw these in groups, surrounded by the same colour. Which is the largest group? Do you think that you behave in a certain way to particular groups?

confusion at first. Infants at school often call the teacher 'mummy' by mistake, or want to sit on someone's knee at story time. They have to learn to adjust their behaviour to fit the relationship.

Once children start nursery or school, their development will be monitored against a set of targets. From the age of 3 to 5 these are called Early Learning Goals (or the Foundation Curriculum). From the age of 5 (the end of reception year) children must follow National Curriculum, Key Stage 1.

As children turn into adolescents, the relationships around them change again. Individuals of the opposite gender can become attractive instead of repulsive. Parental guidance is seen as interfering. Loving grandparents may be stereotyped as ugly. As adulthood is reached, there is usually some kind of equilibrium where individuals are measured on their own strengths and weaknesses rather than by adolescent peer group judgements. Adults sometimes find it easier to have friendly relationships with people they do not like much – for the sake of a quiet life. In childhood, if you don't like someone, it is less easy to hide the fact.

Influences on child development

There are all kinds of influences on the way children develop. Some of these are positive and some are less so (see Figure 8.7). However, it is the differences between people that make people individuals. Some differences are genetic, such as the colour of someone's eyes or of his or her skin. Other differences happen because of events in life. For example, if a child was involved in a road accident and missed school for a period of time, this may affect the child's learning. It might also affect the child's attitude to safety and security: the child may be unwilling to take risks or just be unwilling to cross the road without an adult near by. It might affect how well the child makes friends in later life, because being away from others for a long time might make him or her shy. The effects spread like the ripples on a pond.

Development is also affected strongly by the way a child is brought up at home – a child's **primary socialisation** can alter the way a child behaves, dresses, eats and learns. A household with a high income is likely to produce children who are well nourished, who spend longer in education, have better overall health and are under less stress than a household with a much lower income.

The number of children in a family also affects the way a child behaves. If you are the middle child of five, it is fairly likely you are able to withstand teasing, can look after yourself and value your own personal space. An only child might expect to be the centre of attention, or be uncertain about how to join in with a group of others. The eldest child in a family might feel he or she has the responsibility for younger siblings. He or she might also feel he or she is permanently to blame for the misdeeds of his or her younger brothers and sisters. All these factors affect development.

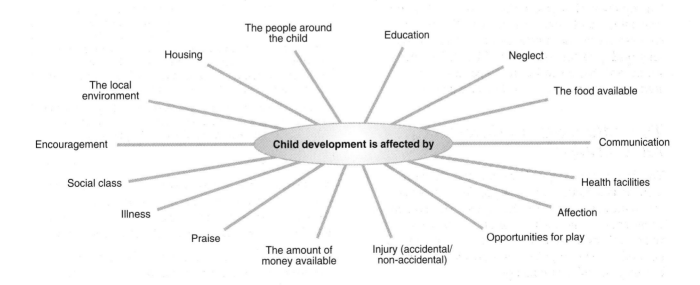

Figure 8.7 Factors that affect child development

CASE STUDIES – Lily and Julius

Using these two studies, draw up a chart showing the influences on each child:

Lily is 9 years old. She is the only child of Hugo and Catherine Thompson. Hugo is an investment banker and Catherine spends a lot of her time organising charity events in support of the third world. Lily goes to a private school. There are nine children in her class and her favourite subjects are French and History. On Tuesday evenings, Lily has ballet classes and, on Thursdays, she is learning to play the piano. Most of her weekends are spent riding her horse, Trigger, which is stabled with some friends who have a riding school and stable.

Julius is also 9 years old. He is the middle child of five and lives with his mother and brothers and sister in a large industrial town. He hasn't seen his dad for a couple of years now. When he first left, it was to find work in another town, but now he doesn't ring up and his mum won't answer any questions about where he is.

Julius' sister is expecting a baby any day now, which will make their house even more cramped. His mum is worried about how they will cope and yells at the boys all the time when they make a mess or want something to eat. She works as a cleaner from 6 am to 8.30 am every day, so Julius has to get himself and his little brother ready for school. There isn't always bread for breakfast and they have to buy crisps on the way to school.

Questions

1 How much time can Lily's parents and Julius' mum spend with their child?

2 How much privacy and personal space does each of the children have?

3 How old do you think each child might be when they finish in full-time education?

4 Who do you think has the best chance of fulfilling his or her potential, Lily or Julius?

People who look after children

You will need to know about the various people who are trained to look after children, how they are trained and how they carry out their jobs (see Figure 8.8).

Nursery nurses

Nursery nurses provide care and support for children up to the age of 8 years, helping and encouraging every aspect of their growth and development. They can work in schools, nurseries, hospitals, holiday centres and can also be employed by families. Nursery nurses usually train in one of two ways, either through a full-time course at college or in the workplace via NVQs or SVQs.

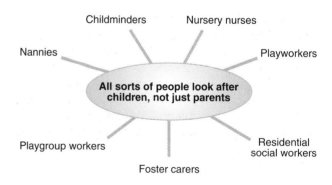

Figure 8.8 The people who look after children

Contact
Professional Association of Nursery Nurses,
St James Court,
Friar Gate, Derby DE1 1BT

Childminders

Childminders are self-employed. They work from their own homes, looking after children whose parents are at work or busy. To be a childminder you must be over 18 years of age and be registered with the social services for your area, who carry out a series of checks on the potential childminder, on any other adults living in the household and on the premises where the childminding will take place.

Many social services departments provide training and support. Although you do not need a qualification in child care to look after children, many parents prefer that their children are cared for by a professional person. There is a National Association for Childminders, which helps to promote training and gives helpful advice on contracts with parents and other paperwork, as well as providing legal support.

'Being a childminder is not simply a case of being paid to play with children. It's a very responsible job: you're totally in charge of the children and their upbringing for the time they're with you'. Nina Bisgrove, childminder.

Contact
The National Childminding Association,
8 Mason's Hill, Bromley BR2 9EY, Kent

Nannies

Nannies look after children in the children's own home. The job can be 'living in' or day to day. Nannies have to negotiate their own contracts with their employers, sorting out their hours, rates of pay, duties and holiday entitlement. A nanny does not have to be qualified or registered, although the government is making moves towards changing this. It is very important if you are working as a nanny that you have proper insurance.

Contact
Professional Association of Nursery Nurses,
St James Court,
Friar Gate, Derby DE1 1BT

Playgroup workers

Playgroup workers often start as volunteers before taking qualifications, which can either be achieved through a college or NVQs/SVQs. They plan and organise activities to help children learn to learn and to develop while enjoying themselves at the same time. Many playworkers are employed by out-of-school clubs or holiday schemes. Special play projects also exist for children with special needs. Playworkers could work in clubs, adventure playgrounds, family centres – in fact anywhere where children will benefit from them.

Contact
National Play Information Centre,
359–361 Euston Road,
London NW1 3AL

Playworkers

Playworkers help children with their out-of-school play. They might be employed by a voluntary agency or by the local council to set up (or work from) an adventure playground, a club or family centre. They work with children to help them learn to be creative or to interact with others. Playworkers are employed both full time and part time.

Contact
National Play Information Centre,
359–361 Euston Road,
London NW1 3AL

Foster carers

Foster carers care for other people's children on a temporary basis until their permanent future homes can be decided upon. This is demanding, full-time work. Prospective foster parents are assessed by the social services in all areas of their lives. Police checks are carried out on the adults living in the house and there are meetings and interviews with social workers. It is important that a child who is already in need of care goes to live with a family who can provide stability and 'an ordinary life' rather than entering into another household where the child's safety is threatened. No formal or academic qualifications are needed to become a foster parent.

Contact
The National Foster Care Association,
Francis House,
Francis Street,
London SW1P 1DE

Residential social workers

Social workers provide care and support for vulnerable members of society. They can be divided into two groups: field and residential workers. Residential social workers are based in residential nurseries, family units, special schools and residential homes. Field social workers visit children and their families in their own homes.

Their job is to help, particularly when there are difficulties. For example, they can help families to collect their benefits, can organise child care and can talk to parents who may be having difficulties with their children. Most are employed by local authority social services units. To work in this area, a Diploma in Social Work is needed.

Contact
Central Council for Education and Training in Social Work,
Information Service,
Derbyshire House,
St Chad's Street, London WC1H 8AD

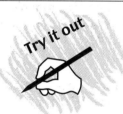

Try it out

Working in groups, look again at Figure 8.6. Do some of your group members have contacts with the people listed there?

Working in small groups or as individuals, arrange to interview just one of the people in the diagram and give your information as a presentation to the rest of the group. You could perhaps use leaflets, show photographs explaining their work or show illustrations of the work the children in their care have produced. Try to find out about their training, their day-to-day work and their opinions of the importance of the work they do, particularly focusing on child development (this interview and presentation will give you evidence for

Caring for children
Children's rights

Every individual has rights. Sometimes these are over-ridden or ignored because the individual concerned has no voice to speak up for him or herself. This could be because the person is ill, is unable to speak the language or because of his or her age. Children's rights are just as important as adults' rights and so it is important they are not

ignored. Legislation helps children with their rights. Since 1991, the UK government has been bound by a piece of legislation known as the UN Convention on the Rights of the Child (Figure 8.9).

Children have the right to:

✓ *Recognition of their value as people now and not merely as adults-in-waiting.*

✓ *Receive physical and emotional care.*

✓ *Feel safe from all forms of physical and mental violence and deliberate humiliation including physical punishment from parents.*

✓ *Express their views on all matters of concern to them and have them taken seriously.*

✓ *Respect for their evolving capacity, including the gradual acceptance of responsibility and decision-making.*

✓ *Information appropriate to their age, both to encourage participation in and to help them understand decisions that affect their lives.*

✓ *Respect for their privacy.*

✓ *Respect for their religious and other beliefs.*

Figure 8.9 The UN Convention on the Rights of the Child

These and other rights are set out in the form of statements, called articles. They all apply to children and to young adults up to the age of 18 years.

Remember: Children are not little adults. They are complex, vulnerable human beings.

In everyday dealings with children, it is very important the children are respected as individuals and given fair treatment (see Figure 8.10).

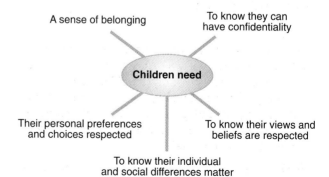

Figure 8.10 Children's needs

Childcare skills

Talk it over

In small groups, brainstorm the sort of skills needed by people who care for children. Remember, these must be interpersonal skills and professional skills, so discuss the day-to-day aspects of the jobs as well as the caring skills.

When you have finished, you could produce a poster that would attract people with the right skills into working with children (see Figure 8.11).

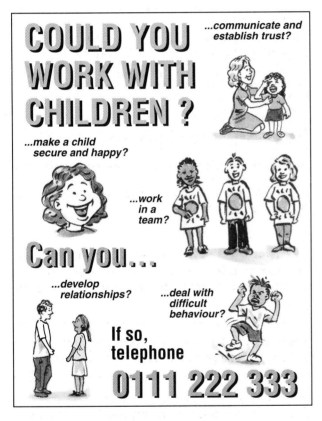

Figure 8.11 The skills needed by people who work with children

You may have been surprised by the range of skills needed. Caring for children isn't just about being able to comfort a crying child or to encourage children to play, it's also about dealing with colleagues and parents and about ensuring the children are happy, safe and able to develop to their fullest potential.

By observing the children in their care, childcare workers are able to check their development. The

communication between the workers and these children establishes trust, and can have positive influences on a child's interest and enthusiasm for a subject. Because of the training and study childcare workers undertake, they understand why children are not always on their best behaviour and can give them the tools they need to handle tricky situations.

Why children need caring for and how this can affect them

There are all sorts of reasons why children are cared for by people who are not their biological parents. Some of these reasons are shown in Figure 8.12. It is very important that the care children receive provides a secure base for them to grow within. The people caring for them are acting as surrogate parents and so are responsible for their care, safety and happiness. Sometimes children who are being cared for by other people may have problems of their own (for example, grief because their parent is dead), which makes caring for them slightly more difficult than it might otherwise have been.

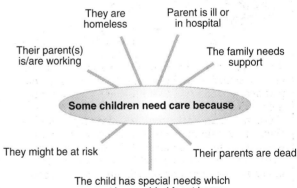

Figure 8.12 Some of the reasons children might need care

Probably the most frequent reason for children being cared for by other adults is because their parents are at work. Occasionally it is possible that the child might be looked after by another relative, such as an aunt or a grandparent, but other options are needed for some people. These include childminders, day nurseries, nannies, mother's helps and *au pairs*. According to research, 'The main form of care for children under the age of three is that given by relatives, followed by childminders, and a long way behind, nurseries and nannies' (Hennessy *et al.*, *Children and Day Care*, Paul Chapman Publishing, 1992).

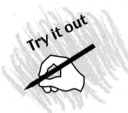

Try it out

Contact someone you know whose children are (or were) looked after by someone else during the day because the parent(s) were at work. How did they choose the carer? Was it difficult to find the person they wanted? Were there any problems? Did the care given live up to the parents' expectations? Was the child happy with his or her carer?

Feed back your findings to the rest of the group. Do others have similar results to the ones you found yourself?

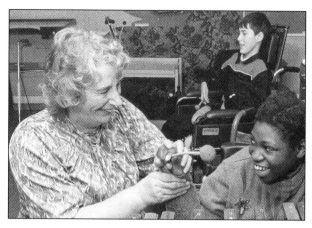

Special needs children can benefit socially and emotionally from being cared for away from home occasionally

If a parent is ill or in hospital, short-term care might be needed for the child. This might include sleeping overnight in an unfamiliar place and staying with people who don't know established bedtime routines. This can be very unsettling for the child, especially if the child is uncertain where

CASE STUDY – Lucas and Ria

Lucas and Ria's mother has been rushed into hospital in the night. When they wake up in the morning, Mrs Williams from next door is in their kitchen. There is no sign of mum or dad. She explains: 'Mummy is a bit poorly, and Daddy's taken her to the hospital. I'm going to look after you today. We'll have a lovely time. Shall we go for a picnic?'

Lucas is 5 years old and feels a bit worried. Surely if Mum and Dad were going out they would have said? He knows that he's not supposed to go anywhere with another adult unless Mum or Dad say it's all right. He can't let Ria go with Mrs Williams on her own, though, because she's only 3 and he's supposed to look after her.

He doesn't know what to do. He'd like to ask someone, but he doesn't know Mrs Williams well enough to explain his problem.

He refuses to eat and knocks his glass over just as Mrs Williams is starting to pour a drink. She says: 'Never mind, dear, accidents happen.' Ria sits down to breakfast. Mrs Williams lets her have sugar on her cereal, and cola to drink. Mum never does. Ria is delighted. This is going to be a good day!

Questions

1   Why do you think these children have reacted so differently to the news Mrs Williams has?

2   How could the situation be improved for Lucas?

3   Why isn't Ria concerned?

4   What sort of day will they have?

5   How might they react when their parents return from the hospital?

mum/dad is and why they have been taken away. Sometimes the child might think it is because he or she has been naughty or because his or her parent does not love the child any more. There can also be uncertainty about whether the separation is temporary or permanent.

Some children are looked after by other carers if they are deemed to be 'at risk'. The care they receive is often focused on rebuilding self-esteem and confidence, and on re-establishing communication and interpersonal skills. Children with special needs are sometimes cared for away from home or by people other than their parents. This could be because special resources or particular types of care are needed. Sometimes the care is long term; sometimes it might just be 'respite care' for a day, weekend or week, allowing the parent or usual primary carer to have a break from his or her responsibility and to rest for a while.

Being cared for by other people can have all kinds of effects on a child's pattern of development, particularly a child's *social* and *intellectual* development.

If a child is cared for at home and in the company of the same people, the way he or she develops could be predicted, especially if there are other children in the family. You might have heard people say things such as 'She's just like her mother – she would do/say exactly the same thing!' **Primary socialisation** – the way we are socialised into the norms of our family and culture – is learnt at home and is taught to us by

CASE STUDY – Lateef, Bianca and Peter

Lateef comes from an 'ordinary' background. His parents are interested in him and his achievements. They try to support him through school and they help him with his homework when they can. There isn't enough spare money to buy computers or the latest technology for the house, but they encourage him to use the library and the facilities at school. They hope he gets a good job.

Bianca's parents think school is a waste of time. They both went – up to a point – but they never got anywhere. Bianca's mum had a job in the local DIY store until she got pregnant, and Bianca's dad has never had what you'd call a career. They get by. Bianca's mum often gets phone calls from school complaining about her daughter's attitude or her lack of attendance. The family laugh about it – Bianca's just got engaged, what does she need with school?

Peter's future is all mapped out. He's going to stay on and take 'A' levels, and then he's applying to Oxbridge to read Law. He'll join the family firm and eventually work in chambers. His parents encourage him in all aspects of his education – he has a study at home, with a computer and scanner, and a laptop which he takes to school with him. He's going to a crammer in the Christmas and half-term holidays to help him achieve the results he needs for a university place. 'Education is expensive these days,' his parents say, 'but you reap what you sow.'

Questions

1 How do you think these students' outcomes will be affected by the attitudes of the people who bring them up?

2 Do you think you need money to get a good education?

3 Is support from other people essential if you are going to succeed, or does self-determination count too?

4 How far do you think these students' attitudes are influenced by their parents?

5 Could you write one further case study showing the connection between social and intellectual development?

the first people who care for us. A child who is cared for outside the home will show the effects of **secondary socialisation** – that is, there will have been other influences on the child's behaviour, ideas and development.

Part of the social and intellectual development process is a child's interaction with the world around him or her. Sociable children are seen as ones who are friendly and outgoing. This could be because of their personalities or because of the lives they have led so far. If everyone around a child has been friendly and happy, and if the child has only experience of a pleasant life with little in the way of upheaval or disruption, then he or she is likely to be friendly. If the same child was a victim of abuse or has lived with extreme poverty and uncertainty then the child is more likely to be less outgoing and happy.

The situations children live in and the experiences they have affect the way they behave. Intellectual development follows a similar pattern. Look at the case studies of young adults (page 267) and how they have developed as a result of the influences on them.

Separation and loss

Being separated from someone you love, even if it is only for a short time, can be upsetting. As adults, we are used to separation. Through life, an individual goes through all sorts of experiences of separation and loss, starting with preschool care, where mum or whoever looked

after the child at home was no longer present all day, through school years when other people started to become more important. Perhaps college or working away from home is the first real experience most people have of being removed from their parents for any length of time. Loss is often thought of as being concerned with physical death, but it can also relate to a change of circumstance (see Figure 8.13).

Talk it over

How many changes have occurred to the people in your group that could now be seen as a type of loss? An example would be moving from one school to another, when we lose a familiar setting and familiar faces.

Working in groups, create a list of 'losses' and a corresponding list of 'gains'. You could use the following example as a starting point:

Situation	Loss	Gain
Changing school	Familiar place, familiar faces	New experiences, new friends, qualifications

Any child who is experiencing change is also experiencing loss. It is the job of the individual caring for the child to help the child through the period when he or she is finding change most difficult. According to age and experience, a child might react in different ways. He or she may become more aggressive or more withdrawn. They might be clingy or throw temper tantrums. Think about the experience of Lucas and Ria given earlier. They did not have the tools of communication and negotiation adults use and so reacted in the only way they could, using their experience of the world so far.

Sometimes change can lead to a loss of self-confidence and self-esteem. When an only child suddenly becomes an older brother or sister because of the birth of a new baby in the household, he or she may feel this new person is a replacement for him or herself because he or she has been bad-tempered or naughty. The child needs to be reassured the baby is an addition, not a replacement, and that he or she is still special and loved. Moving to nursery or a new school might also alter a child's perception of how big and capable he or she is. It's a big difference between being the tallest, oldest child in nursery and the smallest child in infant school.

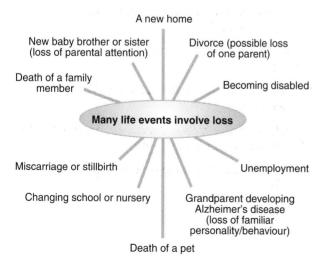

Figure 8.13   Life events that may involve loss

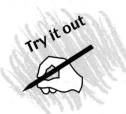

Jordan is feeling miserable. His new baby sister is always crying. His mum is stressed and his dad has left home. He has just had to start with a new childminder where there are two big children aged 4.

Write down ways in which you could help Jordan to feel better – things you could do with him.

The Children Act:

✓ Makes children's welfare a priority.

✓ Recognises that children are best brought up within their families, wherever possible.

✓ Aims to prevent unwarranted interference in family life.

✓ Requires local authorities to provide services for children and families in need.

✓ Promotes partnership between parents, children and local authorities.

✓ Improves the way courts deal with children and families.

✓ Gives rights of appeal against court decisions.

✓ Protects the rights of parents with children being looked after by the local authorities.

✓ Aims to ensure that children looked after by the local authorities are provided with a good standard of care.

Figure 8.14 The provisions of the Children Act 1989

Legislation

You will need to know about the laws, policies and codes of practice concerning the care of children, for example, the Children Act 1989 and the Children Order 1989, Northern Ireland 1989.

Children need legislation to protect them as sometimes the needs and rights of a child are overlooked or disregarded because of the child's age. There are many sections of different Acts that could refer to children, but the most significant piece of legislation is the Children Act 1989. The Act applies to England and Wales. Part X, which relates to nurseries and childminders and other provisions, applies to Scotland. The provisions listed in s.108(12) apply to Northern Ireland.

The Children Act is a wide-ranging piece of legislation that covers all aspects of childhood, from child protection, through the provision of services to the registration of individuals and groups who care for children. It is especially important when a family breaks up. Previously, custody and responsibility for the children was granted to one parent. Now divorced parents are encouraged to remain in touch with the child and be involved in the child's life. Parents are also encouraged to make their own joint decisions, and no orders are made by a court unless needed. Parenthood and responsibility for the child remain, even if the marriage does not (see Figure 8.14).

Codes of practice and policies within child care settings also protect children by ensuring they

receive proper treatment. An example of these would be the CACHE Statement of Values, which applies to all candidates taking the training for either the Certificate or the Advanced Diploma in Childcare and Education. The CACHE Statement of Values requires that CACHE candidates ensure the child's welfare and safety, for example.

Both the Children Act and the Statement of Values uphold the rights children have and promote their well-being. By working within these frameworks, childcare workers are ensuring children receive the best possible start in life. (For more about codes of practice and policies, see Unit 1, pages 50–52.)

Other legislation that affects child care is as follows:

1   The Health and Safety at Work Act 1974 – see Unit 6

2   COSHH (Control of Substances Hazardous to Health) Regulations 1994

3   Fire Precautions (Workplace) Regulations 1997.

Unit 8 Assessment

CASE STUDY – Luther

Luther is three years of age and goes to nursery from 8.30 am until 5.30 pm five days a week. He has been going to nursery for three weeks now, since his mother went back to work. She is a lawyer. Luther's father is a civil servant. They have one other child, Billy, who is seven years old and attends a prep school.

When he first came to nursery, Luther was only there for the mornings, and he cried himself to sleep each time. When his mother came to pick him up he was all tear-stained and clingy, but he seems to be settling in now. Luther has made friends with Jez and Sadie, two other children at the nursery, and he is very fond of Mandi, one of the nursery nurses. On the days when she is not there he is unsettled and miserable.

Luther's mum isn't that worried about him. His elder brother Billy went through the same process when he first went to nursery and he's one of the most sociable children you could ever meet. The fact that Luther has to be with other people during the day will encourage him to be independent and less demanding. Some people's children never leave their side until they go to school, and then they waste time being upset rather than

learning. Luther will get that stage over now, she thinks.

Mandi likes Luther. She encourages him to play with other children, and she enjoys his company. He was very shy at first, but now he's quite a chatterbox. Mandi and Luther often sit and do puzzles together, and Luther likes to sit on Mandi's knee when he is tired so that she can tell him a story. Luther is good at adding bits to Mandi's stories. She doesn't tell him off if he has a 'silly' idea to add in, she just puts that bit into the story, so they have fun together and laugh. On the days when Mandi isn't there, Luther thinks that nursery isn't so much fun. Ceri, the lady who takes her place, doesn't laugh with him as much, and he is often a little bit shy of her.

There are lots of grown-ups in the nursery as well as lots of children. Sometimes they go to the playground, and Luther holds Mandi's hand when they are walking there. It's not very far away, and sometimes Jez goes, too. He doesn't go to the nursery every day like Luther. Once, another little boy fell off the roundabout because he tried to get off when it was moving, so Luther doesn't want to go on that. He is happy with the diggers in the sandpit.

For a *Merit* grade you need to be able to give a clear explanation of how the care a child receives influences his or her development, and suggest other realistic areas of care that could be offered. By reading Luther's case study, can you identify the way Luther and his brother have had influences on their development? Think about:

- influences at home
- influences at nursery
- influences from family members' expectations
- influences from other people (children and adults) at nursery.

When you are looking at the case study, draw a spider diagram to remind yourself what you are looking for. List all the ways people develop, and then try to attach different aspects of Luther's life to each heading. An example would be Social development – making new friends at nursery. When you have found a positive comment to make for each of your headings, try to see if there might be a negative comment you could make. This should help you to work out any areas of development where Luther needs more support. You may have ideas about where or whom the support could come from. To achieve a *Distinction* grade you must take this investigation one step further and look at how health, social and economic factors combine together to affect the development of a child. In Luther's case you can make logical guesses about the sort of social and economic background he has from his parents' employment. Their combined income is enough to fund preparatory school for Billy and full-time nursery care for Luther. Do you think these factors are beneficial to Luther? How do they work? If Luther came from a different background, what effects would that have on his development? Why not write another, different case study about Luther? Try to take away the advantages he has and offer disadvantages instead. Now compare the two and draw up some points about how you could either maximise the good influences on his development, or minimise the bad points. You should be able to give explanations about why you would want to do either of these things.

You need to be able to give an in-depth explanation, with relevant examples, of how the care-worker uses personal or practical skills in caring for the child. How does Mandi help Luther through the day? At the moment his life is going through a period of great change, and she should be able to help Luther in many ways. One way that you might be able to present your explanation would be to create and fill in a table like the one below.

Think about the needs Luther might have in a typical day at nursery. He's there for a long time, so you may need quite a large table. When you have completed it, try to sort out the way that help arrives, and the skills which are needed by a nursery worker. How do they help the children in their care?

To achieve *Distinction* level it is important that you focus on the effect that a care worker can have on another person. Take one aspect of Luther's development and look at the factors which influence that. You might want to look at his emotional development. When Mandi works with Luther, how can she ensure that he develops emotionally to his full potential? Use the negative case study to work with to help you focus on how the external influences on a child can be built on, or worked around to the child's advantage. For example, if Luther was a child who suffered from emotional abuse at home, how would a care worker try to build his self-confidence and esteem? If Mandi could

Type of need	Practical helping skill	Personal helping skill
A cuddle, because Luther's sad		
Shoelaces doing up		
Helping to join in with unfamiliar children		
Sharing with others		

UNIT 8 ASSESSMENT

support Luther when he was at nursery, how would this help him? Remember that children are vulnerable complex human beings, and show that you can see the purpose behind either support or intervention.

You need to understand and be able to evaluate how the legal requirements for child care influence the care the child receives. Explore the way that the law looks after children in day care. You might find that your social services department is very helpful with this. You could persuade a member of

its Family Services team to come to school or college and be interviewed by the group. What sort of registration and inspection procedures need to be followed? How about fire precautions in the workplace? Ask about ratios of staff to children. Think about the accident at the playground in the case study. What sort of repercussions would that have had? Luckily the child only grazed his knee. What if he had broken his wrist? By interviewing a professional about this you will get evidence for communications, as well as for this unit.

Unit 8 Test

1   What is a reflex?

   a   A learned response to a stimulus.
   b   An instant reaction that vanishes in babies when they are about 3 months old.
   c   A controlled movement.
   d   Another term for a fine motor skill.

2   Bonding with a parent or care is part of:

   a   physical development
   b   emotional development
   c   social development
   d   intellectual development.

3   When can babies focus 25 cm away?

   a   At 6 months.
   b   At 3 months.
   c   At birth.
   d   At 9 months.

4   When a child recognises that quantities which look different might in fact be the same, he or she is conserving the volume. This occurs during:

   a   the pre-operational stage
   b   the sensori-motor stage
   c   the formal operational stage
   d   the concrete operational stage.

5   Primary socialisation is learnt:

   a   at primary school
   b   in the pub
   c   at home
   d   when a child reaches puberty.

6   Self-esteem might be damaged by:

   a   not winning every race at sports day
   b   being bullied
   c   coming top in the test
   d   having the same trainers as everyone else.

7   When a child is showing signs of speech delay, who will check him or her?

   a   The midwife.
   b   The doctor.
   c   The health visitor.
   d   A child psychologist.

8   Being able to use a pencil or a pair of scissors is known as:

   a   gross motor skill
   b   self-control
   c   fine motor skill
   d   creative control.

9   Controlling the eyes so they work together is known as binocular vision. Most young children achieve this by:

   a   3 months
   b   2 years
   c   6 months
   d   1 year.

10   Which letters are used to remember the main aspects of development?

   a   TOES.
   b   PIES.
   c   SPUD.
   d   ESTI.

This unit covers the knowledge you will need in order to meet the assessment requirements for Unit 10. It is written in four sections.

The first section discusses the psychological perspectives of human behaviour as these affect our work with people in care settings. Section two outlines the methods we can use to study and to understand human behaviour. Section three explores the types of behaviour we might expect to encounter in care settings. Finally, section four looks at the ways we can evaluate our own behaviour and compare this to the behaviour expected of someone who works in a care setting.

Advice and ideas for meeting the assessment requirements for the unit and for achieving Merit and Distinction grades are at the end of the unit.

Also at the end of the unit is a quick test to check your understanding.

Note: Some important theory needed to understand and evaluate care practice has already been covered in Units 1 and 3. You may want to refer back to these units before taking the test at the end of this unit.

Psychological perspectives on human behaviour in care settings

In the past, psychologists developed different ways of understanding and explaining human behaviour. Four important ways of understanding and explaining human behaviour are listed below:

1   Behaviour is learnt through conditioning and reinforcement.

2   Behaviour is learnt through copying the behaviour of others as well as through reinforcement.

3   Behaviour is influenced by mental processes, such as memory, perception and thinking.

4   Behaviour can be influenced by inbuilt (or innate) tendencies, which are genetically inherited.

Nowadays most psychologists think that all these four ideas (or perspectives) are useful for explaining human behaviour.

Reinforcement and conditioning

Nathanial is 7 years old. At school he will sit quietly for a few minutes and then throw all his work in the air. He will then run round the classroom for a few minutes.

Douglas is a young adult who has a learning disability and who attends a day centre. He often

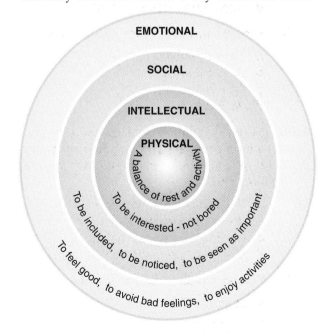

Figure 10.1 Needs

CASE STUDY – Nathanial

Nathanial can easily lose concentration and feels frustrated at having to watch and listen to his teacher. When he first dropped his work on the floor he was noticed – his teacher gave him attention. This attention made Nathanial feel better. He started to drop his work more and more. Whenever the other children or the teacher looked at him, he felt better.

In the end, Nathanial learnt to do more and more extreme things. He discovered the teacher would get upset if he ran round the room. Nathanial didn't want to make the teacher angry, but he felt better when he was receiving attention. Nathanial learnt to throw his work and run because this met his physical need to be active, his social

need to be noticed and his emotional need to feel good.

Nathanial's difficult behaviour happened more and more often and became stronger – because it was 'reinforced'.

Questions

Read the section on 'Reinforcement' below and answer the following:

1 How can reinforcement explain Nathanial's behaviour?

2 Which of Nathanial's needs might be met by him being given attention?

chooses to lie down in the doorway to the centre. This behaviour upsets the other users of the centre.

These two young people might each be seen as 'difficult'. Some people might label or stereotype these clients as stupid or naughty but carers must see beyond labels and try to understand what other people are feeling (see Figure 10.1). People learn to meet their needs in various ways. The way Douglas and Nathanial behave may be due to what they have learnt.

Reinforcement

Reinforcement means that something is made stronger. Reinforced concrete is stronger than ordinary concrete. Military reinforcements make a military base stronger. When a person experiences a good feeling just after he or she has done something, the person will be more likely to do this action again. When we repeat actions, we can say the behaviour is getting stronger or that it has been reinforced. When Nathanial runs round the classroom he feels better than he did before. This means his behaviour is reinforced.

Reinforcement can happen without anyone intending to reinforce behaviour. Nathanial's teacher and the other children all have to give Nathanial attention. Nathanial's difficult behaviour is reinforced because they have to react to the things he does (see Figure 10.2).

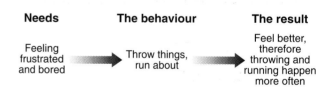

Needs	The behaviour	The result
Feeling frustrated and bored	Throw things, run about	Feel better, therefore throwing and running happen more often

Figure 10.2 How reinforcement works

Spotting reinforcement at work

Carers need to know about reinforcement for the following reasons:

1 It helps to explain why people behave the way they do.

2 It is important to work out how your own actions affect other people.

3   It is important to realise that most 'difficult behaviour' is not planned or reasoned out by clients. People often do any action that will make them feel better. Action is not always caused by intellectual thought; Nathanial may not know why he runs about.

> **Think it over**
>
> Can you use this idea of reinforcement to explain Douglas's behaviour? It may be that he often feels lonely and bored at the day centre. How could lying in the doorway make him feel better? Is it possible that the staff all give him lots of attention and worry about him when he lies down? If the staff do behave this way, might they be making his difficult behaviour stronger?
>
> Without knowing it, the staff may have taught Douglas to lie in the doorway.

What can staff do about reinforcement?

Because attention reinforces Nathanial's and Douglas's behaviour, it is tempting to think that ignoring behaviour would be enough to stop it. If running or throwing things is ignored, Nathanial might stop doing these things – but he might do something even worse instead. Ignoring a person still leaves that person's needs unmet. Ignoring

behaviour does not help someone to develop appropriate behaviour (see Figure 10.3).

Instead of ignoring behaviour, care staff should work out how they can reinforce positive action. Douglas and Nathanial could be given attention before they run about or lie down. Care staff have to work out ways of meeting social and emotional needs before difficult behaviours develop. Perhaps staff could spend more time with Nathanial and Douglas. If a classroom assistant could give Nathanial individual attention it might reinforce study behaviour – he might stop running about if his need for attention could be met in some other way.

Conditioning

Reinforcement is one kind of conditioned learning or **conditioning**. Conditioned learning takes place when we learn to make associations between things that happen. For example, some people cannot eat certain foods. If you eat potatoes and then feel ill a little while afterwards, you might associate feeling ill with eating potatoes. You become conditioned to avoid eating potatoes. This conditioning is not a thought you have – it becomes a very strong emotional reaction that stops you from eating potatoes. Even if you know something else caused your illness and that potatoes are safe and good for you, this knowledge cannot overcome your conditioning.

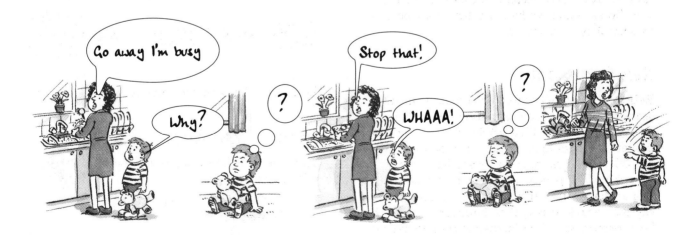

Figure 10.3 Not responding does not teach a child what to do – children will find other ways to get themselves noticed

Learning to associate things together is sometimes called Pavlovian conditioning (named after Pavlov, a famous Russian physiologist who first came up with the idea of conditioned learning). Learning to associate behaviour with 'feeling better' or reinforcement is sometimes called Skinnerian conditioning (named after a famous American psychologist who researched this type of learning).

Both conditioning and reinforcement can influence us without us realising how it has happened. This type of learning influences us on an emotional rather than a thinking level. Psychologists who mainly try to understand people's behaviour using theories of conditioning and reinforcement are called **behaviourists**.

Social learning approaches

Social learning theorists believe that conditioning is important but they also emphasise that people learn by copying what they see other people do. This copying is usually called **imitation learning**.

Care workers need to think about imitation learning because clients will sometimes copy the behaviour they see care workers doing. Children

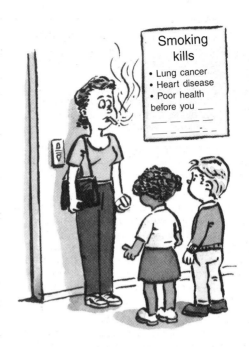

Figure 10.4 People copy the behaviour they see: which would have the greatest influence – medical advice or real-life behaviour?

often learn from what they see other people do rather than from what people say (Figure 10.4).

Cognitive approaches

People learn through conditioning and imitation and through using language and thought. The word **cognitive** means language, memory, perception and thinking. If you learn something from a textbook you will be using your cognitive abilities to enable you to learn.

The way people think about people is very important in care work. The exercise below will help you to explore the importance of cognition in care work.

When used in the UK this story is usually not remembered very well: about 80% of the story is lost altogether! Besides this, the whole story becomes muddled and confused.

It is very difficult for most people to remember this story because the story comes from a culture that most people from a European, African or Asian culture do not understand. Because of this, most people in the UK cannot understand it. You have to be able to understand ideas before you can remember them.

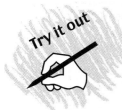

Try a simple experiment with memory using a story. The story below goes back to the psychologist, Frederick Bartlett, who used it in research into memory in 1932.

Explore your 'own' memory by reading 'The Story of the War of the Ghosts' below. Take a break and then come back and try to remember what happened.

Another idea is to use this story as part of a groupwork exercise. In this exercise, read this story to a member of the group without it being overheard. The person who has just heard the story has to repeat the story to one person. This person tells the story to another person. Repeat this process until the story has been retold about six or seven times. Do not take any notes and do not help or prompt or allow people to overhear the story before their turn.

The Story of the War of the Ghosts
One night two young men from Egulac went down to the river to hunt seals, and while they were there it became foggy and calm. Then they heard war-cries and they thought, 'Maybe this is a war-party'. They escaped to the shore and hid behind a log. Now canoes came up and they heard the noise of paddles and saw one canoe coming up to them. There were five men in the canoe and they said, 'What do you think? We wish to take you along. We are going up the river to make war on the people'.

One of the young men said, 'I have no arrows'.

'Arrows are in the canoe', they said.

'I will not go. I might be killed. My relatives do not know where I have gone. But you', he said, turning to the other, 'may go with them'. So one of the young men went, and the other returned home. And the warriors went on up the river to a town on the other side of Kalama. The people came down to the water and they began to fight and many were killed.

But presently the young man heard one of the warriors say, 'Quick, let us go home; that Indian has been hit'.

Now he thought, 'Oh, they are ghosts'.

He did not feel sick, but they said he had been shot. So the canoes went back to Egulac, and the young man went ashore to his house and made a fire. And he told everybody and said, 'Behold, I accompanied the ghosts, and we went to fight. Many of our fellows were killed. They said I was hit but I did not feel sick'.

He told it all and then became quiet. When the sun rose he fell down. Something black came out his mouth. His face become contorted. The people jumped and cried. He was dead.

(Story used by Bartlett, 1932)

When you tape record or video a conversation the tape makes a true record of what happened. You can play it back and hear it time after time. Human memory does not usually work like this. We cannot remember long lists of ideas and we cannot remember stories if they contain unfamiliar ideas. People have to be able to connect what they hear and see to what they already know. It can be hard to remember much more than seven new pieces of information in one go.

The importance of this theory for care work is that people often don't understand other people. If you work with someone with different life experiences from your own you may not understand them. If you had trouble understanding and remembering the story, you may also have trouble understanding people who are different.

Perception

We can remember things clients tell us if we can relate what they say to our own experience. People do not usually have perfect memories; we often alter what we hear to suit what we think! The same is true for what we see. Our brains have to interpret the patterns of light our eyes see. This means we sometimes see what we expect and not what is really there.

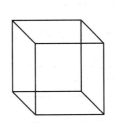

Try this experiment. Look at the two pictures below. Which side is the front of the cube? If you stare at the cube long enough you will see the sides keep changing – yet the visual information your eye takes in does not change.

Do you see a young woman or an old woman in the cartoon, first drawn in 1915? As you stare at the picture your mind will create different interpretations but the picture does not change.

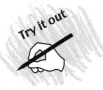

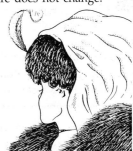

The significance of this theory for care workers is to realise that what we see and what we remember are not simply based on 'truth or facts'. Our culture, our expectations and past experience can alter what we think we see and how we remember events. Two people can experience the same event and interpret it differently. You can experience similar behaviour from a client on different occasions and you can perceive the behaviour differently. Some people look at the 1915 cartoon and see a young woman; some see an old woman. If you stop to think, you can see things both ways. In care work it is vital people stop to think. It is important that care workers do not simply label or stereotype others because they have fixed ideas.

When care workers are busy or tired it is easy for them to misinterpret or fail to understand people with different life experiences. The processes involved in human memory and thinking can create a barrier to communication. Care workers have to develop practical skills to overcome these problems.

Some practical ideas to help you value diversity in others are as follows:

- You need to spend time listening and talking to people from different backgrounds.

- You can remember and learn a few ideas each time you talk with others.

- Use listening skills described in Unit 1 to help you check and develop what you understand.

- Talk with senior staff and take further training to help understand cultural and life experiences that are different from your own.

Inherited behaviour

The things we think and do are mainly learnt through experience, but it would be a mistake to think that all behaviour is caused through learning. When infants learn to speak or walk they are not simply imitating people. Infants 'learn' to speak because they have a genetically inherited 'potential' to develop language. Humans have a genetic potential to walk and talk, but this potential will only develop if children are given opportunities to practise walking and talking. Children who are deaf and who are cared for by deaf people will develop sign language if carers

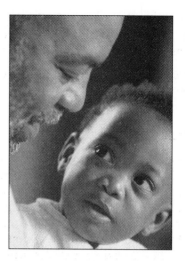

A child's language potential depends on the child experiencing the correct stimuli

sign to them. Our potential for language needs experience if it is to develop.

As well as skills such as walking and talking, some differences between people (such as personality) may be influenced by inbuilt genetic tendencies. But while genetic differences may influence us, our life experience is still a very important influence that will affect the things we do.

Methods of studying behaviour

Care workers need to have skills in understanding other people's behaviour (see Figure 10.5). People are different from each other

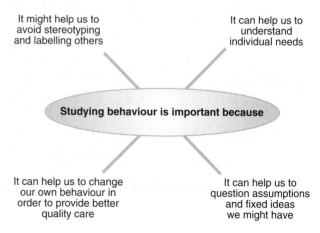

It might help us to avoid stereotyping and labelling others

It can help us to understand individual needs

Studying behaviour is important because

It can help us to change our own behaviour in order to provide better quality care

It can help us to question assumptions and fixed ideas we might have

Figure 10.5   Why studying behaviour is important

– everyone has individual needs. Care workers need to be able to think through different possible explanations of other people's behaviour.

Some of the methods for studying behaviour are listed below.

Observation

Care workers have to be very skilled at noticing details of client needs, such as how happy or miserable a client looks. In health care, workers have to carry out formal observations, such as body temperature measurements or X-rays to check health needs. But sometimes clients cannot explain their needs and so a skilled care worker will have to understand their needs through observation. For instance, people with dementia may not speak clearly, but the look in their eyes, the expression of their face and their hand gestures explain they don't know where they are and are afraid. A skilled care worker may be able to help a client to relax by his or her own actions,

perhaps by being calm, smiling and offering to hold the person's hand.

Care workers need to know about non-verbal communication and to be able to identify the different messages people send with their eyes and faces (details of non-verbal communication can be found in Unit 1).

Care work sometimes involves studying 'challenging behaviours' – behaviours such as disrupting a lesson or lying in the doorway of a centre. One particular observational method is called the ABC method – you have to observe details of A, B and C as set out below:

A = Antecedents (this means what happened before the behaviour).

B = Behaviour (you have to give detailed factual descriptions of what happened).

C = Consequences (what happened after the behaviour).

Below is an outline observation form which uses the ABC method.

ABC method

Student: Chloe, age 7 years.

Context: School art lesson.

Who was involved: Classroom assistant, teacher, other students.

Antecedents (Details of observation before the incident): Chloe worked quietly for 15 minutes, ignored by other students – not seen by staff when she put her hand up.

Behaviour: Chloe threw work and materials on the floor, shouted and ran round the room.

Consequences: Classroom assistant persuaded Chloe to sit with her – talked to her individually for five minutes.

Question

Can you see how reinforcement might be at work just by studying this observation?

By observing behaviour in detail a care worker can make sense of behaviour. Chloe's behaviour may be partly caused by boredom and frustration, but perhaps it is influenced by reinforcement. The classroom assistant gives Chloe attention when she runs around – Chloe does not receive attention at other times. Perhaps if the teacher or the assistant gave more attention to Chloe while she worked it might help her behaviour to change.

Questioning

We can learn a lot about other people by asking them questions. Care workers will spend time talking to the people they work with. More formally, social workers will interview people when they assess their needs for care. Researchers and some homes and hospitals may carry out questionnaires to learn about client views. Interviews and questionnaires require skilled planning. Care workers need to develop questioning skills. This means:

- Using open questions and not too many closed questions.
- Using unbiased questions.
- Planning the interview and understanding the effect it may have on people.

Questioning skills

Carers need to be good at asking open questions. An open question encourages people to talk and explain their thoughts. A closed question is the opposite of 'open'. Closed questions ask for a fixed reply. For example, if you ask the question 'How long have you worked here?', the reply is likely to be a fixed number of months or years. If you ask a question like 'Do you like it here?', the answer will probably be yes or no. Yes or no questions can cause an interview to become boring. Even worse, yes or no questions often create a cold and stressful conversation. Open questions often seem more warm and friendly.

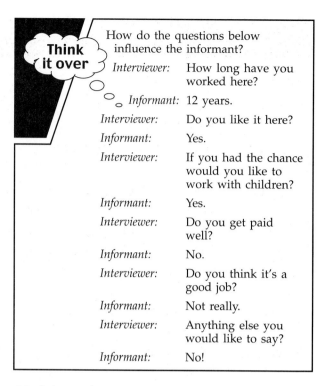

Think it over

How do the questions below influence the informant?

Interviewer:	How long have you worked here?
Informant:	12 years.
Interviewer:	Do you like it here?
Informant:	Yes.
Interviewer:	If you had the chance would you like to work with children?
Informant:	Yes.
Interviewer:	Do you get paid well?
Informant:	No.
Interviewer:	Do you think it's a good job?
Informant:	Not really.
Interviewer:	Anything else you would like to say?
Informant:	No!

Unbiased questions

The way a question is asked will often bias or lead another person into agreeing with your ideas. Biased questions may stop you from finding out what another person thinks. Look at the two case studies below. The first interview biases the informant into agreeing with the interviewer.

The second interview finds out what the person really thinks.

Planning a questionnaire

When care workers research other people's views it is important to work out what questions to ask before starting an interview. It is important to talk about general issues before asking difficult questions. Questions should usually flow naturally from one another and not put pressure on the people who have to answer them. It is important to plan and check questions through before trying to research opinions or design questionnaires. Always check your ideas out with a manager, supervisor or colleague before undertaking interview or questionnaire research.

CASE STUDIES

Interview 1

Interviewer: So was it terrible when you were made redundant?

Informant: Well, in a way I suppose it was.

Interviewer: What was the worst thing about it?

Informant: Well, it was the shock – one minute everything was going Ok and the next minute – I'd lost my job.

Interviewer: Did you feel sad and angry about that?

Informant: Yes, I suppose I did at the time.

Interviewer: So were you treated unfairly?

Informant: Yes, that's right, I did feel it was unfair.

Interview 2

Interviewer: So how did you feel when you were made redundant?

Informant: Well, I was shocked at first. It was unexpected, but then I thought, well, when one door shuts, another one opens.

Interviewer: Could you explain about the doors – I didn't really understand.

Informant: Yes, I was upset, but then I thought, well, I've just got to find another job – there must be something.

Interviewer: So what did you do then?

Informant: Well, I went to the job centre and all that, but then a friend said that there was this job going at the home where she worked and she wondered whether I could do that kind of job.

Interviewer: So how do you feel now?

Informant: Oh well, now I've found this work I'm really happy. I look back on the redundancy and I think – best thing that ever happened to me.

Questions

1 Can you see how **Interview 1** leads the informant to a biased set of answers?

2 Can you see how **Interview 2** finds out what the person really thinks?

Remember: Asking questions is a skilled task if you really want to find out what other people think.

Other methods of studying behaviour

Experiments

Experiments are very rarely used in care settings. Experiments involve controlling situations in order to test theories. If vulnerable people are 'controlled' and tested out, they may be damaged. Nowadays, experiments must only be carried out if they are **ethical**. This means that people must not be disadvantaged or harmed because of an experiment.

Although it is hard to use experiments in care, experiments in other situations have produced important findings care workers need to think about. For example, an important experiment on group behaviour took place some fifty years ago. In 1951 a psychologist called Asch asked people to judge the length of lines. People were shown a line and they had to choose another line that looked similar from a selection of lines they were shown. This is an easy task, but people had to work in groups and Asch had fixed each group so that most people gave deliberately incorrect answers. The experiment was designed to see what individuals would do when the people around them all seemed to see the lines differently.

The results were very interesting. Nearly three quarters of the people who were 'experimented on' agreed with the incorrect answers the other group members gave. It feels uncomfortable to disagree with a whole group of people and it seems that people will often go along with what other people in their group think.

The importance of this experiment is that it shows how powerful social groups can be. People often conform to, or go along with, whatever other people around them believe. In care situations it is important to watch for examples of group pressure or **conformity**. People will sometimes become depressed or angry because other people are depressed or angry – they conform to group pressure. If individuals disagree with the people around them they may be excluded or ignored by others. It can be very hard to not go along with the crowd!

Comparative studies

When psychologists report the findings from experiments it is always important to realise that the culture and social context of the people involved can influence the results. Studies done in the 1950s might not get the same results 50 years later because people live in a different culture. Theories of social behaviour may be more true of certain ethnic or social class groups than of others. It is important to study the differences between different cultural groups.

Comparative studies are designed to see how theories work in different social contexts and cultures. For example, Piaget believed all children had the potential to develop a kind of logical thinking (called 'formal operations' – see Units 3 and 8). Recent comparative studies suggest this stage of intellectual development may only happen when children are taught to think using formal logic.

Animal studies

In the first half of the nineteenth century, many psychologists studied how animals learn. Animals were seen as simple versions of people. A great deal was learnt about how animals can be conditioned and reinforced. Animal studies can be useful in helping us to understand some kinds of learning, but people are always different from animals because of language and the use of language to guide thinking, memory and perception.

Behaviour in care settings

Behaviour in pre-school environments

If you work with young children it is very important to understand how your own behaviour may influence them (see Figure 10.6). Children come into the world with a need to interact with others. In the first weeks of life children take an interest in human faces and soon react by smiling at faces. One theory of the development of thinking in children (developed by the Russian psychologist, Vygotsky) emphasises that children learn because of their social needs. Children learn language and develop their play and moral views because of the need to make relationships with others.

Some other ways of looking at child development emphasise the importance of biological influences.

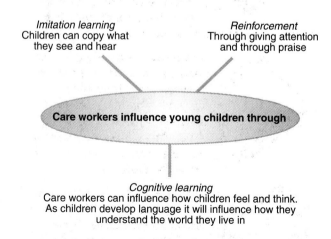

Figure 10.6 How care workers can influence young children's behaviour

Piaget (see Units 3 and 8) believed that abilities, play and moral thinking were strongly influenced by the stage of development a child had reached. These stages of development were influenced by our inherited potential to think and use language.

If you observe young children at play you are likely to see differences between the way boys and girls play. Boys and girls will often choose different types of games and often play in same-sex groups. At the age of 4 years boys might be attracted to construction games while girls might be more attracted to social activities. These gender differences might be partly due to biological differences between boys and girls, but play behaviour will also be influenced by the social learning children have experienced. (Further details of moral development and the role of play may be found in Unit 3.)

Working with people in hospital and residential settings

When people come into care or into hospital, they are likely to be vulnerable. Being vulnerable means you can be hurt or damaged. People may be damaged if their needs are not met. People's needs include the following (look back at Unit 3 and Unit 6 if you need to remind yourself about PIES):

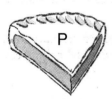

Physical needs: People may be in pain; they may be depressed and find it difficult to respond physically. Because of illness, people may have needs for physical assistance to move or to become comfortable.

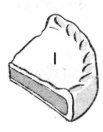

Intellectual needs: People often need to know about how the services work in care or hospital. People sometimes need information and advice about their illness. Supportive conversation can help to meet intellectual needs.

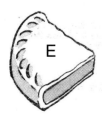

Emotional needs: Coming into care or hospital can threaten a person's self-esteem. Some people have major emotional needs in terms of coping with receiving care. A person's self-

concept can be threatened when he or she comes into a care setting. Supportive conversation can help to meet emotional needs.

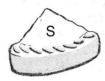

Social needs: Our social role, self-concept and identity are all influenced by the people around us. Care workers have to be sensitive to the importance of helping clients keep in contact with relatives and friends. Care workers may sometimes use communication skills to help meet the social needs of clients. Working within the care value base (see Unit 1) will help to meet these needs.

CASE STUDY
— Sheena

Sheena had been independent and worked in a well paying job for most of her life. At the age of 65 years she had a stroke. At first Sheena tried hard to follow exercises designed for her to improve her speech and mobility. She tried to regain the ability to do housework she had lost because of the stroke. After a few weeks Sheena became frustrated with trying to do daily living activities.

Sheena was assessed as needing home care. Within a few weeks Sheena appeared depressed. She stopped her exercises and said she would never recover. Now that several months have gone by since the stroke, Sheena has become withdrawn and says very little to her carer. Sheena's doctor has been called because she might have clinical depression.

Question

1   How can the theory of learned helplessness explain what is happening to Sheena?

Some people might say that Sheena's stroke has caused her to become depressed but strokes do not cause depression directly. There is a process called **learned helplessness** that can influence a person.

Learned helplessness

A psychologist called Martin Selligman wrote a book about helplessness in 1975. Learned helplessness starts when we feel we cannot control important things in our lives. Sheena's stroke makes it difficult to do everyday tasks: she has lost control of everyday living activities. Carers have taken over the daily living activities Sheena used to do and she has lost her independence. Sheena is anxious about her future and this stress contributes to her depression.

Figure 10.7 outlines some of the stages that can be involved in becoming helpless. Sometimes people who are in pain or people who feel frustrated become aggressive. Sheena will probably feel angry she cannot control her home. When people are angry it is easy for carers to lose their temper and be angry back to them. If this happens it will increase the helplessness a person might experience. An important care skill is to be assertive rather than angry. Figure 10.9

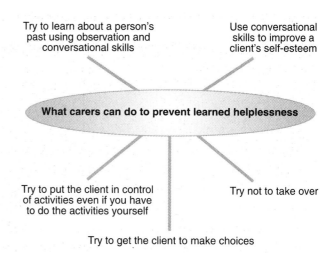

Figure 10.8 Ways of preventing learned helplessness

compares assertive, aggressive and submissive behaviours.

When people give up and become helpless they often just accept what others say. Sheena may become passive and withdrawn, just accepting what doctors or care managers say. If people stop making their own choices and become submissive, this may be a symptom of learned helplessness. Figure 10.8 suggests some things carers can do to prevent learned helplessness.

Group pressure and conformity

It is wrong to think that all the behaviour people do is thought about or planned beforehand. People often just copy or imitate what they see other people doing. People around you can have a major influence on how you think. In care, people often do what others expect them to do. Experiments on group behaviour suggest that people often try to fit in with the expectations of others. Just being in a group may make a person go along with the views of other people (see the section on experiments earlier in this unit for example).

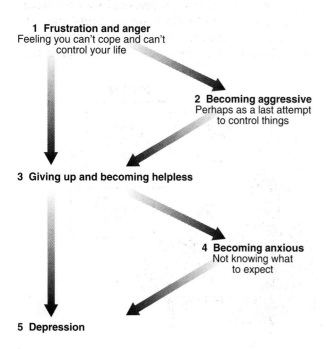

Figure 10.7 The stages in learned helplessness

Figure 10.9 Some differences between aggressive, assertive and submissive behaviour

Aggressive	Assertive	Submissive
Main emotion: anger	Main emotion: staying in control	Main emotion: fear
Wanting your own way	Negotiating with others	Letting others win
Making demands	Trying to solve problems	Agreeing with others
Not listening to others	Aiming at 'no one having to lose'	Not putting your views
'Putting other people down'	Listening to others	Looking afraid
Trying to win	Showing respect for others	Speaking quietly or not speaking
Shouting or talking very loudly	Keeping a clear, calm voice	at all
Threatening non-verbal behaviour, including fixed eye contact, tense muscles, waving or folding hands and arms, looking angry	*Normal non-verbal behaviour,* including varied eye contact, relaxed face muscles, looking 'in control', keeping hands and arms at your side	*Submissive non-verbal behaviour,* including looking down, not looking at others, looking frightened, tense muscles

Self-evaluation and behaviour

Understanding theories of learning and memory is useful because it can help carers to improve their own practice. Working with people creates a great deal of emotions and feelings – some of them nice and some not so nice. Some people we work with will be good to us – they may praise us and tell us they like us. Working with interesting, attractive or kind people may make us feel good.

But many people who receive care will be worried or even depressed or upset; these people may not always be rewarding to work with. Our first emotional reaction may be to want to avoid them. When we have to work with a difficult child it is only natural to feel 'I don't want to – I'd rather do something else' (see Figure 10.10).

If we are to work in a professional way we have to be sure we don't follow the emotional urge to withdraw but instead find ways of coping. Why does the child not want to do the activity? Is the

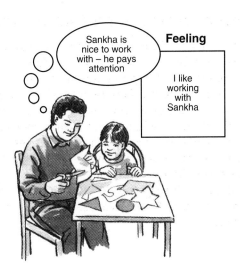

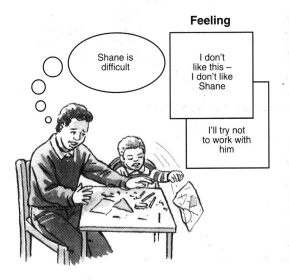

Figure 10.10 We need to review our own behaviour to stop negative emotions from blocking us in our work

child bored, frustrated? If we can think through some answers, we may be able to understand why the child is 'difficult'. If we can understand, we can cope with our emotions. One reason for reviewing your own behaviour is to prevent negative emotions from blocking our professional behaviour.

Thinking a situation through can help us to solve problems. Why does a child throw his or her work on the floor? There could be many different reasons. Talking to other staff or to senior staff may help us to understand. Involving other people will probably help us to understand the people we work with. Talking to the child may help us to understand. Observing what happens during the day may help. Thinking about our own behaviour – how good we are at talking or listening – may also help us to understand (see Figure 10.11). Hence another reason for reviewing your own behaviour is to solve the problems you face.

You will have attitudes and beliefs and ways of understanding people based on your own life experience. It is possible that carers can make assumptions about other people – perhaps that they are bad or dangerous. Assumptions can turn into stereotypes and prejudgements about other people. In the end there is a danger clients can be judged, labelled and discriminated against because they are different. So yet another reason for reviewing your own behaviour is to recognise assumptions in your thinking and to prevent these assumptions turning into discrimination and prejudgements.

It is very difficult to check our own thoughts alone. A good way to check assumptions is to discuss our practice with colleagues, tutors or workplace supervisors. Skilled supervisors may be able to help us question assumptions in our thinking.

How to review your own behaviour

It is often difficult to understand how we influence the people we care for. After we have been working with someone it is useful to stop to think about the work we have done. Sometimes

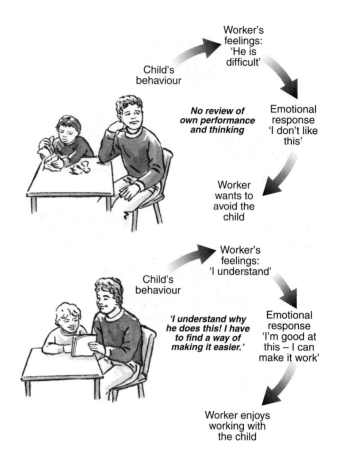

Figure 10.11 Emotions and professional behaviour

discussing our work with supervisors, managers or other staff can be helpful to get new ideas. If we get new ideas they can be tried out in practice to see if they are right. When people have a problem to solve they sometimes go through a process like the one shown in Figure 10.12.

The important thing is to think about your experiences and to learn from them. It is easy to forget our experiences and learn nothing from them if we do not think about them and discuss them. The main ways to review your own performance are to think about your work and to discuss your work. One way to analyse your own behaviour is to rate your own skills using Figure 10.13. You might like to reread the theory on communication in Unit 1 and also the theory on self-concept in Unit 3 to help you think about this task.

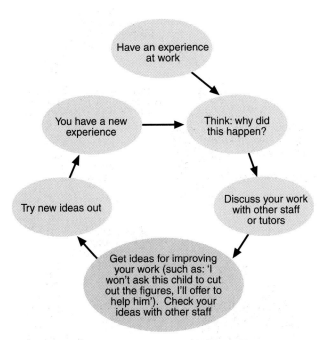

Figure 10.12 The problem-solving process

Figure 10.13 How good are you at each skill? Tick the appropriate column

	Not very good	Good	Very good
• Coping with your own feelings			
• Staying assertive			
• Listening to others			
• Understanding others' non-verbal behaviour			
• Showing respect to other people			
• Understanding how social roles can influence behaviour			
• Understanding the importance of self-esteem and self-concept in influencing behaviour			
• Starting a conversation			
• Keeping a conversation going			
• Working out how reinforcement can affect other people			

Unit 10 Assessment

This unit is tested externally. You will need to answer questions about the ways in which human behaviour can be studied. You will need to be able to explain some of the factors that influence clients and be able to explain how your behaviour can influence clients. An outline test is set out below which may help you with your revision.

The more you understand about communication skills, self-concept, perspectives on behaviour, methods of studying behaviour, influences on behaviour and how your own behaviour affects others, the more chance you will have of achieving a *Merit* or *Distinction* grade.

Unit 10 Test

CASE STUDIES

Mrs Robins

Mrs Robins has recently been admitted to hospital for observation. She lives on her own in a terraced house and has been refusing to take her medication. She has woken her neighbours at night by banging on the walls and screaming and crying. Sometimes she leaves her home and becomes lost. Mrs Robins is disorientated and cannot remember her husband is dead. She only has distant relatives who find it difficult to visit her. Mrs Robins has been assessed as in need of care, but she refuses to go into a nursing home saying she wants to die in her own home.

Questions

1   List some of the needs Mrs Robins may have using the headings below:

Physical needs
Emotional needs

2   What risks of helplessness or giving up might there be if:

a   Mrs Robins stayed at home?
b   Mrs Robins went into a rest or nursing home?

3   Think of three positive ideas for communication skills staff could use to support Mrs Robins while she is in hospital.

Emily

Emily is 5 years old. She often has outbursts of temper at school where she will press her face to the table she sits at and cover her head with her hands. She will stay like this for one or two minutes if left alone, but for longer if staff give her a great deal of attention.

Questions

4   Explain how staff could adapt their behaviour to try to reduce Emily's outbursts of anger.

5   Explain what is meant by learning through reinforcement.

6   What does learning through conditioning mean?

7   Apart from conditioning and reinforcement, explain two other ways in which children learn.

8   In terms of the learning theories you know, explain why care staff should never punish people to try to change their behaviour.

9   Why should care workers know something about the way in which human memory and perception work?

10 If you look after children and they see you acting in an aggressive way, how is this likely to influence their behaviour?

11 If you wanted to learn about differences in the play of 4-year-old boys and girls, what research methods would you choose?

12 Give examples of two different methods of studying behaviour.

ABC of behaviour A way of understanding how reinforcement works.

ABC rule The order in which you should check a casualty: **A**irway; **B**reathing; **C**irculation.

Access Means by which an individual becomes a client of a particular service.

Acute A condition which starts quickly and lasts for a short time, such as a common cold.

Adrenaline Hormone released when the body is anticipating any form of stress.

Advocate Someone who speaks / negotiates on behalf of another person.

Aerobic Needing air or oxygen.

Aerobic respiration Cell respiration in the presence of plenty of oxygen.

AIDS Acquired immune deficiency syndrome, a collection of disorders that result in time from HIV infection.

Anaemia A condition in which the oxygen-carrying capacity of the blood is reduced; there are many types but the most common iron-deficiency anaemia results from a lack of oxygen in the body.

Anaerobic Without air or oxygen.

Animism When children give human thoughts and characteristics to inanimate objects, e.g. 'The naughty mat tripped me up'.

Antecedent What comes before a certain event or behaviour.

Appearance How we look. People use different clothes, hairstyles, cosmetics and adornments such as jewellery to express membership of particular age, class, cultural and friendship groups.

Asphyxiation (or suffocation) When a person is unable to breathe air into his or her lungs.

Babbling A stage infants go through before they can use language. The infant makes sounds which may later help him or her to use words.

Baby talk Adults use a high-pitched voice and slow down their speech when talking to infants. Adults may also use exaggerated facial expressions. Baby talk may help to keep an infant's attention.

Balanced diet A diet that has carbohydrates, fats and proteins in the correct proportions and enough vitamins and mineral salts, fibre and water to ensure healthy living.

Balanced lifestyle Having enough rest, leisure, exercise, work and an appropriate diet to maintain health. Not having too much leisure or work, or inappropriate eating habits.

BASW British Association of Social Work.

Behaviourism A perspective that focuses on studying behaviour. Behaviour is seen as being caused by environmental influences.

Belonging A feeling of identifying with a particular group of people. Feeling safe and supported by a particular group.

Bereavement The loss of a person that you loved. Bereavement often involves strong emotions of disbelief, denial, anger, guilt and resisting change.

Biased question A question that might influence a person to answer in a particular way.

BMI Body Mass Index – a person's weight in kilograms divided by his or her height in metres.

Bonding Developing an emotional attachment to another person. Babies usually make an attachment to carers during their first year of life.

Buffering Partners, friends and family may protect a person from the full stress of life changes and conflicts. Michael Argyle called this protection buffering.

Care Action Plan A plan designed to meet individual needs within a service. It is different from the general Care Plan assessment of needs.

Care Value Base Principles that guide how care workers should behave. Key principles include valuing diversity, promoting rights and responsibilities and maintaining confidentiality.

Career routes The pathway which an individual takes in order to qualify and then move to more senior roles in a certain job or profession.

Carer Anyone who provides care for another person or people.

Carotid pulse The strong pulse from the carotid artery felt in the neck between the windpipe and the neck muscle.

Change Life involves coping with a wide variety of change – some of which is welcome and some of which is not. Change can be classified as predictable or unpredictable.

Charters Documents which set up or explain the rights that people may expect.

Child Support Agency A government agency that deals with setting the level of maintenance money that absent parents are required to pay towards the keep of their children.

Class A group of people who share a common position in society. Class membership is linked to occupation, income, wealth, beliefs and lifestyle.

Client Anyone who receives a service – a general term which covers patient, service user and customer.

Closed question A question that requires a fixed type of answer such as a yes or a no.

Code of practice A set of principles which can be used to guide and measure the quality of care practice.

Cognition A term which covers the mental processes involved in understanding and knowing.

Cognitive development The development of thinking and reasoning ability. Cognitive includes the study of perception, language and learning performance.

Commissioning The process of determining and securing health and social care services.

Communication cycle The process of building an understanding of what another person is communicating.

Community Care Charter Documents which explain what people may expect from community care services within a geographical area.

Community health care Care provided for individuals in the community and, where possible, in their own homes.

Comparative studies A method of research used to compare theories of different cultural or social contexts.

Complementary therapies Therapies such as aromatherapy, reflexology and acupuncture that have not traditionally been available through the National Health Service.

Complexion The colouring and skin texture of a person's face.

Concrete operations The third stage of intellectual development in Jean Piaget's theory. At this stage, individuals can solve logical problems provided they can see or sense the objects with which they are working. At this stage, people cannot cope with abstract problems.

Conduction Heat that is transferred by contact.

Confidentiality The right of clients to have private information about themselves restricted to people who have an accepted need to know.

Conformity People often try to fit in with group opinions if they feel they belong to that group. People sometimes change their behaviour to 'fit in with others'.

Consciousness An awareness of oneself and one's surroundings.

Contracting The process for agreeing the nature, level and standard of service that is to be provided.

Contracts Formal legal agreements to ensure the delivery of services.

Control of Substances Hazardous to Health (COSHH) Regulations, 1988 Requirements to be met by all people who deal with dangerous substances at work.

Controlled drugs Illegal drugs.

Convection The heating of a layer of air close to the source of heat such as the body.

Coronary thrombosis Blockage of part of one of the coronary arteries supplying part of the heart muscle which dies as a result; usually means a heart attack.

COSHH *see* **Control of Substances Hazardous to Health (COSHH) Regulations, 1988**

Cultural differences Differences due to different life and learning experiences which can affect communication and understanding.

Culture The collection of values and norms associated with a group. Culture is intended to describe all the features of a group that make it different and distinct from other groups.

Dehydration The body tissues contain less water than they should.

Dementia A term which covers a range of illnesses involving the degeneration (or wasting) of the brain. Dementia is not part of normal ageing. Most very old people show no sign of dementing illness.

Denial Saying or believing something is not true. Denial is also a defence or stage in reacting to change. People often block unwanted changes and deny that they are real. People may deny that someone has died or deny that the consequences of the death will matter.

Department of Health (DOH) A central government body which administers health and social care.

Department of Social Security (DSS) Government department responsible for the provision of welfare benefits.

Development When a person or system alters how he, she or it functions.

Developmental maturity The degree to which a person or an ability is 'mature' or 'adult like'.

Diabetes mellitus A condition due to lack of the hormone insulin that causes a gross disorder of the body's chemistry and a high blood sugar level.

Dialect Different sounds and words which can result in communication differences.

Differential growth rates While general bodily growth occurs fairly steadily throughout childhood, the nervous system grows rapidly in the first few years of life and the reproductive organs hardly grow until puberty.

Diffusion The movement of molecules of a gas or liquid from a high concentration to a low concentration.

Digestion The breakdown of large complex (food) molecules into simple soluble materials suitable for absorption into the bloodstream.

Dignity Being respected by others, not being controlled or abused.

Dilation The widening of a tube such as a blood vessel or opening such as the iris of the eye.

Direct care Care that is given on a face-to-face basis.

Discrimination Giving a better (or worse) quality of service to some people than to others because of their gender, ethnicity, sexuality, age, social class or other group membership.

Diversity The way in which people are different from one another. Key differences include race, gender, religion, age, class and sexual orientation.

DOH *see* **Department of Health**

DSS *see* **Department of Social Security**

Duty Services that an organisation is required by legislature to provide.

Early Learning Goals A set of targets used in early years education for children aged 3–5 years.

Embryo The stage in development of the new human being between the fertilised egg and 8 weeks of pregnancy.

Emotional development How we learn to develop self-esteem, self-concept and understand and respond to emotion.

Emotional health How people deal with and express emotions such as fear, grief, happiness etc.

Empowerment Giving power to others – enabling others to take control of their lives and make their own choices. The opposite of controlling other people.

Endocrine Producing hormones.

Energy Capacity for activity / work.

Environmental barriers Environmental barriers include noise and poor lighting, both of which can block communication.

Enzyme A biological catalyst that helps chemical reactions to speed up or slow down.

Ethics A system for working out what is morally and socially right and wrong, good or bad.

Ethnicity A word used for 'race'. Some people used to think that biological differences created different races. Nowadays, social scientists use the term ethnicity to make it clear that we are talking about social classification and not physical differences.

Exhalation The process of breathing out.

Experiments A method of research where the researcher controls a situation in order to test a theory out.

Extended family A family which consists of parents and their children, and other relatives such as grandparents, uncles or aunts.

Fieldwork A term used in social care that refers to the work of professionals, usually social workers, in the community.

Fine motor skills Control over small, careful movements, such as when cutting out shapes or picking up tiny objects.

Foetus The name given to the developing life within the mother's womb from week 8 of pregnancy to week 40 (birth).

Formal operations The fourth and final stage in Piaget's theory of intellectual development. People with formal logical operations can solve abstract problems.

Friction The resistance to movement between two bodies in contact with one another.

Gestures Hand and arm movements that can send messages about how we feel.

Goitre Swelling of the neck due to a lack of iodine in the diet.

GP fundholders General practitioners who hold budgets with which they can buy health care for their patients.

Gross motor skills Control over large movements, such as when running or jumping.

Growth When the body or an organ of the body gets bigger.

HA *see* **Health Authorities**

Haemoglobin The iron-containing red pigment that carries oxygen and is located in red blood cells.

Haemorrhage Another name for bleeding.

HASAW *see* **Health And Safety At Work Act (HASAW) 1974**

Hazard A danger which threatens health and safety.

Health And Safety At Work Act (HASAW) 1974 Deals with the health and safety of people at work.

Health Authorities (HA) Regional departments within the NHS which have responsibility for commissioning and purchasing health care within their area.

Healthy lifestyle Daily activities and routines which promote physical and mental health and well-being such as a balanced diet, enough exercise, enough rest, work and leisure. The term usually includes an avoidance of unhealthy habits such as smoking and substance abuse.

Helplessness Learned helplessness is where people learn to 'give up' and stop trying to control or influence what is happening to them.

HIV Human immuno-deficiency virus that infects people who exchange body fluids with infected persons.

Holistic Treating a person as a whole individual by looking at all relevant issues and not just the details of certain symptoms.

Home Life A code of practice for residential care.

Homelessness Not having a home in which to live.

Hyperthyroidism A medical condition in which too much of the hormone thyroxine is produced, resulting in a speeding up of the body's chemical reactions and processes.

Hypothermia A life-threatening medical emergency when the body is cooling down too much.

Hypothyroidism A medical condition caused by insufficient thryroxine hormone being produced, resulting in a slowing down of the body's chemical reactions and processes.

Imitation learning People can learn to copy the activities they see other people do. We can learn to copy or imitate others.

Impulse A tiny electrical charge cause by chemical ions that can be transmitted along nerve fibres.

Income Money received as wages, interest on savings or profits from business activities.

Independence Being able to function without being dependent on others. Adolescence is seen as a time of growing independence in Western culture.

Indirect care Services provided to support direct care, e.g. the ambulance service.

Infectious diseases Diseases usually carried by bacteria and viruses that are passed from one person to another.

Informal care Care given by people who are not paid for the care they give, e.g. family or friends.

Inhalation The process of taking air into the chest or breathing in.

Inherited behaviour Our genetic inheritance may influence how we behave. Behaviour is not fixed by genetic inheritance; it can always be influenced by environment.

Intellectual development The development of our ability to think, reason and understand. Here, the term covers use of language, remembering, thinking and the development of knowledge.

Intellectual health How people think and organise their thinking.

Jargon Technical talk which is hard to understand.

Kilojoules (kJ) SI units that measure food energy. They have replaced calories and kilocalories (Calories).

Life chances The opportunities which are really open to individuals. People are born into different social class and wealth categories. These categories may restrict or enhance the opportunities that people have to be healthy or wealthy.

Life changes Major changes in life include starting school, starting a new job, leaving home, marriage, retirement. These changes usually alter a person's self-concept.

Life stages Infancy, childhood, puberty and adolescence, adulthood and old age. Life stages are ways of looking at people's life-span and breaking it into sections.

Lifestyle choice A choice made by individuals about the way in which they lead their lives.

Listening Trying to understand the messages that other people send us. Listening is an active process which involves more than simply hearing what is said.

Local Authority Social Services Departments which provide social care to meet the needs of people in the community.

Lone-parent families A family consisting of one parent and children.

Maternal deprivation John Bowlby's theory that children would become emotionally damaged if separated from their mother during a critical period of their early life.

Mean average This is the average value found when all the numbers are added together and divided by the number of units.

Means testing This is when an individual's income and savings are taken into account when deciding on the cost of a service to a client, or whether he or she is eligible to receive the service.

Median average This is the average value which is found when all the figures are put in ascending order – the median is the one in the middle.

Menopause Cessation of menstruation, usually occurring naturally between the ages of 45 and 55.

Metabolism The chemical reactions taking place in the body.

Micro-care plan A plan of action designed to meet individual needs after more general needs or services have been assessed.

Micro-organism Living things such as bacteria and viruses that are too small to be seen by the naked eye.

Mixed economy of care Care provided by a mixture of statutory agencies, voluntary and private organisations and informal care givers.

Monitoring Checking how an activity or process is working – checking how a care plan is working.

Mono- and unsaturated fats Vegetable and fish oils considered less likely to lead to heart disease.

Mood The frame of mind a person is in, such as happy, sad, angry, aggressive etc.

Moral development People's views on what is right or wrong are influenced by their cognitive development and how they have learned to think. Adults usually have more complex ways of understanding right and wrong than do children.

Motor development How muscles co-ordinate and pull together to allow more and more complicated movements to happen.

Multi-disciplinary team A team consisting of people from different professions, e.g. doctors, nurses, occupational therapists and social workers.

Muscle tension Our muscles – particularly the muscles in the hands and face – can send messages about how we feel.

National Health Service (NHS) In England the Secretary of State for Health has overall responsibility for the NHS.

National Health Service and Community Care Act 1990 An Act of Parliament which aims to allow more vulnerable people to live as independently as possible, within their own homes or in a homely setting in the community.

National Society for the Prevention of Cruelty to Children (NSPCC) Charity founded in 1889 to act in the interests of children's safety.

Negotiation Discussion to achieve agreement between people.

Neonate A new-born baby.

NHS *see* **National Health Service**

NHS Trust A free-standing body within the NHS that has responsibility for determining its own structure and spending.

Norms The rules of behaviour which are followed by members of groups. Norms are what is expected as being 'normal' things to do.

NSPCC *see* **National Society for the Prevention of Cruelty to Children**

Nuclear family A family consisting of parents and their children who share a residence and co-operate economically and socially.

Oedema A build-up of tissue fluid surrounding body cells.

Oestrogen A female sex hormone (actually a group of hormones) responsible for secondary sexual characteristics.

Open question A question that could result in many different types of answer.

Opportunistic infections Infections that occur when immunity is low, as in HIV and AIDS cases; normally the immune system would prevent opportunistic infections from happening.

Osteomalacia The adult version of rickets; the bones are soft and weaker than normal so more fractures occur.

Over-the-counter drugs Drugs such as cough medicine and aspirin that do not require a prescription; they can be bought in any chemist or pharmacy shop.

Passive smoking Inhaling unfiltered smoke from other people's tobacco materials.

Patient's Charter A document which sets out the rights and standards people can expect from the NHS. A new charter will probably be mainly concerned with standards of service rather than rights as such.

PCG *see* **Primary Care Group**

Peak flow The maximum speed at which air can be forced out of the lungs.

Perception The ability to see or take notice of the events and people around you.

Physical health Health related to the functioning of the human body.

PIES This stands for physical, intellectual, emotional and social. It is a way of understanding the different aspects of human development.

Play Play enables children to learn by exploring, to practise skills, to learn to use imagination in order to understand how things work and to understand social roles. Play also helps people to meet emotional needs and adult 'recreation' often involves 'play'.

Polyunsaturated fats Fats usually found in animal and dairy products that are considered more likely than mono- or unsaturated fats to lead to heart disease if taken in excess.

Posture The position of parts of the body at any one time, e.g. the way we sit or stand. Our posture can send messages about how we feel.

Poverty Not having enough wealth or income to be able to live like the majority of people in this country.

Pre-linguistic When babies and toddlers are able to communicate their needs to their primary carers without language. Babbling and making happy noises are part of the pre-linguistic stage.

Pre-operational The second stage in Jean Piaget's theory of intellectual development. At this stage a child is not able to use logical reasoning.

Prescribed drugs Drugs that require a prescription from a doctor.

Primary care Health care provided in the community, e.g. GP services and dentistry.

Primary Care Group (PCG) In England, a PCG is comprised of GPs and community nurses, covering a population of approximately 1000,000, and having responsibility for commissioning primary and secondary health care.

Primary socialisation The influential socialisation that takes place during early childhood. This is when we are socialised into membership of our families and our culture.

Private organisations / services Services offered by businesses which are intending to make a profit.

Procedure A set way for carrying out a task. Procedures are often set up to protect clients' rights and safety.

Prognosis A prediction of the probable course and outcome of a disease.

Provider An organisation that sells its services to a purchaser.

Puberty The period of change leading towards being capable of sexual reproduction.

Public health services A branch of the NHS that deals mainly with the prevention of ill health.

Purchaser An organisation that buys in necessary care.

Pyrexia Another name for a fever or raised temperature.

Radiation The transfer of heat from a hotter body to a cooler one.

Recommended dietary intake (RDI) The quantities of each nutrient that will maintain a healthy lifestyle for most people.

Reconstituted families A family which is made up of children from previous family groups. The couple are not both the parents of each child in the family.

Recovery position The safe way to lie a person down to protect the airway.

Referral Methods by which a client is referred or passed to a service.

Reflexes Automatic muscular responses to stimuli; for example, a light stimulus shining in the eye causes the muscle of the coloured iris to contract making the pupil small.

Reinforcement This means making behaviour stronger. A behaviour becomes stronger and more likely to be repeated when it is followed by a pleasant outcome.

Respiration The breakdown of molecules (mainly glucose) to released stored energy.

Resuscitation Restoring breathing and the beating of the heart.

Review Checking over and looking back on a situation. Seeing how well a care plan has worked.

Rickets A medical condition of children in which bones and cartilage are not hardened correctly; weight-bearing causes the bones to bend – resulting in bowlegged legs. The condition is caused by inadequate Vitamin D intake.

Rights Services and standards that people may expect. General agreement as to how people may expect to be treated.

Risk The chances of people being injured by a hazard.

Secondary care Health care that is often curative in nature and is given in hospitals, clinics and surgeries.

Secondary socialisation The influence on us from our peers and the media, which helps us to accept society is made up of lots of different kinds of people with different ideals and beliefs.

Seebohm Report Government report published in 1968 which resulted in the amalgamation of the children's and welfare departments within local authorities.

Self-concept The way we use concepts to understand who we are. A clear understanding of self may be necessary for independent functioning in Western society.

Self-confidence An individual's confidence in his or her ability to achieve something or cope with a situation. Self-confidence may influence and be influenced by self-esteem.

Self-esteem How much a person values him or herself and his or her life. High self-esteem may help a person to feel happy and confident. Low self-esteem may lead to depression and unhappiness.

Self-help groups Groups which meet to help individuals with particular concerns.

Self-image The way we imagine and visualise ourselves – similar to self-concept.

Self-worth The value or esteem we place on ourselves. A sense of worth is a more general feature of development which may exist before adolescent and adult self-esteem needs develop.

Sensorimotor The first stage in Jean Piaget's theory of intellectual development. Infants learn to co-ordinate their muscle movements in relation to what they think makes sense, such as when reaching out for a toy held out to them.

Services Help which is provided to support individual and community needs.

Sexual maturity A stage of physical development that results in the ability of males and females to reproduce.

Slang Informal terms which some people may not understand.

Social context A setting where social influences affect an individual's learning and development.

Social development How people make relationships and interact with others. Learning to relate to family, friends and wider society.

Social exclusion People who are excluded from opportunities to have a healthy and economically comfortable life. Some factors which create social exclusion are poverty, discrimination and stressful living conditions.

Social health How people form relationships with other people.

Social inclusion Including people in opportunities to lead a healthy and economically active life.

Socialisation The process of learning the norms and values of a group, and developing a role within it. Through socialisation people become part of a group or culture.

Socioeconomic The interaction of social (relating to the society in which a person lives) and economic (to do with money) factors.

Status A measure of the rank and prestige of a person. Status helps to explain how people see themselves.

Statutory services Services set up because of a legal requirement to provide a service.

Stereotyping Seeing members of a group as all being the same.

Sterilisation A procedure to prevent the fertilisation of eggs by spermatozoa usually by cutting and sealing the oviducts in females of the vas deferens in males.

Stress management Finding ways to reduce stress or cope with it.

Sub-culture Group values and beliefs which are shared by a particular set of people, but which differ in some way from general values and beliefs within a recognisable culture.

Suffocation *see* **Asphyxiation (or suffocation)**

Tertiary care Health care often provided in specialist units, or units that are rehabilitative in nature.

Threat Something which is understood as a danger to physical, social or emotional well-being.

UKCC The United Kingdom Central Council for Nursing, Midwifery and Health Visiting.

Unified structure The combining of health and social care at an organisational level, e.g. the Northern Ireland Department of Health and Social Care.

Unsaturated fats *see* **Mono- and unsaturated fats**

Unstable condition When the condition of the casualty is liable to change.

Value base The values which guide professional behaviour in health and care work. Current NVQ standards identify valuing diversity, promoting rights and responsibility and confidentiality as key values.

Values Principles which guide practice and day-to-day decisions in care.

Vegans People who eat or use no animal products at all.

Vegetarian people who eat no slaughtered (killed) meat or fish but who will eat milk, eggs and dairy produce.

Verbal Communication that uses words.

Voluntary organisations These provide services to bridge gaps in statutory provision. Some services are provided free of charge. They are non-profit-making organisations.

Wealth The value of the property owned by a person. Wealth includes the value of houses, cars, savings and any other personal possessions.

White Paper A government document setting out its proposals for the provision of services.

Answers to tests

Unit I

Answers to the 'Think it over' features in this Unit follow the answers to the Unit 1 Test.

1 Statutory services.

2 Any three of the following: planning services within its area; assessing primary health care needs; developing services within its area; commissioning primary care; arranging community services; managing community services; monitoring the quality of services; providing information for the public; registering and dealing with complaints.

3 **b**.

4 Three examples would be a nursery school, a crèche and a playgoup.

5 Direct is used to describe those jobs where the worker has face-to-face contact with the client. Indirect is used to describe those jobs where the worker supports those who come into face-to-face contact with the clients but where the workers may not come into contact with the clients him or herself.

6 Three skills might include: communication skills (verbal and written); the ability to take in large amounts of information and to be able to analyse; the ability to work flexibly – both alone and in teams.

7 0–8 years.

8 Values are basic principles that guide practice in care work. Values help care workers to protect vulnerable individuals.

9 Practical ways of valuing diversity include: using listening skills to build an understanding; treating everyone as individuals and offering choices; finding ways to show respect and value for individuals; respecting the rights of others; avoiding making assumptions about people; following policies on equal opportunities.

10 Rights and responsibilities include: freedom from discrimination; a right to be independent; a right to make choices; a right to receive respect and dignity; a right to safety and security; a right to confidentiality.

11 Codes of practice and charters are needed to provide a definition of good quality care that can be measured.

12 Communication skills are used to understand the needs of others, make relationships, show respect and value for others and meet emotional and social needs.

13 Non-verbal communication is communicating without using words. Non-verbal communication includes body language and tone and volume of voice.

14 Listening is an active process, where your own non-verbal communication and conversation skills show the other person that you have understood what they are saying. Listening forms part of the communication syle. Hearing just means that you have received the sounds that another person makes. Listening is about understanding.

Answers to Think it over questions on pages I7 and 48

Page I7

The organisation which uses this symbol is ChildLine, a voluntary organisation which provides a free national helpline for children and young people in trouble or danger. It was founded by Esther Rantzen in October 1986.

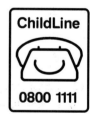

Page 48, Safety hazards in the kitchen

Crockery is left unwashed, with particles of decaying food around.

Electrical safety – the kettle lead is near water, creating a risk of electric shock. The electrical point might be overloaded with too many connections. The toaster is too near the sink and water supply.

Fresh food is left uncovered – flies can land on it and spread micro-organisms from the decaying food in the sink and bin. Micro-organisms from the air can also contaminate the food.

Bleach can be hazardous – it should not be stored near food. Here the lid is off and there is a risk of spillage or even food contamination.

Food preparation surfaces have not been cleaned, allowing micro-organisms to build up and transfer to fresh food.

Knives are not stored in a safe way.

Decaying food is left in a broken pedal bin, encouraging flies and the spread of micro-organisms.

Fresh food is placed near decaying food, encouraging the spread of micro-organisms.

The dishcloth is contaminated with micro-organisms from the (dirty) floor area – separate floor and dishcloths should be used.

The dirty floor might create a hazard of slipping and falling, as well as encouraging the spread of micro-organisms.

The mop and bucket might be tripped over.

Unit 2

1 **a.**

2 **a** and **b.**

3 **c.**

4 **d.**

5 **b.**

6 **c.**

7 **d.**

8 **b** and **d.**

9 **a.**

10 **c.**

11 **d.**

12 Carbohydrates; fat and protein (in the correct proportions) to provide energy, growth and repair; sufficient vitamins, mineral salts, water and fibre to sustain a healthy lifestyle.

13 Any three of the following. Eat less salt; more fibre; less fat; more vitamins and mineral salts; more fresh fruit and vegetables.

14 Fibre stimulates bowel movement; prevents constipation; gives us a feeling of fullness; prevents bowel disorders.

15 Proteins for growth and repair, fats and carbohydrates for energy.

16 We need energy to manufacture cells when we are growing. Adolescents are growing rapidly, old people are not.

17 People in professional classes (1.1, 1.2, 2) may consume diets rich in animal fats and may be overweight. They may take less exercise due to pressure of work. Stress at work is likely to be great, with no time for stress management techniques. All the above can combine to cause heart attacks and strokes. This group of people may abuse alcohol in the form of wine and spirits.

18 To provide fibre, vitamins and mineral salts.

19 Health education units, doctors' surgeries, dentists' surgeries, health centres, etc.

20 Any four of the following: addiction; force of habit; lack of motivation; low self-esteem; too busy; lack of child care; low income.

Unit 3
Scenario one

1 Any one of the following. *Physically*: growth, reflexes, development of muscle control; *intellectually*: muscle control; babbling; learning how physical objects work; *emotionally*: attachment to carer (bonding), guided by carer's behaviour; *socially*: recognise carer, respond to carer.

2 Sitting, crawling, bear-walking, walking alone, toilet training.

3 Spend time playing with Anil. Encourage social and language development through talk and interaction. Provide good-quality toys and activities that will encourage his intellectual development.

4 Anil may be able to bond or build an emotional attachment with the people who provide attention. Anil may feel safe when familiar people are around him.

5 Any one of the following: in her grammatical use of language; a much larger vocabulary; her play will imitate social behaviour; her muscle co-ordination skills will be more developed (such as climbing, running and jumping).

6 The parents spend less time with Anil. This may influence Anil's intellectual development

– less practice with talking, less encouragement with play. If his parents became emotionally withdrawn, this may upset Anil's attachment to them – he may feel less emotionally secure.

7   Any three of the following: impairments of hearing and vision; problems with her heart, breathing and circulation; less efficient muscle strength; the onset of arthritis; slower reactions; risk of brittle bones; her kidneys and liver may be less efficient. (*Note*: dementia, loss of memory or senility are incorrect answers – these problems only happen to a minority of older people.)

8   Family and friends provide relationships. Relationships prevent social isolation and protect people from stress. Relationships may create a positive sense of 'self-esteem' or 'self-worth'. Relationships may create a sense of belonging and they meet social and emotional needs. Living with the family may help the grandmother maintain a positive self-concept.

9   Praise will encourage the development of a positive self-concept and of positive self-esteem.

10 Gender role.

11 Any three of the following: secure attachments in infancy; friendships; family relationships; positive feedback from other people; success with activities or with school work or sports; positive opportunities and environment; belonging to a clear culture shared by his family and friends; being popular.

12 Going with his family to worship at the local temple; mixing with other children at school.

Scenario two

13 Any four of the following: parents stressed by money worries; overcrowding; poor diet; more hazardous housing; fewer resources to help with school work; less chance of keeping up with the latest styles of clothing; low expectations of success in life; pollution; noise; petty crime.

14 There are no eggs left in the woman's ovaries.

15 Any two of the following: onset of menstruation; increased fat deposited under her skin; pubic and under-arm hair growth; enlargement of her breasts.

16 It will affect her self-concept because it will have a positive effect on her self-esteem and self-worth: she may feel more independent, more adult, may have a higher status among her friends and may feel more in control of life.

17 Any two of the following: understanding herself as a member of a partnership or couple; being independent; being responsible for the home.

18 Failing eyesight, particularly at night; bones may have become more brittle; their sense of balance may be impaired; their sensitivity to heat, cold and pain could all be reduced; their smell and hearing could be impaired.

19 Any one of the following. *Physical*: enough sleep and rest; coping with stress and pressure; *intellectual*: learning about new people, new tasks, new routines; learning how to cope with new activities; *emotional*: self-esteem needs – the need to feel competent, the need to keep a positive self-concept; the need for positive feedback from others; *social*: the need to belong, fit in; the need for respect; the need for inclusion in social activity.

20 Any three of the following: denial, anger, resistance to change, guilt, withdrawal, trying out new ways of coping.

Unit 4

1   Aorta – high, pulmonary artery – low, coronary artery – high, pulmonary vein – high.

2   Cartilage – to protect the bone ends against wear, synovial fluid – to lubricate the joint and reduce friction, ligaments – to prevent the joint from bending too far in a direction.

3   Muscles cannot contract without receiving impulses from the nerve fibres supplying them.

4   At eight weeks of pregnancy.

5   Regular turning, ripple mattress (water bed), sheepskin pads.

6   Evaporation of sweat is the main method of heat loss, and this could be artificially simulated by cool showers. Radiation from

exposed skin surfaces would also help, providing that the environmental temperature was below body temperature; if not, seek shade which is cooler.

7   An accumulation or build-up of fluid around body cells.

8   Effort, fulcrum and load or load, fulcrum, effort.

9   The small intestine is extremely long with an inner surface covered with microscopic projections known as villi (each villus also has very, very small projections known as microvilli).

10 Hypothyroidism or athletic training.

Unit 5

1   Proteins, carbohydrates, fats, vitamins, mineral salts, fibre and water.

2   Fat.

3   Fish.

4   a.

5   c.

6   True.

7   See Figure 5.14.

8   *Listeria, Salmonella, Campylobacter, E.coli.*

9   Sugary foods need to be avoided but complex carbohydrate may be eaten. Do not miss meals and stagger the intake of carbohydrates.

10 Meat 12 o'clock, potatoes 6 o'clock, vegetables 3 and 9 o'clock.

Unit 6

1	c.	6	c.
2	a.	7	b.
3	b.	8	b.
4	b.	9	a.
5	c.	10	d.

Unit 7

1   Employers, employees, the general public.

2   Recent fall or knock, pain at the site of the injury, swelling and bruising, deformity, some shock.

3   The Fire Precautions (Workplace) Regulations 1997.

4   Place the client in the recovery position, monitor closely, insist that he or she sees a doctor. If recovery does not occur within a few minutes, send for the emergency services.

5   Clear a space around the child and cushion the fall, if possible. Check the child is not in physical danger. Loosen clothing to aid breathing. Maintain the child's dignity.

6   Check the nature of the hazard, investigate the market to see if there is a less hazardous substance that would do the same job, inform the staff who will use it of the hazards, hold a training session, perform a risk assessment, keep a record of this risk assessment, and update it regularly.

7   Hypothermia.

8   Milly should sit up in bed for 5 minutes before putting her feet to the ground. This will make her get up more slowly and avoid the dizziness. Inform other carers: ask them to encourage her to remember this and to monitor her awakening until the routine is established.

9   Wet floors are slippery, and this might cause falls to others or himself. Urine is unhygienic and unpleasant to others. It is also a source of infection.

10 Explain what is happening with great tact and care. See if he can avoid doing it. If not, provide a urine bottle for early morning use, and have the client checked by his doctor to see if there are any physical causes for the spillage.

Unit 8

1	b.	6	b.
2	b.	7	c.
3	c.	8	c.
4	d.	9	c.
5	c.	10	b.

Unit 10

1   *Physical needs:* needs to take medication regularly; memory needs; does not feel safe; becomes lost when she leaves home.
    Emotional needs: for others to help with her memory and orientation needs; increase self-esteem; the need to be valued and treated with respect.

2   **a** Mrs Robins may 'give up' and become helpless at home because she is disorientated. Her memory problems may cause her to lose control of daily activities – she may withdraw from people because they are never there to help her when she needs them.
    b Mrs Robins may 'give up' and become helpless in a care home because she may feel it is not her choice to go there. She may be unfamiliar with people and routines in the home and feel she cannot control anything. She may feel devalued as she cannot choose or control her own life

3   Listening, showing respect and value; talking about Mrs Robins' past in order to build self-esteem and maintain a positive self-concept. Being good at keeping conversations going; using reinforcement skills to keep conversations going. Coping with own feelings and building an understanding of Mrs Robins' past. Being 'warm' and friendly.

4   Staff could provide positive support and attention before Emily 'withdraws'. Staff might try to reinforce positive social behaviour. Staff might be caring and assertive but try to spend more time with Emily when she is behaving than when she withdraws.

5   Learning reinforcement means a person's behaviour changes because he or she experiences a nice or pleasurable feeling after he or she does an action. If a child misbehaves but then gets lots of attention, this can create a nice feeling which reinforces or strengthens the misbehaviour. Reinforcement works on animals as well as people. No thinking or language needs to be involved for reinforcement to work.

6   Conditioning means that one behaviour becomes associated or linked with another one. If you eat something and later you feel sick you might become conditioned to feel sick whenever you try to eat that food again. Reinforcement is a special kind of conditioning where nice feelings become associated with a behaviour.

7   Children learn by imitating or copying others. Children also learn through language and through developing concepts and ideas they can share with others.

8   Punishment can block or stop a behaviour, but punishment does not guide a person towards alternative actions. Punishment does not teach new constructive behaviours. People need positive learning experiences in order to grow and develop. Reinforcement, imitation or cognitive learning can create positive learning.

9   Understanding how memory and perception work can help care workers to understand and review their own behaviour. This understanding may help care workers to be able to avoid labelling and stereotyping others.

10 Children may imitate or copy the behaviours they see others doing. Children may copy aggressive behaviour they see.

11 It would be important to use observation to study the play of children. Watching behaviour might enable a researcher to classify what he or she sees. We might be able to tell how much time boys and girls spent in different kinds of play. Questioning could be useful, but young children might not be able to explain what they do very easily. Observation might be the best method to choose.

12 Methods of study include: observation; questioning (questionnaires, surveys and interviews); experiments; comparative studies; animal studies.

Suggestions for further reading and useful websites

Books

Body fitness and exercise, M. Rosser (Hodder & Stoughton, 1995).

The First Aid Manual (Dorling Kindersley, 1999).

A handbook for care assistants, S. Benson (Care Concern, 1995).

Human life, D. G. McKean (John Murray, 1988).

Human biology and health studies, Martin Rowland (Nelson, 1996).

Investigating health, welfare and poverty, P. Trowler (Unwin Hyman, 1989).

NVQ Level 2 in Care Student Book, Yvonne Nolan (Heinemann, 1998).

Website addresses

www.active.org.uk An interactive website which helps you to analyse how much exercise you are getting, and comes up with ideas for how you can become more active.

www.avert.org.uk AIDS Education and Research Trust – information and education about HIV issues.

www.lifesaver.co.uk Offers support and motivation to help people stop smoking

www.lovelife.hea.org.uk Sexual health website for young people.

www.quick.org.uk How to check whether you can trust the information you find on the Internet.

www.thinkfast.co.uk Helpful advice on how to make healthy choices when eating fast food.

www.trashed.co.uk Website offering information about drugs and their effects.

www.wrecked.co.uk Facts about the effects of alcohol and alcohol abuse.

Index

The page numbers in brackets refer to Fast Facts.